THEORIES IN PSYCHIATRY

BUILDING A POST-POSITIVIST PSYCHIATRY

NIALL McLAREN

Future Psychiatry Press

Ann Arbor, MI

Contents

Preface.

> You never change something by fighting the existing reality. To change something, build a new model that makes the existing model obsolete.
>
> Richard Buckminster Fuller (1895-1983),

In my other work, *Natural Dualism and Mental Disorder: the biocognitive model for psychiatry,* I build a dualist model to replace the existing, reductionist-biological concept of mental disorder [1]. My goal in this book is to provide the intellectual basis to dispose of biological psychiatry forever.

This book replaces my four earlier books with a tighter focus on theories in the field of mental disorder. In the fifteen years since the first volume was published, there have been many developments which need to be brought into any discussion of psychiatry, psychology and social work. However, the field of mental disorder is so large that all I can hope to do is start a long-overdue debate, one that psychiatry itself has carefully avoided throughout its history.

My starting position is that mental disorder is real, which also meanst the mind is real. Mental disorder means something yet, despite anything you may see in the media, there is no explanation. Most psychiatrists today believe mental disorder is always and only caused by a disturbance of brain function at the level of neurotransmitters, hence the widespread trope, "a chemical imbalance of the brain." After a hundred and fifty years, this remains an unproven hypothesis. Most emphatically, do not be swayed by biological psychiatrists who proclaim that we are "on the cusp of a breakthrough in mental disorder." That's just public relations.

There are still a few psychiatrists who say mental disorder is wholly a matter of psychology, including faulty learning, faulty parenting or faulty life experiences. The remainder hedge their bets by saying it is caused by a mix of biological, psychological and social factors, but they can't be more specific than that. In an ideal world, treatment would flow from the model of mental disorder but because there isn't an agreed model, almost all mentally-troubled people who come in contact with psychiatry will be given drugs and other physical forms of treatment. Why? Because drugs (and the belief system that goes with them) now define psychiatry, separating it from psychology.

Despite this lack of a formal theory of mental disorder, psychiatrists have a peculiar grip on the public mind. Thirty years ago, the lawyer and historian, Eric Dean raised the question of psychiatrists as "moral entrepreneurs." The term comes from the 1963 book, *Outsiders: Studies in the Sociology of Deviance,* by the sociologist Howard Becker. He defined a moral entrepreneur as "an individual, group or organization that seeks to influence a group or society to maintain a particular norm or adopt a new one, the goal being either to reinforce or alter the boundaries of morality, including altruism, deviance, duty or compassion." Dean continued:

> This impression of scientific certitude in the midst of substantial and potentially crippling problems is a tribute to the ability of psychologists and the psychiatric profession to acquire and wield power ... the salient point is that the mental health professions have a track record of advancing diagnostic categories that lack clear underlying unity based on scientific evidence, but that, nonetheless, have the effect of responding to popular needs and aggrandizing the power and authority of mental health professionals [2, pp200-202]

In his series entitled *Can't get you out of my head,* the remarkable documentary maker, Adam Curtis (2021, *BBC Film*), looks at the life of a man in the 1970s who decided on the then-radical step of trans-itioning from male to female. Having already lived as a woman for some time, she was referred to a psychiatrist for assessment and management. After endless delays and fiddling around, she decided to have breast implants performed privately. At the next appointment, when she revealed the operation, the psychiatrist was furious. Starting at about 23 minutes, the unseen psychiatrist speaks in a cold and demeaning voice, bitterly critical of his patient's action, before abruptly terminating the interview. His parting words were "Come back and see me in a month," the clear implication being "... when I've had time to get over your effrontery."

What comes through loud and clear is the psychiatrist's fury at the patient taking things into her own hand, of not doing exactly as she was told. It was about the psychiatrist's anger over not being in control, over not getting what he wanted—in other words, the psychiatrist's personality disorder on full display. People who have seen this shrug dismissively: "Yeah, so what? All shrinks are like that, control freaks one and all." And they're right. The history of psychiatry is one of very gross abuse of the civil process [3]. All too often, mentally-disturbed people are grabbed without warning from the streets or from their own homes, handcuffed, thrown in a police van and taken to a mental hospital. There, they are wrestled to the ground, stripped, injected and locked in solitary confinement, sometimes before anybody has actually asked why they are there.

Once in the system, psychiatric patients have essentially no civil rights, or certainly fewer than convicted prisoners. They are detained after a quasi-judicial process which admits unsworn and hearsay evidence; they generally they have no knowledge of the material on the application forms; they are usually denied the right of cross-examination of the hospital staff or police who signed the application; most have no legal representation; and they have practically no rights of appeal, even if they knew of them, which most don't, and could afford it, which they can't. Caught in the machinery of the psychiatry industry, it is all but impossible for detained people to extricate themselves. Everything they do, every time they object or resist, is taken as evidence of mental disorder and therefore leads to more, not less, "treatment." In particular, people caught up in the forensic system can effectively kiss their lives goodbye.

Even though this is legally permissible, it represents the most profound and widespread breach of human rights. It takes place every day in every country of the world, in systems that operate outside public sight—and far from public concern. All this is done by order of "a caring community working within the moral constraints of the science of mental disorder for the benefit of the patient." So how is this justified? Is this just tradition, akin to the way we butcher animals or we used to treat slaves or, all too often, still treat indigenous populations and women, or is it rational, justified by some science of mental disorder? If tradition, it needs to be examined right now but if we claim it's rational, it needs to be irreproachable, far more so than even the scientific justification of Covid restrictions.

Part I of this book starts by looking at the fundamental belief systems which underlie discusssions of mental life, the Cartesian dualist model and the positivist reaction to dualism (see Part II Preface). These set the scene for psychiatry as it is practised, specifically the theoretical authority for the various forms of treatment. My goal is to find an articulated, publicly-available model of mental disorder of a form that permits predictions to be made and tested. We look at each "brand" of psychiatry to see what it says about the nature of mental disorder and how it arises in the normal course of events. What we find is that, stripped of its self-justifying verbiage, psychiatry has no theory or model of mental disorder that justifies either today's forms of treatment of the mentally-troubled, or the wholesale and indefinite removal of their civil and human rights when they have broken no laws.

Since psychiatrists are manifestly operating in a theoretical vacuum, Part II looks at a range of philosophies of mind to see if any of them can be developed to the point of justifying society's treatment of mental disorder. At many points, I emphasise that any model for psychiatry must show a *mechanism* that can explain mental disorder. In the final analysis, the activity and output of any complex system is governed by three features: by the mechanism by which the physical structure does its job (the matter-energy interchanges of its workings); by the medium in which that activity takes place; and by whatever its managers have planned for it (the informational states governing its physical activity). To understand mental disorder, we need solid explanations of each of these points.

Of course, this is also true of the question of the nature of mind. People may object: "Oh but the question of mind is entirely metaphysical, it can't be resolved by empirical facts." True, but empirical facts set the boundaries of discussion. Because they tell us firmly what *can't* be the case, they soon eliminate some ideas. Facts tell us the mechanism by which we can expect the mind to emerge or be reduced (the question remains open for now), and the medium in which mental activity is implemented. Just as the heart functions as a pump, the liver functions as a chemical factory, and skin functions as a barrier, so the brain works as a high-speed, multi-modal information processor. That's its role, that's what it does. Our job is to relate that role to the emergence of mental properties, and thence the development of mental disorder.

Given this role and the macro- and microstructure of the brain, **any theory of mind must start with, and ultimately be defined within, a**

theory of information. Apart from magic, there isn't anything else at this stage. Now information isn't something grafted on or channeled through the brain, it is implemented in the brain's physical architecture via a rational generative mechanism that we can understand [1]. Lacking an adequate explanation of that structure and mechanism, all talk of minds and mental disorder is descriptive, not explanatory. This point is important: in the physical realm, we are accustomed to descriptions amounting to explanation, just because of our immense implicit knowledge of how the physical world works. For example, by describing a shaft joined to a wheel, we immediately understand that turning the shaft will turn the wheel, and vice versa, because we know implicitly that that's how the world works. In the physical world, our implicit knowledge means that description amounts to an explanation; we then assume that **all** description serves as explanation but this is **not true of the informational realm.**

An explanatory model based in a theory of information shows that mental disorder can arise wholly through disturbances at the level of the information processing in the brain. While physical disturbances at the level of the brain's microstructures are potentially sufficient for mental disorder, they are neither necessary nor likely. Brain disorders are profoundly different from mental disorders because, in a perfectly healthy brain, there is a additional level of function, the informational, at which errors can arise. Given the complexity of human psychosocial development, disturbance of normal function at the informational level is far more likely than biological disorders of the brain. **In recasting mental disorder as a primary psychological disturbance, a disorder of mind but not of brain, we move to an explanatory model which, in turn, dictates treatment.** This is the key to understanding mental disorder, and opens the path to rational treatment.

Part II will look at the work of a number of philosophers who dominated their field during twentieth century. A clear theme will emerge, dividing them in two groups. The larger group simply accept that the mind is a real, causally-effective thing, and they proceed forward from there, trying to work out the rules that govern it. However, with the positivists breathing down their necks, they are all careful avoid the woolly metaphysical excesses of the great historical names, such as Spinoza, by sticking to a pruned-down version of the mind, essentially, the mind as a cognitive organ. In fact, we will come across several authors who use just that expression. While they accept the reality of the mind, they make no attempt to explain how it arises from the physical brain or the medium in which it is implemented. I conclude that all of these philosophies are only half a program which, while interesting, can never succeed.

The other and much smaller group looks at the mind, then turns and tries to work back to how it arose. Most will simply try to eliminate the mentalism of the mind by arguing one or other version of the physicalist doctrine. Their plan is that the mind will reduce to the brain such that a thorough knowledge of the brain will answer all questions of mind, with no interesting questions remaining. One author, David Chalmers, tries to give an account of the mind as a mental thing with interesting results, but even his work leaves very large gaps in the explanatory sequence from brain to mind and drifts toward a very unsatisfactory conclusion. Once again, I am forced to conclude that philosophy as it stands today can contribute nothing to the idea of mental disorder [1].

A final comment: Starting as a child in a small town far from anywhere, collecting shells, bones, flowers, stones and anything that caught my eye, I have been deeply immersed in biology and the world of science for almost my entire life. Some children collected toys or stamps, I collected little skulls and looked at them. Some boys had model aircraft, I had a tiny microscope that opened a new world. Some children learned music, I sat on rocky headlands overlooking the mighty Southern Ocean and tried to work out the order governing the waves as they crashed on the rocks below. Long before space flight, I loved to see the mysterious full moon high in the sky but, more than that, I loved moonless nights with the huge southern Milky Way sprawled overhead, drowning me in its sense of the infinite. I think I was very lucky growing up where I did.

Over a period of about twenty-five years, I first went through high school, then spent six years in medical school followed by four years training in psychiatry, topping it off with two years back at university to study philosophy. At no stage in my education did anybody tell me that what they were teaching was the positivist version of science and philosophy. Even in the course on philosophy of science, it wasn't mentioned. The teachers and professors simply accepted that this is it, there is only one conceivable version of these fields, learn it and shut up. Which, of course, was also how religion was taught. Only recently did I discover that all of this (long and expensive) education took place within the very tight confines of the positivist view of the world. That was liberating: it allowed me to see how it has had a pernicious effect on psychiatry, and on philosophy of mind in general. All this will become clearer in the body of this work.

References

1. McLaren N (2021): *Natural Dualism and Mental Disorder: The biocognitive model for psychiatry*. London, Routledge.

2. Dean ET. *Shook over hell: Post-traumatic stress, Vietnam and the Civil War*. Harvard: University Press, 1997.

3. Scull A (2022) *Desperate Remedies: Psychiatry and the mysteries of mental illness*. London: Penguin.

Part I:

Mental disorder:

the practical possibilities.

1   Setting the scene: philosophical foundations of psychiatry

> Good sense is the most fairly distributed thing in the world; for everyone thinks himself so well-supplied with it, that even those who are hardest to satisfy in every other way do not usually desire more of it than they already have .
>
> Descartes, *Discourse on Method*, Part 1

1.1. Descartes' "substances."

The Big Question that towers over psychiatry is this: "Is the mind the sort of thing we can talk about rationally, or is it not?" Oddly enough, most psychiatrists aren't aware of this question: as far as their daily work goes, the matter is settled and they're definitely on the right side of the answer. In fact, it's not settled, giving us branches of psychiatry based in incompatible perceptions of the nature of mental disorder that don't even talk the same language. Nonetheless, we can trace them back to their historical origins. It's important to understand these otherwise we end up with a scientific tower of Babel, meaning a pseudoscience.

The default position is that yes, the mind is real and yes, we can talk meaningfully about it and its disorders. While there have been ten thousand philosophers in dozens of cultures over thousands of years who have had opinions on this question, from the point of view of modern psychiatry, the most influential was the French polymath, René Descartes (1596-1650). Descartes has the distinction of having his name applied to two entirely different fields, Cartesian geometry and Cartesian dualism. However, as will be seen, it is now fashionable to deride his contribution to philosophy as the very worst primitivist-spiritualist nonsense imaginable.

I don't agree with that at all and see that attitude as "the very worst pseudosophisticated relativism imaginable." For example, I once gave a talk on Descartes' contribution to a group of psychiatrists but it was clearly not going over very well. When it came time for questions, one psychiatrist, who claimed to have studied Descartes at university, said: "I don't take any notice of him, he had no education and hadn't studied any of the great books." The next said: "He knew nothing about neuroanatomy." The last said: "His stuff wasn't original. The work of the great skeptic Marcus Aurelius had just been rediscovered and Descartes simply rehashed it."

OK, where do we start? First, Descartes had an outstanding education, starting at home in his father's library (he could read Latin and classic Greek by age six). At the age of ten, he attended the foremost Jesuit college in France (and probably in the world), the *Collège Royale Henri-le-Grande*, at La Flèche, from which he graduated as an exemplary student. He then studied law for several years at the University of Poitiers but he wasn't happy with the idea of practising law as he was more interested in mathematics and philosophy. At the time, the best way to study maths was to enlist in the military and train as an engineer, so this is what he did. Along the way, he met some influential mathematicians and wrote a treatise on music.

Of the Great Books, at the age of about twenty-three, he decided that they didn't add up to much. He realised that for any opinion expressed by a great author, he could go to another book and find exactly the opposite opinion:

> But I had become aware, even so early as during my college life (high school), that no opinion, however absurd and incredible, can be imagined which has not been maintained by some one of the philosophers ... the ground of our opinions is far more custom and example than any certain knowledge ... a plurality of suffrages (majority vote) is no guarantee of truth ... I entirely abandoned the study of letters. Resolving to seek no knowledge other than that of which could be found in myself or else in the great book of the world, I spent the rest of my youth travelling, visiting courts and armies, mixing with people of diverse temperaments and ranks, gathering various experiences, testing myself in the situations which fortune offered me, and at all times reflecting upon whatever came my way to derive some profit by it (*Discourse on Method*, 1637).

By this means, he shifted attention from received truth (from God by way of the ancients) to discovered knowledge, which is the basis of modern science. The impact of this simple but totally revolutionary move cannot be overestimated. As for anatomy, he practised what he preached. Descartes was an accomplished anatomist and dissectionist and was quite clear that the best way to learn about mind and brain was to get the head of a large animal and dissect it—oneself. His work, *The Passions of the Soul* (1649) is a detailed analysis of emotions and mental processes based on his knowledge of neuroanatomy and the workings of the brain, although it's difficult to read now as we don't use terms such as 'passion' in the sense he did. It's clear, however, that, in an era when human dissection was generally prohibited, he knew a great deal about the human brain and that this factual knowledge guided his thinking. After detailed arguments and evidence, he concluded the only difference between animals and humans was the immaterial soul. The vegetative functions, including sensation, were common to all animals, including the human animal.

Finally, the work of the great Stoic, general, and later emperor, Marcus Aurelius, was never lost. Only the classic Greek authors were "lost" until the Renaissance, but Descartes was very familiar with them, and didn't think much of skepticism: "Not that in this (self-critical method) I imitated the skeptics who doubt only that they may doubt, and seek nothing beyond uncertainty itself."

Quite clearly, my psychiatric audience were not applying Cartesian skepticism to themselves. René Descartes made a major contribution to Western thinking and it is difficult, if not impossible, for us moderns to escape his shadow. There is a huge secondary literature but his formulation of the status of the mind *vis a vis* the body needs no interpretation: mind and body are separate and distinct substances with no commonality, as: "Each requires nothing other than itself to exist." The essence of "mind substance" is thought, while the essence of material substance, such as the body, is extension in space. There is, of course, a third element in his universe, divine substance, whose essence is perfection but, having created them, the divinity doesn't interfere further with the other two substances.

Together, mind substance and body substance form an interactive duality, hence the name Cartesian dualism, but this leads immediately to the major problem: How do they interact? Although he was fully aware of the problem, and suggested a point at which they interact (the

midline pineal gland, the only non-duplicated cerebral body), he was
unable to provide any details, as he grumpily admitted:

> ...the most ignorant people could, in a quarter of an hour, raise
> more questions of this kind than the wisest men could deal with
> in a lifetime; and this is why I have not bothered to answer any
> of them. These questions presuppose amongst other things an
> explanation of the union between the soul and the body, which I
> have not yet dealt with at all (letter to Clersellier, 12 January
> 1646).

This intractable question, generally known as the mind-body
problem, has never gone away. Every waking person knows that
something goes on inside the head which is related to the world but not
of the world: I look at a tree outside my window and see an expanse of
green but there is not a trace of green inside my brain. Starting in about
1880, and propelled by the remarkable research of another heroic
figure, the neuroanatomist Santiago Ramon y Cajal (1852-1934), it
became clear that empirical science had no points of contact with
Descartes' proposed "soul stuff." Therefore, the only sensible conclusion was that science should not bother itself with the mind; it
should stick to hard facts and leave the ghostly mind or spirit to poets,
priests and charlatans. Thus, western science as it is understood today
is not just dismissive of concepts of mentality, it is often openly
contemptuous. The quickest way to be shown the door at a scientific or
philosophical conference, including psychology and psychiatry, is to say
something like "I'd like to talk about healing the soul ..."

1.2. Positivism and eliminating substances.

But first, why would anybody want a non-mentalist theory of
human mentality? There have been many contributors to this idea but
one of the most influential was the French philosopher, mathematician
and author, Auguste Comte (1798-1857). Among other achievements,
Comte developed the field of sociology and, in the process, wrote a
grand plan for human progress. He was greatly influenced by the
disruptive effects of the French Revolution on society and hoped to
chart a formula for progress. Society, he said, is searching for truth, and
proceeds through stages. In the first, which he called the theological
stage, truth is seen to come from on high. Truth is what the priesthood
says it is and it is the duty of all to fall into line without arguing.
Society as a whole believes in the power of the supernatural realm to
influence daily life and a large part of everybody's life consisted of

following the myriad rules to keep on the right side of the unseen powers and their earthly representatives. Especially their earthly representatives. People were told what to believe and they questioned it at their peril, as witchcraft trials showed.

The theological stage was followed by what Comte called the metaphysical stage, in which divine authority is replaced by man's perception of universal laws of nature and of morality. Universal rights are seen to occupy a higher plane than human authority, including the priesthood's interpretation of divine authority. In this stage, Comte believed, people start to question what they had been taught, to the extent of rebelling against the older power structures, even though they often weren't sure how to replace them. The idea of investigating the natural world to discover truth took over from simply accepting what the ancients had to say about it, but there would not be much progress beyond sorting out the nature of the problems to be investigated and the means. Full understanding would come in the third and final stage, which he termed the scientific stage. In this, people free themselves of all pre-existing beliefs in order to study the world as it is using rational methods of enquiry devised by their unbiased intellects. The whole program was positive in the sense of moving positively, away from prejudice and stagnation, toward enlightenment and progress, hence the name of "positivism."

One of the most important steps in the transition to the scientific stage was to strip from science all traces of metaphysical thinking, i.e. all unproven concepts on the nature of reality. Instead of wondering how magic spells made wine go bad, Louis Pasteur put some under a microscope and discovered germs. Instead of asking why God had made so many species, Charles Darwin went to the Galapagos Islands and looked at finches for the answer. Instead of accepting that only living entities could produce biological chemicals via their "life force," Friedrich Wöhler synthesised urea in his laboratory. In Chapter 4, Behaviorism, we will see how Wilhelm Wundt applied Helmholtz's science of biology to the mind, and how, in 1913, John B Watson finally launched a rational science of psychology when he broke free of the chains of mentalism.

All of this was taking place piecemeal in many different centres of the world, including in Vienna, where a group of mathematicians, physicists and logicians had formed a society dedicated to the work of the physicist and philosopher, Ernst Mach (1838-1916). A smaller group of them were committed to his idea that science and philosophy had to eliminate all unobservables from their fields of study. Published in 1929, their manifesto [1] declared that science must be built only on what can be seen or measured. Philosophy itself had to undergo some fairly radical pruning until all that was left was what they called logical analysis. Religious and other undefined metaphysical notions had no place in their hard-headed view of the world. Known to history as the Vienna Circle, these thinkers have had a profound effect on the direction and conduct of science over the past century.

The Vienna Circle's manifesto was a brief but uncompromising statement intended to direct science, mathematics, philosophy and all other fields of rational enquiry to a novel "scientific world-conception." Biology, psychology and sociology are mentioned but the thrust is empirical investigation of the universe according to their strict logic. Their goal was to build a unified system of science on reliable knowledge which, to them, meant knowledge derived from sense data alone. A great deal of their motivation was anti-religious, so they had no time for metaphysical musing: "Neatness and clarity are striven for, and dark distances and unfathomable depths rejected. In science there are no 'depths,' there is surface everywhere ..." [1, p 9]. They firmly believed that the old ways, of trying to *reason* how the world must be, were going nowhere. Their methods, and *only* their methods, exemplified in the rapid progress in physics, would forge ahead:

> Everything is accessible to man; and man is the measure of all things ... The scientific world-conception knows no unsolvable riddle. Clarification of the traditional philosophical problems leads us partly to unmask them as pseudo-problems, and partly to transform them into empirical problems and thereby subject them to the judgment of experimental science. The task of philosophical work lies in this clarification of problems and assertions, not in the propounding of special 'philosophical' pronouncements. The method of this clarification is that of *logical analysis* of it ... [1, p 9; their emphasis].

In his reliance on studying the world, Descartes beat them by about three hundred years. When it came to practice, the method of science was reductionism, the idea that to understand something was to understand what it was made of, how it was made and how it functioned as a processor of matter and energy. Formally, reductionism says that the behavior and properties of a higher order entity are fully explained by the behavior and properties of the lower order entities of which it is composed. While the concepts embraced by positivism were not new, they essentially redefined and justified the direction of many fields of science, including biology, economics, history, linguistics, psychology, philosophy, and, of course, medicine:

> We have characterised *the scientific world-conception* essentially by *two features. First* it is *empiricist* and *positivist*: there is knowledge only from experience which rests on what is immediately given. This sets the limits for the content of legitimate science. *Second*, the scientific world-conception is marked by application of a certain method, namely *logical analysis*. The aim of scientific effort is to reach the goal, unified science, by applying logical analysis to the empirical material. Since the meaning of every statement of science must be statable by reduction to a statement about the given, likewise the meaning of any concept, whatever branch of science it may belong to, must be statable by step-wise reduction to other concepts, down to the concepts of the lowest level which refer directly to the given [1, p 12; their emphasis].

This radicalism became the guiding light of twentieth century science and rationality. No, it was much more than a guiding light, it was the searing sun that dispelled the cloying tendrils of ignorance and prejudice drifting in the darkness of religiosity. In other words, positivism is a itself a faith [2]. A central part of that faith was to eradicate any and all traces of spiritualism, including, naturally enough, human mental life.

In no time, positivism became the foundation of science, mathematics, engineering, philosophy and logic, so basic, indeed, that most students were not actually taught it. Today, few people working in fields cast entirely in the positivist framework would even know about it. As a medical student in the 1960s, as a trainee psychiatrist (resident) in the 1970s, and as a philosophy student in the 1980s, I was never taught anything about it. It was not that it became just part of the furniture, positivism was the very air we breathed, and nothing has changed. There was only ever one form of rationality, and that was the form specified by the Vienna Circle in the 1920s. People who lived and worked before the Age of Positivism were groping in the dark; nice people, for sure, but only we moderns have a solid grip on the universe.

The next year, Moritz Schlick published a brief essay on what he saw as "the turning point" of philosophy. Echoing Wittgentstein's opinion that "anything that can be said at all can be said clearly, and what we cannot talk about we must pass over in silence," Schlick shoved philosophy in a new direction:

> There are consequently no questions which are in principle unanswerable, no problems which are in principle insoluble. What have been considered such up to now are not genuine questions, but meaningless sequences of words. To be sure, they look like questions from the outside, since they seem to satisfy the customary rules of grammar, but in truth they consist of empty sounds, because they transgress the profound inner rules of logical syntax discovered by the new analysis ... There is, in addition to it, no domain of "philosophical" truths. Philosophy is not a system of statements; it is not a science. But what is it then? Well, certainly not a science, but nevertheless something so significant and important that it may henceforth, as before, be honored as the Queen of the Sciences. For it is nowhere written that the Queen of the Sciences must itself be a science [3].

This has been called the "linguistic turn" in philosophy, away from formulating metaphysical structures in some undefined space, to a process of careful analysis of language itself, later known as ordinary language or analytic philosophy. This was the basis of the split between Anglo-American or analytic philosophy and what is known as Continental or phenomenological philosophy, which dominates the field today. Somewhat surprisingly, early positivists were sympathetic to Freud's psychology. As late as 1949, in his classic monograph, *The Concept of Mind*, philosopher Gilbert Ryle (1900-1976) referred to Freud as "psychology's one man of genius" [4, p305].

Under this astringent influence, biology eagerly rid itself of all considerations of sentiment, prejudice, hope and so on: in other words, of all humanity. Because their training was thoroughly biological, physicians accepted without demur what was actually an ultra-radicalist policy [5]. Without the distraction of searches for the invisible *élan vitale* and other metaphysical notions, the life sciences powered ahead, their success constantly reinforcing the idea that positivism was the correct policy. Recasting itself as "applied bioscience," medicine transformed daily life for the masses but, while physicians occupied an exalted position in society, not everybody was happy. Instead of the caring family doctor, we had enormous hospitals working as production lines, staffed by "clinical consultants" and "biomedical technicians." By the 1970s, even physicians themselves were starting to realise something was missing [6] but medicine as clinical bioscience was on a roll, and psychiatry eagerly joined in.

1.3. Conclusion: psychiatry without the evangelism.

Philosophy, as we will see, isn't ready to surrender to the siren song of mentalism. The brief survey of some philosophies of mind in Part II will emphasise that a great deal of philosophising on the question of mind could be eliminated if philosophers knew more about the physical brain. Some do claim that they know a great deal and garnish their work with biological stuff to prove it but biology won't tell you what the mind is, it can only tell you what it is not. All too often, philosophers cherry-pick the biological evidence to justify positions they adopted before they knew any biology—and, just as often, before they knew any philosophy.

As a preliminary, I will suggest that positivism's evangelical zeal to eradicate "magical thinking" is overdone. Firstly, while in English, we only ever read about "thinking substance," Descartes himself used the terms "thinking substance" and "thinking thing" more or less inter-changeably: "*Je suis une chose qui pense ... et qui sent...*" I am a thing that thinks... and senses. The thinking soul was composed of thinking substance which, because it didn't follow the laws of physics, has always been regarded as necessarily magical. But... substances have no internal structure, they are isotropic. For example, regardless of where you start in a fog and in which direction you proceed, there is no difference in what you come across. It's all foggy. That is, there are no energy or chemical gradients in a substance so, in material terms, it can't *do* anything. If Descartes' "thinking thing" does achieve an output, it is *either* a magical entity and should be dismissed, *or* it has an internal structure, and therefore isn't a substance *per se*.

However, *things* or entities can and do have an internal structure, so they can instantiate properties which a substance can't. In terms of their inner mechanisms, the properties of things can be reductively explained whereas the properties of a substance can't. It's not possible to add to them or subtract from their properties, they are blobs that simply *are*. Any change in the properties of a substance changes it to a different substance. However, as long as the thinking thing is explained in terms of thinking elements, no laws are breached. The only breach is when we try to explain immaterial thinking in material terms [7].

The second point flows from this: the crucial feature of the thinking thing was not that, beyond immortality, it had magical properties but that it was not governed by the laws of the physical realm. As it didn't have space or mass, the laws of space and mass couldn't and didn't apply. The concept of dualism must not be restricted to mean two incommensurable *substances*. More precisely, the notion of "incommensurable substances" necessitates two sets of laws. If they both obeyed the same set of laws, they wouldn't be incommensurable; they are incommensurable just because they are governed by two sets of laws. In contrast, the distinguishing point of "magic things" is that they acquire new, anti- or non-physical properties *within* the physical realm. This is what renders them unacceptable. Tinker Bell's pixie dust acted on ordinary bodies to give them extraordinary properties, that's why it was magic. Dualism does not imply magic. It means "domiciled in a non-physical realm and governed by an alternative set of laws while exempt from the laws of the physical universe" [7]. That is how the incommensurability arises.

That puts an entirely different light on it: Can we imagine a "thing" which occupies a realm existing in parallel to the physical realm, which can be reductively explained in its own terms but not in physical terms, which is both causally effective in the physical realm and yet operates independently of the laws of gravity and thermodynamics? Yes, we can. Most people have one in their pockets right now. We call it a telephone but it's actually an informational space governed by the laws of binary algebra [7]. We will come back to this topic but the essential point is this: stripped of centuries of misperceptions, dualism means two sets of laws.

In the chapters that follow in Part I, we will see how the endless and unresolved conflict between Cartesian dualism and positivist anti-dualism has bounced psychiatry from one extreme to the other. In Part II, we will see how an anti-mentalist philosophy of mind, along the lines envisaged by John Watson in 1913, and by the authors of *The Scientific Conception of the World* in 1929 [1], has not just failed but can never succeed [8]. There has never been a plausible monist account of mind and there never will be. When it comes to the mind, positivism and its sterile offspring, antidualism, necessarily fail, and there is a perfectly obvious reason: given two sets of laws in the universe, *materialist* reduction only works on one of them. Materialist reduction does not work on non-material entities. Since there cannot be a material explanation of mental phenomena, that means biological psychiatry inevitably fails. Despite the array of "key opinion leaders" who have sternly marched behind the positivist banners, it is simply not true that everything about us is "statable by reduction to a statement about the given." As we will see, that's lucky for us.

References

1. Hahn H, Neurath O, Carnap R (1929). *The Scientific Conception of the World: The Vienna Circle*. Ernst Mach Society, University of Vienna.

2. Kolakowski, L. (1968). *Positivist Philosophy: From Hume to the Vienna Circle*. New York: Doubleday.

3. Schlick M (1930). Die Wende der Philosophie. *Erkenntnis* 1: 4-11. Translated as *The Turning Point in Philosophy*. Available online.

4. Ryle G 1949 *The Concept of Mind*. London: Hutchinson. Reprinted Penguin University Books, 1973.

5. Guze SB, 1992. *Why psychiatry is a branch of medicine*. New York: Oxford University Press.

6. Engel GL (1977). The need for a new medical model: a challenge for biomedicine. *Science*; 196:129-136.

7. McLaren N (2021): *Natural Dualism and Mental Disorder: The biocognitive model for psychiatry*. London, Routledge.

8. Stoljar D (2010). *Physicalism*. Oxford: Routledge.

<table><tr><td>

2

</td><td>

Biological Psychiatry:
Reductio ad Absurdum

</td></tr></table>

Medicine and science will be *just that much different* because we have lived.... Treatment and understanding of (mental) illness will forever be altered.... and in our way, we will persist for all time in that small contribution we have made toward the Human Venture.

Nathan Kline (psychiatrist).
Conference on biological psychiatry, Baltimore, 1970

Explanations exist; they have existed for all time; there is always a well-known solution to every human problem — neat, plausible, and wrong.

Henry L Mencken.

2.1. Setting the scene for biological psychiatry.

As mentioned in the Preface, the concept of mental disorder as a special form of brain disorder goes back a long way, definitely long before Benjamin Rush. Modern psychiatrists are perfectly clear where they stand. David Kupfer, chairman of the committee charged with writing the fifth edition of the American Psychiatric Association's (APA) Diagnostic and Statistical Manual of Mental Disorders (DSM5), stated emphatically: "Psychiatric disorders are brain disorders ... Psychiatric disorders *are* medical disorders" [1, his emphasis]. In the US, the National Institute of Mental Health (NIMH) provides the great bulk of psychiatric research funds, about $1.5bln each year. From about 2010, its former director, Thomas Insel, supervised a new orientation in research, the Research Domain Criteria (RDoC) project. Their starting position was explicitly biological:

> First, the RDoC framework conceptualises mental illnesses as brain disorders... Second, (it) assumes that the dysfunction in neural circuits can be identified with the tools of (standard laboratory) neuroscience... [2].

This didn't come out of the blue. Insel, who trained in neurophysiology and built his reputation on his research on voles, had often made similar claims:

> The good news is that we now have the tools to enable a new science of mental disorders... this science will revolutionize the diagnosis and treatment of mental illness and... transform psychiatry, ultimately realigning it with neurology and potentially creating a new discipline of clinical neuroscience... [3]
>
> Mental disorders are brain disorders ... By Congressional proclamation, the 1990s were designated the 'Decade of the Brain'... that decade marked an end to a three-century division between mind and brain. Increasingly, the most complex aspects of the mind were being addressed through studies of neural activity ... the focus on mental activity as neural activity has widened to include a focus on mental disorders as neural disorders [4].

In 1984, Nancy Andreasen, former editor in chief of the *American Journal of Psychiatry*, recipient of the National Medal of Science and a host of other awards and honours, published her views in a book entitled *The Broken Brain: The biological revolution in psychiatry* [5]. Her position was unshadowed by doubt: "Psychiatry is moving from the study of the "troubled mind" to the "broken brain" ... the biological revolution in psychiatry has already occurred" (pviii). This credo is repeated throughout the book:

> The person who wants to discover the causes of major mental illnesses... must proceed from a medical model and assume they are diseases (p151-52) ... Mental illness is truly a nervous breakdown—a breakdown that occurs when the nerves of the brain have an injury so severe that their own internal healing capacities cannot repair it (p219) ... The various forms of mental illness are due to many different types of brain abnormalities, including the loss of nerve cells and excesses and deficits in chemical transmission between neurons... (p221).

The psychiatric geneticist Kenneth Kendler has made similar claims. He believes mental disorders are real and of essentially the same nature as "classical physical-medical disorders," thus explicable in biological terms [6]. He sees psychiatry as "a legitimate biomedical discipline," its scientific status not in doubt, but psychiatric disorders are "probably inherently multifactorial" which creates considerable problems in understanding "the pathophysiologies of major mental health disorders."

There are many, many quotes like these but psychiatrists are not alone in this view. After a long career in basic research, Nobel Prize-winning neurophysiologist Eric Kandel published two books, a collection of his papers [7] and his autobiography [8], in which he explicitly stated that biological reductionism will answer the problems of mind and of psychiatry. The first lines in his autobiography spell this precisely:

> Understanding the human mind in biological terms has emerged as the central challenge for science in the twenty-first century. We want to understand the biological nature of perception, learning, memory, thought, consciousness, and the limits of free will [8].

It should be clear he was not saying "understand the biological mechanisms of consciousness etc." Throughout his career, Kandel was sympathetic to Freudian psychoanalysis (as a child in Vienna, his family lived near the Freud household) and was sure that what he called "radical reductionism" could provide a solid basis to this theory. He saw no limits to the capacity of biology to explain human behavior. Such statements are liberally scattered throughout both these works:

> ... my insistence that ... biology can transform psychoanalysis into a scientifically grounded discipline [7, xxi] ... in the near future, neurobiology will address a matter of more general and fundamental importance: the biology of human mental processes... Psychology and psychiatry can illuminate and define for biology the mental functions that need to be studied if we are to have a meaningful and sophisticated understanding of the biology of the human mind [7, 7] ... to understand behavior, one had to apply to it the same type of radical reductionist approach that had proved so effective in other areas of biology [8, 236] ... the underlying precept of the new science of mind is that *all* mental processes are biological ... Therefore, any disorder or

alteration of those processses must also have a biological basis [8, 336, his emphasis].

Philosopher Paul Thagard is equally clear as to the nature of mental disorder:

> Psychiatry assumes that mental disorders are as biologically objective as diseases like infections and cancers ... Neuroscience is beginning to provide the biological basis for the view that mental illnesses are just as objectively real as infections, cancers, and other diseases ... Attacks on the objectivity of mental illness will become even more ridiculous if mental illnesses can be effectively classified on the basis of the causal mechanisms that produce them, if these causal mechanisms provide detailed pathways from genetic and environmental conditions to mental symptoms, and if biological understanding paves the way for improved therapies. I expect that advances in theoretical and experimental neuroscience will satisfy all these requirements [9].

We can take it as read: the great majority of psychiatrists, including the most influential, along with many other scientists and philosophers, are committed to the idea that a full explanation of mental disorder will automatically flow from a full knowledge of the brain as a physical organ, with no questions unanswered. Biology will tell us all we need to know about mental disorder because there is nothing else to know. As our understanding of the brain progresses, all accounts of mental disorder as a primary psychological phenomenon will fade away, just as casting spells to cure illness faded away under the relentless advance of modern science.

Now, given the immense sums of money spent on basic brain research in psychiatry, you might think psychiatry would have something to show for it, that things are actually getting better for the mentally-troubled of the world, but that's not happening. In an interview after he left the NIMH, Thomas Insel appeared to be having second thoughts about the hard line he had followed:

> I spent 13 years at NIMH really pushing on the neuroscience and genetics of mental disorders, and when I look back on that I realize that while I think I succeeded at getting lots of really cool papers published by cool scientists at fairly large costs—I think $20 billion—I don't think we moved the needle in reducing suicide, reducing hospitalizations, improving recovery for the

tens of millions of people who have mental illness ... I hold myself accountable for that [10].

And well he may. From 2009-20 inclusive, the US spent an additional $620billion or so on prescription psychiatric drugs, presumably in the hope they would actually do something, although Insel doesn't seem convinced it was money well spent. But it was he who set the trajectory of psychiatric research for the biggest funding agency on earth; if he had doubts at any stage in his 13 year career at NIMH, surely he would have voiced them? Not so, because in 2010, he said:

> ... the biological model (of mental disorder) is sufficiently entrenched to ignore criticism and commit psychiatry to a new reductionist program ... [2].

However, criticism is the engine that drives scientific progress, so ignoring criticism as he recommends is a fairly gross breach of the scientific ethos. The trouble for "key opinion leader" Thomas Insel, and all who are influenced by his opinions, is that, absent criticism, there is no way of knowing whether their program is failing. That's the role of criticism. His advice was similar to disconnecting the temperature guage in your car: you will always feel you're doing well, until one day, you aren't.

With their new RDoC project, Insel had pushed the hardest of biological lines, wholeheartedly committing the NIMH to a new and very long term program of fundamental brain research in the belief it would give us all the answers about mental disorder. Despite anything the public had been told by psychiatrists and drug companies, he announced, mental disorder is not a "chemical imbalance" of the brain. Instead, we need to look at brain circuits because that's where the problem lies. And again, it sounds impressive, just as the "chemical imbalance" meme did in its day. Still, the question remains: Can biology tell us anything interesting about mental disorder, or is Insel's RDoC just throwing good money after bad in the search for the end of a rainbow? Since people's lives depend on them, these are important questions.

When somebody says "mental disorders are neural disorders," or "psychiatric disorders are brain disorders" or decides to "recast psychiatry as clinical neuroscience," what are they actually saying? Unfortunately, there is no clear answer to that question because the people who routinely make those statements have never actually sat down and worked out the full implications of their claims. Some people find this a bit shocking. "Surely," they say, "all these clever and responsible professors have worked out the details of their program?" That, in fact, has never happened. A lengthy survey in 2013 showed that no psychiatrist, or philosopher, or psychologist or neuroscientist had ever written anything that could justify these claims [11]. The "reductionist medical model" doesn't exist. "Aha," comes the reply, "that must be because it's self-evident, what they mean is so obvious that it doesn't require justification." Nothing in science is self-evident; that opens the door to prejudice so, in this chapter, we will investigate the claim "Mental Disorder is Brain Disorder." Can reductionism tell us anything about the mechanisms of mind, and of mental disorder, or is that just academic conceit?

2.2. The ontology of mental disorder.

Nothing in science is self-evident. If you fly in an aircraft or undergo an operation, you want to be certain that everything has been proven ten times over. Thus, before claiming that routine laboratory science can tell us all about mental disorder, as Insel did, he and his supporters need to show how they plan to investigate the mind using microscopes and gene probes and scans. And prior to that is the question of whether the human mind is the type of thing that can be pinned to a bench and dissected or seen in a scanner? This question is actually not science, it is a question about the fundamental nature of things, otherwise known as metaphysics, an ancient part of philosophy.

But questions of metaphysics cannot be determined by empirical evidence, meaning evidence derived from experience. The statement by David Kupfer, "Psychiatric disorders are brain disorders," is not scientific in any sense of the word. It is wholly ideological, a statement of his ontology, meaning his *opinion* about the fundamental nature of things. What he should have said was: "In my opinion, psychiatric disorders are brain disorders." As an unproven opinion, it carries no scientific weight. So at the outset, the search for a biological cause for mental disorder runs into major difficulties. If a physicist or geologist or ecologist tried to get a research program approved based just on their opinions, they would be laughed out of the room. However, since a lot of influential people seem to think that's fine for psychiatry, we need to look at it a little more closely.

The traditional view is that mind and body are utterly different, meaning the universe is of a dual nature. Dualism says there are two forms of being, and thus two of causation: physical (as in hailstones knocking the fruit off my trees) and non-physical, such as when I decide to move my chair. Richard Watson summed it up neatly:

> The crux of dualism is an apparently unbridgeable gap between two incommensurable orders of being that must be reconciled if we (wish to justify) our assumption that there is a comprehensible universe… [12, p210].

As we will see, the devil lies in the details of the dual natures which produce the "apparently unbridgeable gap." Convinced that this ancient problem cannot be resolved, many people have looked at the alternative, monism, the doctrine that despite appearances, the universe is actually of a single nature. Here, we have a number of choices:

Option 2.2.1: Neutral monism says that the universe only seems to be of a dual nature. In time, its supporters say, we will discover that mind and body are just different manifestations of the same fundamental stuff and we will stop seeing them as different in nature. Neutral monism doesn't have many followers these days, not least because it exists as an idea only, with no indicators as to where to start looking for the mysterious stuff.

Option 2.2.2: Idealism, the notion that the universe is actually some form of mental construct, perhaps just a dream or an idea in a cosmic mind. We will come across this notion again in Chapter 10.

Option 2.2.3: Physicalism, the idea that the universe consists of no more than matter and energy interacting in time and space according to the standard laws of physics, all of which exists independently of any minds that may perceive them. For anybody who is deterred by the uncertainty of dualism, this has considerable appeal as it is both an all-encompassing doctrine and a research program in one package. Physicalism dispenses with the supernatural and encourages people to take a hard-nosed view of the world, while its hugely successful research program, reductionism, has given us the modern world.

To reiterate, reductionism says that the behaviour or properties of a higher order entity are fully explained by the behaviour or properties of the lower order entities of which it is composed. There are no supernatural elements, so it appears the path is open to a full understanding of the higher order entity's behaviour. This concept is the foundation of Western science as it exists today. If you want to know how anything works, take it apart and examine how its physical structure mediates the matter-energy flows that it manipulates in producing its output. If you want to know why it stopped working, take it apart again and sort out where the matter-energy flows were interrupted (because you forgot to connect the widget to the thingo). If you want to know why some natural event happened, look at all of its contributing physical factors in turn and watch how they interact to produce the outcome.

This is how we've come to understand photosynthesis, normal body function and disease, volcanoes and earthquakes, phases of the moon, black holes and so on. It's also how we've been able to build machines that fly, travel underwater or harness energy and, of course, machines that transmit information. Behind it is the idea that the universe is a rational, rule-governed place that we can understand by diligent and objective application of our intellects. There is no magic in the universe, nothing supernatural, and we are obliged to leave God out of the equation. This doesn't exclude God (lots of scientists are believers) but it says that He (*sic*) created the universe with all its laws, set the whole thing running and sat back to watch.

Physicalism lends itself to scientism, the notion that the only things that matter are those that can be measured and handled by laboratory science. It says that unverifiable subjective experience is too unreliable to be of any value in science and must be discarded. Psychiatrists, psychologists and philosophers have therefore attempted to "write mentalism out" of their explanations of human behaviour. Instead of saying "He wanted to X" or "She felt like Y," devout physicalists were required to say "He was conditioned to X" or "Her reward centres were stimulated by Y." For the past century, this has been a powerful influence in psychiatry and psychology and has led to many dead-ends. I will revisit this point a number of times.

Scientism can also mean the inappropriate application of scientific methods and principles to questions of no empirical content, i.e. metaphysical questions. I will argue that that is just what psychiatry is doing in its endless and hugely expensive search for what has been called "the elusive schizococcus." This is a scornful term for the original search for a germ that caused schizophrenia but it raises an important point about people hoping to find something important. Any reduc-tionist research program starts with the expectation that the method will yield results, except sometimes it doesn't. By rights, that should lead to a reappraisal of the whole program but this rarely happens. All too often, the researchers keep promising results that just need more time and more money, and the program degenerates into what is called promissory materialism. As one target after another is missed, the researchers keep finding new ones to chase but they never question their fundamental beliefs, as Paul Thagard made clear: "I expect that advances in theoretical and experimental neuroscience will satisfy all these requirements" [9].

Promissory materialism pops up unbidden all the time, partly because nobody starts a research program without some expectation of success but mainly because people fall for the idea of quick, simple answers and can't admit they could be wrong. This is true of all life: we don't go to the shops without the expectation that they will be open. However, it can be difficult to distinguish promissory materialism from a genuine research program that has run into difficulties until after it has failed. More commonly, our taxes end up paying for a program that is later shown to be seriously flawed or even impossible just because its proponents eagerly skipped across the difficult patches, hoping they would sort themselves out.

In essence, this is what happened to the precursor of the NIMH RDoC project, its "Research Diagnostic Criteria" (RDC) plan from about 1980. The first step was to sort all mental disorder into discrete categories, meaning distinct groups with carefully defined inclusion criteria. This was the goal of the third Diagnostic and Statistical Manual of Mental Disorders (DSMIII) issued by the American Psychiatric Association (APA) in 1980. It was hoped that each disorder would then be shown to be the result of a specific defect or disturbance in brain chemistry (the "chemical imbalance of the brain" theme) which, in turn, would map down to a unique error in the genome. Finally, a full knowledge of the brain would allow a drug to be developed to rectify each genomic defect, and so the scourge of mental disorder would be conquered by rational science.

As we know, the RDC program with its ancillary "brain chemistry" project failed [2] but this was not unexpected. Critics were ignored and it is now clear that the RDC project was a classic example of promissory materialism, of ambitions which did not, could not, mesh with the reality of the world. Nature was too complicated for such a simplistic program goal. This is why the NIMH felt it needed a new plan: it couldn't keep going to Congress year after year asking for its

$2billion budget without something to show for all the money. But Insel's RDoC program is no better. All talk of finding causes of mental disorder in "brain circuits" is undiluted promissory materialism just because we have no idea what the term means in practice. Moreover, we certainly don't have even the inkling of a technology to understand what the circuits may be doing. Granted, "brain circuits" sounds very sophisticated but sophistication can conceal a host of failures. In this case, it conceals the fact that, as it stands, the program is irrefutable and is therefore non-science [13]. One way of avoiding falling into the trap of promissory materialism is to listen to critics and not ignore them, even—or especially—when you're head of the NIMH.

2.3. Mind-brain identity theory.

With those warnings in mind, we turn to Kupfer's claim: "Psychiatric disorders are brain disorders." How could it be true that mental disorder is brain disorder? One possibility is to nest the claim in a larger but consistent belief system so that it reads:

> Psychiatric disorders are brain disorders *just because* all mental events are brain events.

The larger concept is known as mind-brain identity theory (MBIT) which had its heyday in the 1950s and '60s. Rather unusually, it was pushed along by a group of materialist philosophers working in Australia. Starting with an uncompromising materialism, Smart [14], Armstrong [15], Place [16] and others argued that mental events certainly occur but, as a matter of contingent fact, they are nothing more than brain events. In this construction, the troublesome junction of mind and body is eliminated, so the problem of causal significance loses its impact. Smart confidently expressed the group's optimism:

> … it seems that even the behaviour of man himself will one day be explicable in mechanistic terms … (there is) … nothing in the world but increasingly complex arrangements of physical constituents [14].

Armstrong agreed: "…the sole cause of mind-betokening behaviour in man and the higher animals is the physico-chemical workings of the CNS" [15] (by 'mind-betokening,' he meant the sorts of actions that would make us think there is a mind behind them). As a case of strict identity, he said, sensations and all other mental events just are brain events.

Naturally enough, this has immense appeal to psychiatrists who, as physicians, are trained in the reductionist world of biology and ordinary laboratory sciences and, with rare exceptions, have no philosophical training (or inclinations). The biological psychiatrist wants to see minds as real but capable of a complete physicalist analysis. By real, biological psychiatry means "of the same nature as the rest of the universe, not magic, not a mistake and not made up." This is important because if minds aren't real then mental disorder also isn't real and psychiatrists would be out of a job. Sixty years ago, it appeared that only MBIT could satisfy these restrictive requirements. However, powerful arguments against MBIT quickly appeared. Philosopher Norman Malcolm argued that as an empirical fact, MBIT would be unintelligible as it is irrefutable. The only convincing test of whether thoughts and brain events are identical would be to identify thoughts positively, i.e. independently of the subject's reports of them [17]. Clearly, that would be impossible.

Second, he demonstrated that there are emergent (i.e. irreducible) laws and properties in the universe, such as the rule that hearsay evidence is inadmissible, the annualised national current account deficit, or the doctrinal beliefs underlying Holy Communion. These matters govern human behaviour yet they cannot be identified with molecules or fundamental particles bumping around in the dark. They are something more, something above and beyond the physical brains with which they are associated. A complete account of these and a host of similar notions relies on the concept of an intelligent observer to close the explanatory chain. Supporters of MBIT would have to show that the mind is not an emergent entity, which can't be done because they are themselves the intelligent observer making the judgement about their own minds i.e. they cannot escape begging the question. The fact that the properties of mind and the properties of brain are not identical, i.e. some mental properties are not also brain properties and vice versa, is strongly supportive of emergentism. If mind and brain were identical, meaning they each had the same set of properties, we wouldn't have separated them in the first place.

Third, Malcolm argued that even if, as MBIT asserts, it is true that thoughts and brain events are one and the same thing, it is not correct to extend the argument by saying that explaining the brain event necessarily explains the thought event since that further step confuses the thought with the mechanism that caused it. More generally, this means that a computation is independent of the mechanism that brought it about, be it by human brains, computers or extra-terrestrials. While the computation is encoded in the physical substrate, the informational content exists independently of its physical medium and, unless an observer knows the code (which requires the mental ability called intelligence), nobody can know what the mechanism is doing. This is not a trivial point. It implies that unless we know the codes the brain uses, we may never understand how the experience of mental events arises.

The question of computation raises another point on the inadequacy of MBIT. The number of arithmetical computations (sums) which the human brain can compute is infinite, whereas the number of neurones involved is finite. It is not possible to establish a relationship of identity between the elements of a finite series (the neurones) and those of an infinite series (the sums). It could be argued that while there can be no relationship of identity between sums and neurones, there is potentially one with the approximately infinite combinations of the billions of neurones involved. However, this attempt at a solution runs into the same sort of problem. Is there a fixed relationship between a particular combination of neurones and a particular sum? If so, how does the brain 'know' just when to send a sum to that particular set of neurones? Or, were these neurones determined genetically? There isn't enough genetic material in the human genome for this purpose.

These sorts of objections spell the end of the line for MBIT, and the end of the line for Kupfer's bold claim that "Psychiatric disorders are brain disorders." Anybody looking for a physical cause of mental disorder will need to do more than try to rub mental events out of the equation.

2.4. Practical reductionism.

We can grant Dr Kupfer a second chance by allowing that what he meant was "Regardless of the nature of mind, as a matter of empirical fact, all psychiatric disorders are *caused by* brain disorders." This avoids the problems of normal mental function and gives him a lot more scope because, as an empirical fact, it's quite feasible. It's a claim of the same nature as "As a matter of empirical fact, heart attacks are caused by occlusion of the coronary arteries." Thus, in an emergency department, one can hear conversations like this:

> Patient: "Help me, I'm having a heart attack."
> Medical Officer: "OK, so let's have a look at your coronary arteries."

> P: "But I'm having a heart attack, don't you understand?"
> MO: "I do, so our first step will be to check your cardiac perfusion."

As a matter of empirical fact, the clinical picture of what people call a heart attack (chest pain, sweating, pallor, collapse, loss of consciousness etc) is the predictable result of reduced cardiac perfusion. The patient wants his heart attack treated and the MO wants to look at his coronary arteries. They are talking different languages but, as a question of physiology, the phenomena which the patient identifies as a "heart attack" are caused by or reduce to impaired cardiac perfusion. As a case of reductionism in action, improving cardiac perfusion relieves the "heart attack" (a term with no meaning in medicine).

Meanwhile, the patient in the next cubicle has been referred to a biological psychiatrist:

> Patient: "My life is going badly and I can't see it getting better so I may as well end it now."
>
> The biological psychiatrist replies: "OK, so you have a brain disturbance and when we fix that, you'll feel fine and able to cope with your life."
>
> P: "But I feel depressed. I hurt my back at work and I've lost my job. I'm in constant pain, I have no sexual interest so my wife thinks I'm seeing somebody else and now my poor old budgie has died. Don't you understand?"
>
> BP: "I understand perfectly but your life events have nothing to do with it. You're depressed because you have a chemical imbalance of the brain. Take these tablets and come back in a month."
>
> P: "Will that make my wife sympathetic to my back pain?"
>
> BP: "You also have somatising disorder. Take these tablets as well and we'll see you in a month."
>
> P: "What about my job, and my budgie?"
>
> BP: "Indeed, so pop along to the social work department, they'll sort that out. Next please."

Biological psychiatrists agree with this statement:

> As a matter of empirical fact, the clinical picture of depression is caused by a particular brain defect. While we do not yet know the nature of the defect, there are drugs that can improve mental disorders.

We could even propose a modification of Koch's Postulates to cover mental disorder, for example:

> The particular brain defect must be found in all or most sufferers but not in the mentally well;

> Inducing the defect in a healthy person must cause the clinical syndrome;

> Reversal of the defect must relieve all symptoms, and...
> A rational cause for the defect must be conceivable.

Unfortunately for biological psychiatry, these finer points have never been filled in. It has long been known that most mental disorders are related to psychological stressors, either recent or long past, but the relationship is not understood. In the case of schizophrenia and other major mental disorders, the cause is seen purely as a matter of biology. Life events may be noted in the case history but are not given any weight. To a biological psychiatrist, they are as irrelevant as the patient's star sign at birth. Emotions are stripped of their empathic significance and reduce to markers of brain pathology.

In the case of depression, psychiatrists may take a similar view, dismissing adverse events as insignificant or, more likely, saying that they occurred *because* the patient had developed a biological illness of the brain. That is, the patient above had his accident because he was withdrawn and not paying attention, the depressive illness caused loss of sexual function and preoccupation with pain, and his self-involved behaviour caused his wife to withdraw her support and sympathy, etc. When the tablets reverse his primary mental disorder, all his mental symptoms will disappear, the pain will improve, his sex life will recover, his wife will be happy, they will choose another budgie together and all will be well. There is no attempt to explain how this came about; all that counts is that the presence of certain mental symptoms leads to a unique biological diagnosis for which modern science has developed specific and curative drugs. Because of his genetic predisposition (a "depressive diathesis," in medical terms), the patient is highly likely to have further bouts so, as depression is a serious illness, he should take medication for life.

Just as, for example, searching the blood films of patients with a severe febrile illness led to the discovery of the malaria parasite, the biological approach to mental disorder leads to a valid research program, albeit hit or miss. For nearly a hundred years, psychiatrists have examined the body fluids of patients, conducted post mortems, scanned their heads or analysed their genomes, all at enormous cost. There was Insel's $20billion, plus all the NIMH money spent since its inception in 1949, plus all the money spent in other countries, plus all the money spent by drug companies, plus the private charities and foundations, plus all the rest, and what has it shown? Nothing. After a century of blind screening for Dr Kupfer's empirical cause of mental disorder, there is no consistent evidence that any primary mental disorder is caused by a provable brain defect. More to the point, nor is there any clue as to where such a program could go (we can exclude mental symptoms arising in the course of proven physical illnesses such as Huntington's Disease, or following drug intoxications such as amphetamines, etc, as they tell us nothing about similar cases with no biological illness). All it shows is that psychiatrists are hanging on to their unproven biological convictions with a tenacity that is immune to evidence and, indeed, common sense. That is, they meet the definition of ideologues, not scientists (11, 13).

This raises a further question from the philosophy of science: Can we refute the claim "As a matter of empirical fact, psychiatric disorders are *caused by* brain disorders"? If not, it is not a valid scientific statement and should not be used as the basis of a research program. I don't believe it is valid just because a formal theory or model of mental disorder must derive from a theory of mind, which we don't have. Remember this is not the same as searching for the cause of AIDS, for hominid fossils, for gravity waves or the Higgs boson [1]. In each of these, the search was generated by a *pre-existing model*. The search for a physical cause of mental disorder is not anchored in a physicalist model of mind. It exists independently as a statement of belief, but it has no basis in an articulated theory, and there is not a shred of empirical evidence to support it. It turns out that "evidence-based psychiatry" is based in no evidence and is immune to lack of evidence, i.e. the "evidence" is evidence only of the psychiatrist's prejudices.

So what evidence would refute it? Committed biological psychiatrists believe there is no possible evidence that would refute the claim because they believe it is correct and they will prove it "one fine day." Granted, absence of proof of a physical cause of mental disorder

---

1   Actually, SETI, the search for extraterrestrial intelligence, has similarities to the search for the schizococcus: the model is humans ourselves; the search technology is available; the idea is attractive; there is money to burn, so let's go, the details will sort themselves out.

is not proof that there is no such cause, but there comes a point in every unproductive search where the searchers have to ask themselves (and explain to the taxpayer) "How do we know we're on the right track? What would tell us this is wrong?" Let's consider the possible answers:

2.4.1 "We just know we're on the right track, there's no way we could be wrong so stop asking stupid questions."

> This attitude is not compatible with science. A person who says this may be a good researcher but should not be in charge of a research program because this level of commitment cannot be distinguished from fanaticism—or delusion. Funding agencies should reply: "You're in breach of the most elementary rules of science, call us when you've lifted your game."

2.4.2. "We know we're on the right track, our model of mental disorder predicts it."

> That would be fine. It would be like Columbus searching for China by sailing west—his model was that the world is round, not flat—and like the search for gravity waves or the Higgs boson, which are predicted by the standard model of physics. Except psychiatry doesn't have a standard biological model of mental disorder, or any model [11]. Funding agencies should reply "That's fine, call us when you have one and we'll reconsider."

2.4.3. "We're probably on the right track, it's always worked in the rest of medicine."

> This is a low-grade inductivism. Funding agencies should reply "That's fine but can you convince us that what works in the rest of medicine will also work in psychiatry, that mental disorder is of the same nature as physical disorder? Call us when you've sorted it out."

2.4.4. "We hope we're on the right track, we don't have any tools for investigating unobservables."

> This is like the drunk man who searched for his lost key under the street light because that was where the light was. Funding agencies should reply "Would you pay a plumber who didn't have the right tools for the job? You're scientists, is it asking too much that you develop some? Call us when you've sorted it out."

2.4.5. "This has to be the right track. We can't conceive of a non-physical cause of mental disorder."

> Funding agencies should reply "Philosophy 101: don't mistake your lack of imagination for the limits of science. The correct answer to the cause of mental disorder is likely to be counter-intuitive so you should ask around, especially ask all those critics you don't like. Better still, why don't you tell them to apply for funds, we'll give them some of yours."

2.4.6. "We've invested our careers, our reputations and our egos in this search, there's too much at stake, we can't possibly be wrong."

> Funding agencies should reply "We feel for you, take some tissues to wipe your noses. Next please."

A neutral observer would be inclined to say that the existence of post-traumatic states argues against the idea that all mental disorder is biological in nature. It stands to reason: a person with no previous history of mental disorder experiences a severe psychological shock and develops long-lasting mental symptoms. Even that doesn't convince the true believers. They will argue that, for some unknown genetic reason, the subject was predisposed to react badly to intense psychological stressors, and this induces long-lasting changes in brain biochemistry, possibly epigenetic, which themselves cause the continuing symptoms. If the chemical changes can be reversed, then the symptoms will disappear. For them, it is biological even though the proximal trigger was psychological.

The problem is the lack of anything like a formal theory of mind to guide the research. Regardless of the evidence put forward to say one disorder or another is wholly psychological in nature, the reductionists will always argue that, in the final analysis, all mental disorder is biological in nature (and here they quote people like Insel and Kandel) because the brain. However, that statement is irrefutable, which means that the whole of psychiatry's biological research program is non-scientific.

Over the past century, hundreds of suggestions have been investigated as "the biological cause of mental disorder" but not one of them has survived. There is hardly a month goes past without somebody somewhere finding a new idea to study, or a miraculous new drug or physical treatment that will transform our lives but, beyond spending a lot of money on pointless research and making drug companies rich, they go nowhere. Why will the psychiatric establishment not call a break to reconsider its research program? You would need to ask the researchers or the people who control the funding but I think the answer will boil down to something like option 2.4.6 above: "We've invested our careers, our reputations and egos, and all this money in the pursuit of the elusive schizococcus and we can't bring ourselves to consider we may have been wrong. Worse still, we would have to admit our enemies have been right all along."

That, of course, is exactly what fanatics do (*n.* a person filled with excessive and single-minded zeal, especially for an extreme religious or political cause). Is it reasonable to refer to a specialist branch of the medical profession as fanatical? Let's look at each of the features of the definition of fanatic:

Zeal? Yes, they are certainly zealous in their pursuit of their goal. They have journals and conferences and networks; they teach it, study it, research it; they talk to anybody who will listen and anybody with money; and there are even signs in public toilets asking: "Are you depressed? Go and see your doctor" (who will give you a prescription but won't ask about your terrible job, your unhappy marriage or your dreadful childhood, etc. Or your budgie).

Single-minded? As per the quotes in Section 1.1, there are no doubts in the mainstream as to the validity of the biological research program. Granted, a few psychiatrists, mostly in the UK, Canada and Australia, say they follow something called the biopsychosocial model but they're a minority (see Chap. 5).

Excessive? After a hundred years of not budging the needle, as Insel put it, I believe it is excessive, particularly when measured against the time and money spent on researching the alternatives, meaning practically none.

Religious? It is often said, e.g. by Thomas Szasz [18], that psychiatry has many of the features of a cult but that is a sociological phenomenon, not scientific. While this complaint is outside the scope of this work, I don't believe it can be dismissed lightly.

Political? Psychiatry is most definitely intensely political in a way that, for example, cardiology is not [19]. Even its main diagnostic manual, the APA's DSM system, is the result of a prolonged and often bitter political process. The higher one goes up the institutional/academic ladder, the more political it becomes. The ultimate proof is the political power granted to psychiatrists to detain people indefinitely and force them to take treatment against their will. Even among those who claim to practice an "evidence-based psychiatry," there is no medical evidence whatsoever to support involuntary treatment, on either an individual or on a population basis, but psychiatry bitterly resists any efforts to change it.

So to look at the question again: Is it reasonable to refer to a specialist branch of the medical profession as fanatical? Answer: If the cap fits, wear it.

I should add that every time I make an observation like this, a wave of hostility sweeps my way. What *never* happens is an anxious call from the higher echelons of the profession asking whether there should be a discussion of the topic, would I like to submit a paper to the journal to start it, or perhaps a session at the next conference where I could present my case? That's how scientists respond to criticism but zealots never do, because they're never wrong. Ask them.

2.5. Panpsychism.

It seems then that the search for a direct physical cause of mental disorder is on shaky grounds, which leads to the bigger question: Is the mind itself reducible to its physical substrate, the brain, or is that not possible? The first question is: Where does the reduction stop? If we're trying to explain the sense of humour, do we find its causes in specific brain centres, or in neurones, or molecules, or in subatomic particles? Perhaps the mental property of humour, or consciousness, whatever, is evenly distributed through the universe, with each physical particle also having a tiny bit such that when it comes together, the whole structure gains a mental ability. This is the concept of panpsychism, which has been around for a long time but it quickly gets out of control. If the human body contains enough atoms of consciousness to form a mind, then what about elephants? Sperm whales, which have the biggest brains of any creature that has lived? The earth? OK, then obviously what counts is the way the atoms with their tiny bits of consciousness are assembled. They have to be in the form of a human brain before they create human consciousness. But that still leaves whales with a form of whale consciousness, and cows, so perhaps we shouldn't eat them? Philosopher Thomas Nagel explored the possibility of panpsychism in his monograph *Mind and Cosmos*:

> Everything, living or not, is constituted from elements having a nature that is both physical and nonphysical—i.e. capable of combining into mental wholes. So this reductive account can also be described as a form of panpsychism: all the elements of the physical world are also mental [20, S.3.4].

There are people who believe this but it's an opinion so, even though it's presented as an established scientific fact, it isn't. The counter-argument is that simply stating that physical elements also have mental properties does not advance our knowledge, it merely moves what requires explanation from one explanatory dimension to another. Consequently, Nagel saw little prospect of a rational account of such a model:

> The protopsychic properties of all matter, on such a view, are postulated solely because they are needed to explain the appearance of consciousness at high levels of organic complexity. Apart from that, nothing is known about them: they are completely indescribable and have no predictable local effecs, in contrast to the physical properties of electrons and protons, which allow them to be detected individually. So we have no idea how such a compositional explanation would work… panpsychism does not provide a new, more basic resting place in the search for intelligibility—a set of basic principles from which more complex results can be seen to follow. It offers only the *form* of an explanation without any content… [20, S.3.5; emphasis added]

We can try different options but the answer is there are no quarks of consciousness hidden in physical atoms, no mental properties nestled among the physical. A molecule is a molecule, be it in a dog's brain or human; if it has no moral value or properties in the dog brain, it has none in a human brain. It is the *arrangement* and then the *performance* of molecules that gives human brains their moral capacity; that is, morality emerges from one particular arrangement of molecules and its associated actitivity but not from another. It's not the actual molecules that count, it's what they're doing. Human consciousness, humour, morality, etc are entirely the result of the unique form of the human brain, of how it's put together and what it can then do. Its structure determines its function, meaning its function emerges from its specific structure. We can take panpsychism off the list of possibilities.

2.6. Physicalism.

The broader question of physicalism, the view that the ultimate nature of all that is consists of the physical elements of the universe with nothing left over, is fraught. Today, physicalism in one form or another is more or less the default position of philosophers the world over. Historian and philosopher Richard Carrier states the position unambiguously:

> ... the sciences have converged on just such a discovery: more and more it appears that all of sociology can be reduced to psychology; all of psychology can be reduced to biology; all biology to chemistry, and all chemistry to physics, which is the study of matter and energy in space-time. Therefore everything is matter-energy in space-time. This is called "reductionism" [21, III.5.4.2] ... the view that everything can be reduced to matter and energy in space and time: quarks and other sub-atomic particles and their behaviors are all that there is, out of which everything without exception is made... societies can be reduced to sub-atomic particles ... theoretically, all of sociology and psychology can be described entirely by physics [21, III.5.5; for the unacknowledged ambiguity in his position, see Chap. 14].

There are plenty of authors who are openly contemptuous of the notion that in talking of human affairs, we need to take account of a causally-effective, non-physical mind. Boston philosopher Daniel Dennett is one such and we will look at his work in Chapter 8. At first glance, Carrier's almost brutal reductionism seems to offer consistency, if nothing else. However, philosopher Daniel Stoljar has sounded serious warnings:

> The first thing to say when considering the truth of physicalism is that we live in an overwhelmingly physicalist or materialist intellectual culture. The result is that, as things currently stand, the standards of argumentation required to persuade someone of the truth of physicalism are much lower than the standards required to persuade someone of its negation. (The point here is a perfectly general one: if you already believe or want something to be true, you are likely to accept fairly low standards of argumentation for its truth) [22].

So what is Carrier's argument in favour of his radical physicalist reductionism? Well, that's the problem, he doesn't give one. His case is no stronger than "more and more it appears that societies can be reduced to sub-atomic particles." Presuming he doesn't mean by nuclear warfare, then his "appears" carries no more weight than, say, a psychoanalyst who says "It appears his ego functions have been swamped by id impulses," or an atrologer who says "It appears Mars is in the ascendent; be ready for conflict," meaning no weight at all. But assume his case is correct: Where in the physical hierarchy, for example, should we locate a sociological matter such as the annualised rate of change of unsecured per capita national debt? Or the theory of evolution? Or a belief in ghosts? Indeed, where in the physical realm can we locate belief in the first place? What would it mean to say "My brain molecules believe in fairies." What is there about sub-atomic particles that determines truth or falsity? No idea; in fact, "the standards of argumentation required to persuade someone of the truth of physicalism" are here so low they don't exist. We are pushed to accept his case on the single basis that nobody has come up with an alternative. But that's not an argument at all: The lack of a good answer doesn't compel us to accept a bad answer.

Following his exhaustive analysis of physicalism, Stoljar [22] concluded that there is no possible version of the physicalist thesis which is both true and worthy of the name. The claim that the ultimate nature of the universe is physical is either true but boring and of no scientific or philosophical value, or an interesting idea that seems helpful but just turns out to be wrong.

The central problem for naive physicalism (which includes biological psychiatry) is that when coded systems interact in a suitable substrate, they are not constrained by the ordinary laws governing the interaction of matter and energy in the physical universe [23]. Codes operate by their own laws, formalised as the logic of that particular system. Necessarily, the logical is independent of the biological, which physicalism states is impossible. MBIT, for example, was devised to overcome the problem of codes (language, mental events, etc.) simply by declaring it a 'non-problem,' according to Moritz Schlick. In order to be able to claim success, its supporters (if there are any left) must be able to map the higher order human functions such as language, mathematics, music, etc. directly to a lower order material element, i.e. to its mechanism. But the whole point of a code written in symbols is that it is *not* directly related to its mechanism. If it were, it wouldn't be a code, it would be a physical system akin to a door key. In the case of humans, those code-users par excellence, mental events such as wanting to be a poet or planning genocide cannot be reduced to a matter of neurones firing off in our skulls. Merely watching cerebral neurones fire will give as much information as looking at the surface of a CD as it spins around, meaning none at all (if anyone still uses CDs).

All mental events, including everything abstract that we regard as distinctively human, involve choices, and choices are made by manipulating symbols. Necessarily, symbols are independent of the material base in which they are coded. At the level of meaning, there is a disjunction between a symbol and its material substrate, the brain. There has to be. That's what 'symbol' means: something that stands for or represents an entity or process but which is not itself that entity or process. Reductionism cannot bridge that gap because, by definition, it's unbridgeable, it represents the leap from the material realm to the immaterial. These are "incommensurable orders of being," and necessarily so. If there were not an epistemological gap between information and its substrate, I would never be able to *imagine* a mind-body problem or even what my brain would look like.

Almost as an afterthought, and bearing in mind Kandel's ambition of "understanding the human mind in biological terms" or gaining "a meaningful and sophisticated understanding of the biology of the human mind," what would a genuinely reductionist model of mind or mental disorder look like? This is a separate question from Stoljar's point of whether it is possible. The first point to remember is that, as normal mental function, consciousness is a product of the whole, intact, healthy brain operating within its biological parameters. Reductionism is off to a bad start: we can't take the brain apart to find the mind, any more than we can, as they say, take a cow apart to find the moo. This is because not all functions or properties of a higher order entity are entailed by the functions or properties of its constituents. Some functions, and this includes all the interesting ones, are not the direct product of the physical constituents but of how they operate together.

Take a simple example. I have on my work bench seven items, including four wheels, two shorter pieces of metal rod and one longer. They are jumbled together and their only property is their combined weight. However, by putting the wheels on the ends of the short rods, now called axles, and fixing one axle crosswise at each end of the long rod, I have made a trolley which has the novel property of transport (actually, it's a performance but we won't split hairs). The new property of transport is a higher order property which comes into existence or *emerges* wholly as a product of the particular arrangement of the seven items on the bench. That is, higher order functions are dictated by the geometry of the object and cease to exist when that geometry is interrupted. This is the concept of emergentism [23]. The only ways we can claim that reductionism can explain my little trolley's property of transport is either by fiat (essentially what Insel and all the other influential psychiatrists have done), by promissory materialism, or by concealing that which needs to be explained somewhere in the environment. This ploy was used by the behaviorist, Burrhus F Skinner, as will be discussed in Chap. 4.

The second objection to materialist reductionism is: Where does it stop? Should we look to the level of the brain's complex molecular structure or should we keep going down? And down? But it becomes silly. I have a sense of humour but molecules don't. I can decide to make a cup of tea but a single neuron can't. I don't think we need to go any further. Materialist reductionism works on pulleys, it works on piston engines and power stations, on chloroplasts and hepatocytes, but it doesn't work on information, i.e. everything that makes us human. Reductionism is a tool, not an ontological statement, but, like all tools, it should only be used on the correct job. There is a tool called informational reductionism but Thomas Insel and his friends aren't up to that page yet.

In the case of simpler machines, we can understand the matter-energy flows within them just by inspecting their layout, and impaired output can also be explained this way. When the matter-energy flows are controlled by informational flows, it becomes much more difficult as we need to understand them first; in the case of our brains, we don't have any such understanding and may well never have it. So we don't have any indication of what a "radical reductionist" model of mind would look like, not least because radical reductionism will necessarily destroy the brain we are trying to study. Putting that aside, biological psychiatrists could claim that while mind is indeed an emergent phenomenon, totally dependent on the intact brain, disorders of mind are always and only caused by physical disturbances of the brain: an unhealthy brain is necessary and sufficient to produce an unhealthy mind. That, however, leads straight to promissory materialism and all the problems listed in S2.4, above. But that's not surprising: even Kandel's reputation as a neurophysiologist couldn't prevent him from falling into the trap of promissory materialism.

2.7. Conclusion: no physical way out.

The claim "Mental disorder is brain disorder" is either an empirical claim or a logical statement. If it's offered as an empirical claim, there's no evidence to support it. Zero. It is entirely a matter of promissory materialism, of people mistaking their hopes and ambitions for a scientific program. And now that the massive investments in psychiatric genetics are coming up empty-handed, there are no other avenues to explore. I see no evidence to suggest the current biological research program in psychiatry will ever achieve its goals, nor that the latest project to emerge from NIMH, the Research Domain Criteria program, will fare any better than the last one. The reasons are basic, often not much more than common sense, just like the reasons that sank psychoanalysis and behaviourism. As with those two failed programs, the reasons for their failure were built in from the beginning but everybody was so excited that they forgot to look at the details. Only philosophers did.

If, however, "Mental disorder is brain disorder" is offered as a logical claim, it is either true but boring and of no scientific or philosophical value, or an interesting idea that seems helpful but just turns out to be wrong. Either way, it's no way to run a scientific program.

Unfortunately, as will be shown, the institution of psychiatry has no other plan. Biological psychiatry just is their Plan B. Fifty years ago, they scornfully rejected the concept that mental disorder may be *sui generis*, a thing unto itself. Caught in the grip of positivism, but not aware of it (see Chap. 1), there didn't seem to be a way of investigating the mind. So they declared it *res non grata*, off limits for real scientists, and slammed the door shut, thereby locking themselves into a dead end. But where is the argument to say that primary mental disorders can't exist? There isn't one, nobody bothered. Just like John B Watson in 1913, they decided that ignorance of the mind-body problem was the path to the future. Well, the future has arrived and we're still ignorant.

References

1. Kupfer DJ, Kuhl EA, Wuisin L (2013) Psychiatry's integration with medicine: the role of DSM5. *Annual Review of Medicine* 64: 385-92.

2. Insel TR, Cuthbert BN, Garvey M, et al (2010). Research Domain Criteria (RDoC): toward a new classification framework for research on

mental disorders. Commentary. *American Journal of Psychiatry,* 167: 748-751.

3. Insel TR (2009). Disruptive insights in psychiatry: transforming a clinical discipline. *Journal of Clinical Investigations* 119: 700–705.

4. Insel TR (2010). Faulty Circuits. *Scientific American* April 2010, p45.

5. Andreasen NC (1984). *The Broken Brain: The biological revolution in psychiatry.*New York: Harper and Row.

6. Kendler K (2016). The nature of psychiatric disorders. *World Psychiatry.* 15(1): 5–12. doi: 10.1002/wps.20292

7. Kandel ER. *Psychiatry, psychoanalysis and the new biology of mind.* Washington, DC: American Psychiatric Publishing. 2005.

8. Kandel ER. *In search of memory: the emergence of a new science of mind.* New York: Norton, 2006.

9. Thagard P (2008). Mental Illness from the Perspective of Theoretical Neuroscience. *Perspectives in Biology and Medicine,* 51(3): 335-52.

10. Rogers A (2017). Star Neuroscientist Tom Insel Leaves the Google-Spawned Verily for ... a Startup? *Wired Science* May 11 2017.

11. McLaren N (2013). Psychiatry as Ideology. *Ethical Human Psychology and Psychiatry* 15: 7-18.

12. Watson RA (1995) in Audi R (Ed.). *The Cambridge Dictionary of Philosophy.* Cambridge: University Press.

13. McLaren N (2011). Cells, circuits and syndromes. A critique of the NIMH Research Domain Criteria project. *Ethical Human Psychology and Psychiatry* 13: 229-236.

14. Smart JJC (1959). Sensations and brain processes. Reprinted in: Borst CV, Ed. *The Mind/Brain Identity Theory.* London: Macmillan,

15. Armstrong DM (1980). *The Nature of Mind.* St Lucia: University of Queensland Press,.

16. Place UT (1956). Is consciousness a brain process? Reprinted in: Borst CV, Ed. *The Mind/Brain Identity Theory.* London: Macmillan,

17. Malcolm N. Scientific materialism and the identity theory. Reprinted in: Borst CV, Ed. *The Mind/Brain Identity Theory.* London: Macmillan,

18. Szasz TS (1977). *The Theology of Medicine: the Political-Philosophical Foundations of Medical Ethics.* Baton Rouge: Louisiana State University Press.

19. Whitaker R, Cosgrove L (2015). *Psychiatry Under the Influence: Institutional Corruption, Social Injury, and Prescriptions for Reform.* New York: Palgrave MacMillan.

20. Nagel, T 2012. *Mind and Cosmos: Why the materialist neo-Darwinian conception of nature is almost certainly false.* New York: Oxford University Press.

21. Carrier, R. (2005). Sense and Goodness Without a God: a defence of metaphysical naturalism. Bloomington, IN: AuthorHouse.

21. Stoljar D (2021) Physicalism. *Stanford Encyclopedia of Philosophy.* At: https://plato.stanford.edu/entries/physicalism/ Accessed April 5th 2022.

22. Stoljar D (2010). *Physicalism.* Oxford: Routledge.

23. McLaren N (2021): *Natural Dualism and Mental Disorder: The biocognitive model for psychiatry.* London, Routledge.

3   The Disorder of Mentalism

Whenever a theory appears to you as the only possible one, take this as a sign that you have neither understood the theory nor the problem which it was intended to solve.

Karl Popper (1902-1994), *Objective Knowledge: An Evolutionary Approach* (1972)

Progress is slow partly from mere intellectual inertia. In a subject where there is no agreed procedure for knocking out errors, doctrines have a long life. A professor teaches what he was taught, and his pupils, with a proper respect and reverence for teachers, set up a resistance against his critics for no other reason than that it was he whose pupils they were.

Joan Robinson (Cambridge economist) (1903-1983)

3.1. Setting the scene for psychodynamic psychiatry.

If you ask people in the street what they understand by the word "mind," they will look at you in surprise and reply along the lines of: "Mind? I don't think about it much, I just get on with things but it's what goes on inside my head. You know, thinking, deciding, remembering, what I see and hear and feel, the senses and all that sort of stuff."

If you then ask: "And how does it all get there?" you'll likely get a dismissive grin: "I dunno, that's the brain's job, isn't it?" Other people may say something like: "Well, that's the soul's job I suppose, as long as my body's healthy, it keeps things on track."

Biological reductionism says that "all that sort of stuff" is of no real interest, all the action takes place at the level of the brain as a biological organ. Reports of mental events are of interest only insofar as they indicate the underlying and unseen biological pathology. The opposing view, mentalism, says that the mental life, as in "thinking, deciding, remembering, what I see and hear and feel, the senses and all that sort of stuff," is both real and causally significant. Mental life is real in the sense that there is a difference between the taste of chilli and the taste of icecream, between choosing to turn right and choosing to turn left, and that these differences must be explained, not explained away. And mental life is causally significant in that if I decide to add chilli to my icecream, that's what will happen.

Once the existence of the mind is explained, which is philosophy's job, then the whole of the mental contents can be understood in the context of the mind itself: the cause of a mental event is a prior mental event, not a physical event. This also applies to mental disorder. For a mentalist, there is no contradiction in saying that a mentally-disordered person has a perfectly healthy brain whereas for a reductionist, that statement is absurd.

The most far-reaching and influential mentalist model of mental disorder was psychoanalysis, founded by Sigmund Freud (1856-1939). Freud was a Viennese neurologist and researcher who studied at the Salpetriere Hospital in Paris under the renowned Jean-Martin Charcot. Charcot used hypnosis to treat and also to provoke the symptoms of the condition known as hysteria, which was generally thought to be a form of hereditary degeneration of the brain. This sparked Freud's interest and on returning to Vienna, he decided to specialise in this field. However, he was not very good at hypnotism so, working with another physician, he developed the idea of a "talking cure." The physician listened non-judgementally to the patients and gradually helped them see how their symptoms were the result of suppressed psychological trauma, mostly of a sexual nature. Bringing the forbidden material to consciousness encouraged the patients to deal with it in a more mature manner than simply locking it away, and thus allowed the symptoms to resolve. Freud soon gathered an international following which, almost as quickly, splintered into squabbling groups. Over decades, the notion of unconscious causation developed into the most elaborate theory of mental life in history.

The history of the psychoanalytic movement is very much part of the twentieth century. In his historical critique of psychiatry, Andrew

Scull [1] gives a balanced and readable account of the development of this most influential of theories, how it arose and why, inevitably, it fell. Freud declared that as a model of mind, of mental development and of treatment, his theory was entirely original, it was scientific and it was universal, applying to all people at all stages and in all walks of life. Each of these claims has since been refuted. However, it must be remembered that Freud's followers reacted savagely to criticism of their demigod and even at this distance, any criticism of psychanalysis still provokes arguments. Before we say anything about his theory as an exemplar of mentalist theories, we need to settle these points.

First point: Freud's work was not original. Freud was Jewish and was raised in a traditional religious family in a provincial city. His wife was the daughter of a prominent rabbi in Hamburg but Freud was pointedly secular and played down his religious and ethnic background. Vienna, where he trained and worked, was relatively liberal but Jews were still restricted in some ways. However, it seems most of his patients and his colleagues were members of the Jewish community so it should be no surprise that, in many respects, Freud's basic concepts are consistent with his background. In particular, many of the ideas he developed seem to be derivative of the Kabbalah, the traditional mystic beliefs of Ashkenazi Jews.

The second point is more important: his work was not scientific. With a background in laboratory research in human and animal brains, Freud clearly saw himself as part of the scientific establishment. At the time, late nineteenth and early twentieth centuries, science was racing ahead and if at any stage he had said that his work was not entirely scientific, it would have been the kiss of death. In brief, psychoanalysis ran headlong into the problem that had dogged dualist systems since Descartes' time, how to differentiate convincing evidence of mental life from spiritualist fantasies. Until psychoanalysis could reliably separate itself from metaphysical, absurd or frankly insane beliefs, it could not gain wide acceptance within the scientific community. Within the movement, however, Freud's word was law. This, more than perhaps anything, led to the endless arguing and schisms that are so characteristic of the psychoanalytic movement—and, of course, of any religious or political cult.

The philosopher, Karl Popper (1902-1994), who knew some of the first psychoanalysts in Vienna, decided very early in his career that their doctrine was little better than nonsense. In his autobiography, he recounted a conversation with Alfred Adler (of "inferiority complex" fame) in 1919, in which he began to suspect the ease with which analysts believed their theories were confirmed in daily clinical experience:

> It was precisely this fact—that they always fitted, that they were always confirmed—which in the eyes of their admirers constituted the strongest argument in favour of these theories. It began to dawn on me that this apparent strength was in fact their weakness [2, p35].

In time, Popper expanded on the crucial difference between valid empirical science and metaphysical systems [2, p41-43]. He was looking for some reliable means of distinguishing a valid scientific theory from nonscience, some demarcation criterion that allows us to draw a line between the two, as it is now known. For Popper, the specific feature was that empirical science can always be refuted by further evidence whereas non-science can't: there is an asymmetry between the value we attach to supporting evidence vs. disconfirming evidence [3]. If a scientific theory makes a prediction which turns out to be right, we don't know whether it was because the theory is a general truth or it was only true by chance. If, however, the prediction turns out to be wrong, we can be certain it is not a general truth. When a non-scientific theory such as a religion, a political movement or pseudoscience makes a wrong prediction (e.g. the Church's insistence that the earth is the centre of the universe), its supporters can always "explain away" any findings they don't like. Scientists don't have that luxury.

Popper's choice of a demarcation criterion between science and nonscience was the concept of refutability, that science can always be refuted whereas nonscience can't. If a theory is in principle irrefutable, it isn't science. Psychoanalytic theory impressed its followers as it seemed able to account for everything, but that was its undoing. Nothing that anybody said or did could ever prove it wrong. Any prediction or statement could be turned around to conform with the theory. The reason was just because psychoanalysis had no basis in a theory of mind, no mechanism of its origin or emergence, and no medium of implementation of the processes of mind. His work was thus wholly descriptive with no explanatory capacity.

To a large extent, this intellectual plasticity came from the concept of ego defence mechanisms, which allowed the analyst to "prove" that everything the patient said and did confirmed his opinion of the patient. If the patient felt guilty about something, it was due to bad impulses; if he didn't feel guilty, that was also due to repressing bad impulses by one defence mechanism or another. Nobody could escape the analyst's dire "interpretations" as the analyst was never wrong.

Within psychoanalysis, the situation was worse than that, much worse, as the movement came more and more to resemble a cult. Starting in 1984, this was exposed by Jeffrey Masson, a non-medical analyst who had been appointed director of the Freud Archive. After exhaustive studies of the voluminous material in the archive, Masson concluded that Freud had actually falsified his results to produce a more socially-acceptable theory [4]. Needless to say, Masson's claim provoked a furor and he quickly lost his job. In 1990, in his autobiographical memoir, he added insult to injury by his revelations of the often quite appalling conduct of psychoanalysts [5]. Today, well into the new century, there have been further critiques [6, 7] so that practically the whole of Freud's work now seems quaint and irrelevant. However, the lesson reverberates through psychiatry in its open hostility toward anything that smacks of mentalism [2, 7]. The violent swing in the decade of the 1970s, which opened with psychoanalysis dominant in the US and ended with the publication of the biologically-based DSMIII in 1980, still has a long way to run but the significance must not be underestimated: in equating mentalism with the cultish movement of psychoanalysis, psychiatry has put all its eggs in the biological basket with nowhere to turn.

The final claim for psychoanalysis was that it was universal, a theory of mind and mental development for all humans in all cultures. In fact, Freud's theories were based on his experience of a limited range of mental disorders among a minuscule subsection of the human race, essentially well-educated, predominantly secular, upper middle class Jewish (and therefore white) Viennese prior to the Great War. As clinical experience, it doesn't get much more limited. There was never any evidence to support the claim of universality: psychoanalytic theory was a classic example of an unthinking and very restrictive Eurocentrism.

3.2. The many failings of mentalism: psychoanalysis.

The problems with psychoanalytic theory fall into three groups: how to deal with what the patient is saying; the mental structure that determines it; and the process of development of that structure. We will leave aside what I consider to be the most important question for any mentalist theory, the nature of the medium in which the mental activity takes place, meaning the nature of mind, because psychoanalysis never addressed it. Freud believed it would all be biological but had no idea how this would come about. By mental, I mean everything that the ordinary person would ordinarily understand by the word. This is the private world of sensory experience, knowledge, memory, emotion, decisions and so on that fills my head from waking to falling asleep, and again in dreams. While I have the impression that I have a large measure of control over my actions, I'm also aware that it isn't perfect, that a lot of things I do, decisions I make or emotions I experience, aren't entirely rational.

So we have to make sense of this but the major difficulty is sorting out what's real from fantasy. Freud said that a very large part of what counts in mental life is not conscious in the ordinary sense of the word. In addition to the private but very obvious circus in my head, there is also a large, dark world where all sorts of scary or forbidden ideas, emotions and impulses bump around. The three rings of the circus were called ego, id and superego, Ego roughly corresponded with the ordinary, conscious self; id with the dark impulses of sexuality, violence and death; and superego represents the conscience.

Complicating matters, a significant part of mental life takes place outside awareness. Some of it is preconscious, meaning we could become aware of it if we wished, but a great deal, especially id impulses, is entirely unconscious. Even though the id influences conscious decisions, mostly badly, we can't access it ourselves. Similarly, a person may suffer because of an excessively strict or punitive superego, meaning the set of rules that were absorbed in early childhood were strict and were never modified as part of the normal process of adolescence and early adult life. Freud believed the unconscious material could be brought to full awareness through his process of "free association," in which the patient simply verbalised without censorship whatever came to mind. The analyst then interpreted this back to the patient so that the mental events could be fully understood and resolved.

Early critics of Freud's theories were quite blunt: the Russian author Vladimir Nabokov is said to have called psychoanalysis the worst sort of quackery and Freud himself a charlatan. During the 1920's, a few positivist philosophers attacked the theory but by then it was too well-established—not the least because there simply wasn't anything that could compete. The problems were manifold. On the one hand, nobody, including the patient, could be sure that what the patient was saying was factually correct. Most of Freud's patients were members of the *haute bourgeoisie* of imperial Vienna. It emerged that during their sessions, large numbers of the women with "hysteria" were recounting incidents of sexual molestation during childhood. If this sort of material become public knowledge, lives and careers would be ruined.

Freud resolved this by saying it was all fantasy based in infantile needs. But this was the source of Masson's complaint: if a patient recounted being sexually molested as a child, did it happen or did it not? Psychoanalysts resolved it to their satisfaction ("Blame the victim") but the question recurred in the 1980s with the notion of "recovered memories" ("The victim cannot be wrong"—also known as false memories, see later). In simple terms, we can never be sure whether a person is recounting fact, fantasy, falsehood or delusion. In a mentalist theory, that matters.

The second group of problems for psychoanalysis lay in the elaborate model of mind Freud and his followers developed. The theory was based in science as Freud understood it, meaning hydrodynamics. In his model, forbidden or threatening material from the id was actively resisted and kept from consciousness but it seeped through. The analyst's job was to interpret this to the patient but if the patient objected (e.g. "Excuse me, I never had sexual feelings for my mother"), that too was put down to resistance and required further analysis. The analyst was never wrong, which went back to Popper's point that psychoanalysis was irrefutable and thus non-scientific. The mental structure itself could never be refuted (how do you prove the id doesn't exist?) and the content was open to interpretation. This lop-sided system was wide open to abuse of patients by dominant or intolerant analysts, which Masson described in detail. Freud was himself a dominant character so it's not surprising that he wrote a theory of this type.

Third, his theory of infantile mental development was completely fanciful. His proposed stages of mental development, later greatly elaborated by his followers, were based not in what infants showed (there is no evidence he analysed an infant and anyway, they can't talk) but in what his theory needed to make sense of what patients were saying. That is, he worked backwards. He didn't start with observable facts and then try to connect them with a testable theory, he started with the conclusions he had already reached and "discovered" that his method confirmed his claims about infantile development.

Finally, nobody knew where to stop. The Swiss analyst, Carl Jung, for example, developed his ideas in the setting of his extensive knowledge of mythology, anthropology and languages. Jung soon fell out with Freud over concepts such as personality types and his peculiar notion of the "racial unconscious." Unlike Freud, Jung travelled quite extensively, including lecture and study trips to the US, and lengthy trips to East Africa and to India. His ideas were arcane to the point of incomprehensiblity and while he was educated in diverse fields such as archaeology and linguistics, his inventiveness was unrestrained. He was greatly interested in spirituality and the occult and how this was expressed in different cultures: one of his last works before he died in 1961 was an analysis of the psychological significance of UFOs. His impact has faded since his death and it's unusual to meet a millennial who has heard of him but that's partly a sign of the times: social influencers are now more important than spiritualists.

As a result of these problems, the idea that psychoanalysis had anything reliable to say started to fade and, by the late 1970s, it was becoming outdated and irrelevant. Nonetheless, some of Freud's ideas have had lasting effects on the idea of psychology. The first was the concept of the active unconscious, the idea that material such as memories, impulses, etc. can exist outside of awareness yet still be psychologically-significant. It's actually an old idea but psychoanalysis shifts it to centre-stage. Memories and emotions that are seen as too threatening can be actively repressed in the very long term. However, they don't die from lack of sunlight; they stay in the unconscious and cause trouble.

One way in which repressed material exerts its baleful influence is through transference, the distortion of relationships in the present by unresolved conflicts from the past (emotions from past conflicts are transferred to similar figures in the present). Thus, a person who had bad experiences of authority figures during childhood may have trouble relating to authority in adulthood. One person may react aggressively while the next may be excessively timid and submissive. What counts is that in dealing with bosses, managers, senior officers, etc, such people act irrationally and not as adults should. The analyst's role is to bring these forbidden memories and emotions to consciousness so they can be dealt with in a mature manner (reprocessed, as people now say). However, the patient often resists this actively so the analyst must work hard to overcome this pathological esistance, which lends itself to the analyst forcing ideas on the patient that have no basis in fact.

Perhaps the most valuable part of Freud's legacy was the concept of ego mechanisms of defence. He apparently developed the notion that the sense of self is unconsciously protected from unpleasant or embarrassing material but his daughter, Anna, a lay analyst, wrote the definitive account of them [8]. She paved the way for others and before long, concepts such as projection, intellectualisation, rationalisation and reaction formation had entered common language (well, among the chattering classes). However, the notion also fails as science because each defence mechanism functions as a self-contained mental entity in an unknown medium with no conceivable explanation in a formal theory of mind. Freud described them as "watchmen" that guard the door to consciousness but didn't break them down any further. Anna Freud used military metaphors of soldiers peering over ramparts in order to repel hostile attacks. That is, ego defence mechanisms functioned as "little men" in their own right, with little minds making decisions on how to protect the conscious ego from assault. And what makes their decisions? Why, another little man or homunculus inside the little man's head, and so on. That is, the descriptive model of unconscious ego mechanisms of defence immediately sets up an infinite regress, which is never scientific, and thus has no explanatory content. Granted, it gives us a convenient way of describing processes but it wasn't scientific and it wasn't original.

But that aside, it's still a valuable idea in psychotherapy and in ordinary life. It's handy to recognise when somebody is protesting too much, when their supposed intellectual interest conceals a seedy motive or their generosity is a cloak for self-interest. The trouble is, the concepts are slippery. Regardless of how noble the patient's motives, a clever therapist can make any decision look bad and use it to dominate the patient inappropriately, which Masson [2] and others [4] have described at length.

The final complaint against psychoanalysis was that it was occupational therapy for the self- involved rich, pandering to their narcissism but not doing anything for the great mass of the mentally-troubled. Treatment consisted of daily fifty minute sessions "on the couch," which meant that even in the wealthiest country on earth, it could never touch the lives of more than a tiny proportion of the population in the biggest cities. It simply licensed the time- and money-rich to indulge their favourite hobby, sitting with a captive audience and talking endlessly about themselves. Some have said psychoanalysis was treatment masquerading as entertainment but the reality was entertainment masquerading as treatment. Anyway, to nobody's great regret, it's now gone to its rightful place in the history books.

3.3. Modern mentalism: Cognitive psychology.

Regardless of what philosophers of science have to say, there is one fact that cannot be refuted: I know there is something going on inside my head right now. The question is not *whether* it's there but *how* the experience arises, whether it controls my behavior (as it seems to) and, crucially, whether science can say anything reliable about it. Unlike behaviorism, which we will discuss in the next chapter, modern psychology accepts that mental events are real and causally effective. Cognitive psychology studies the processes of cognition, the various mental processes that underlie knowing and knowledge. This is a broad field including intellect, memory, attention and concentration, perception, decision-making, language, personality, etc. In the laboratory, cognitive psychology studies these processes separately and together, and is thus closely associated with computational models of mind, and with neurophysiology, neurology and so on. It leads to fields such as educational, industrial, social and developmental psychology and, of course, studies of personality, both normal and abnormal. Clinical cognitive psychology uses all these fields to attempt to make people's lives better. It has wide application, not just in routine counselling for mental disorders but also in schools, prisons, rehabilitation services and so on.

For a non-specialist, the central question is: What unites these diverse topics? What do they have in common, with each other or with clinical psychology? The problem is that neither academic nor clinical cognitive psychology starts with anything like a formal model of mind. Disciplines like physics, chemistry and cosmology are united in the sense that they start with a standard atomic model of matter. All of modern biology starts with DNA and the synthetic theory of evolution. Psychology doesn't have anything like that, there is no agreed or core model of mind to underpin the discipline. Cognitive psychologists accept the reality of mind, that we can, for example, make decisions or experience emotions, and they proceed from there. Thus, there can be no demarcation criterion separating the science of psychology from psychological fantasy. This means it can and often does stray into pseudoscience, which can be dangerous.

The academic study of cognitive processes is important but it is highly abstruse and doesn't have much relevance to mental disorder except at one point: the matter of inherent biases. While we humans, especially we white male humans, would like to believe we are entirely rational and can coolly make balanced decisions based on carefully-marshalled evidence, the fact is we're not, and we generally don't. Research in inherent cognitive biases has been dominated by the work of Daniel Kahneman and Amos Tversky, which resulted in Kahneman being awarded a joint Nobel Prize in Economics in 2002 (Tversky was already deceased, at the age of 59). Kahneman has published a popular account of his work, *Thinking Fast and Slow* [9], which should be required reading for all senior high school students (and certainly for all politicians).

Clinical cognitive psychology takes all of this as reality and, as the C in CBT, tries to use it to better people's lives. As such, it is heir to the rationalist-moralist theme in mental health management but despite evidence of its efficacy, it is fighting a losing battle against the immensely powerful axis of the drug industry and its eager ally, institutional psychiatry. Part of the trouble is that cognitive psychology is not nested in a larger theory of mind. The eminent behaviorist, Burrhus F Skinner, outlined this point in a chapter entitled *Why I am not a cognitive psychologist* [10] published in 1978, almost at the end of his career. Just as with the model of ego mechanisms of defence, the central notion in any cognitive psychology leads directly to an infinite regress and is therefore nonscientific. However, Skinner wasn't unbiased in his appraisal, as the opening sentence in that chapter shows:

> The variables of which human behavior is a function lie in the environment.

That is, he did not accept that mental elements could play *any* part in controlling behavior, meaning he had made up his mind before he examined the evidence. Nonetheless, his case against cognitive psychology was detailed and was essentially correct. Unless cognitive psychology is based in a formal model of mind (which Skinner said was impossible), there is no demarcation criterion separating it from flights of fancy, so it can't be brought into the scientific arena. CBT has some success in evading this problem because it is deliberately limited in scope and uses only established behaviorist methods. However, that imposes severe restrictions on its practice and people are often tempted to venture outside the limits, with dire results. One such example was the bizarre case of the "recovered memory syndrome" but it would be unfair to dump the blame on cognitive psychology. It is a textbook example of feral mentalism unburdened by any awareness of the concept of the limits imposed by demarcation criteria—or by decency.

3.4. Mentalism unleashed: False memory syndrome/RSA/alien abduction.

In any attempt to talk about the mind or its contents, the central problem is to find a reliable method of establishing whether mental contents have (a) any basis in fact and (b) any significance in the person's life. There are, however, people who aren't bothered by these concerns. To them, if it's in the mind, it's definitely factual and significant but if it's not in the mind, it's repressed and has to be brought to mind so it can be found to be significant. The central idea is that unpleasant or frightening events generate intense emotions but, because these are so threatening to the child, they are actively repressed. However, they haven't gone away: as a legacy of Freud's hydrodynamic model, the bad emotions are locked away in memory as a packet of mental energy which constantly causes trouble. It's a bit like how a pocket of pus from an old infection in the physical body can cause persisting trouble. Treatment consists of the therapist actively working to bring the memories and their associated emotions to full consciousness so they can be "reprocessed," leading to relief of the symptoms.

The act of expressing strong emotions associated with past events in order to relieve distress is strongly associated with Freudian theory and is known by analogy as catharsis. This term originally meant the event of being relieved of the catamenia, the monthly discharge of the uterine contents, but was borrowed by psychiatrists to mean cleansing or purgation of harmful contents of the mind. There is no clearer example of this than the continuing furore over the psychiatric effects of sexual molestation during childhood and adolescence. As in Freud's time, this is a charged issue; some people take the view it never happens, or that it is rare but harmless, or children provoke it, while others believe it is the cause of all adult mental disorder. As a matter of criminology, sexual contact between adults and children does take place; Western society regards this as repugnant and worthy of punishment; children are legally incapable so the adult is deemed the offender; but very often, the only witness is the child, whose evidence may not be admissible.

In personally assessing and managing well in excess of 12,000 cases in a variety of settings over nearly half a century, I have never once heard a person say something like "I'd completely forgotten this but I've just remembered that I was sexually abused as a child." My experience has always been that people who experienced it are perfectly aware of it and there has never been any question of their having forgotten it. Generally, they won't reveal it unless specifically asked for details of their childhood, including relationships with significant people, then they recount it in a fairly matter-of-fact or even dismissive tone. The great majority are not interested in pursuing the matter and often resist reporting it to police; they're not keen on talking about it but will do so to get their symptoms settled so they can get on with life. They come across as plausible, sensible, consistent (their stories don't change) and with no ulterior motives.

There is no reason to believe that these people will be improved by forcing them to relive the experiences, and a lot of evidence that says that it can actually make them worse. These are the routine cases; then there is a completely different type of case:

> A 23yo single woman was referred for psychiatric assessment after she took an overdose following the latest breakdown of a stormy relationship extending over several years. Her history showed a pattern of impulsive and rather destructive behavior since early in high school. While reasonably intelligent, she left school at age sixteen to have an abortion. She had never held full-time, permanent work and had never completed any of the various courses she had started. She tended to drink to excess on weekends and regularly used a variety of drugs, mostly amphetamines as they allowed her to mix socially and talk to people.
>
> Her family background was unsettled as her parents separated when she was fourteen when her father had moved interstate and had another family. She had little contact with him and felt he wasn't interested in her, only in her younger sister who had joined the military. Her mother had had numerous relationships over the years and also drank quite heavily. While she had moved back to stay with her mother, they often had quite ferocious arguments, especially when they had both been drinking, meaning most weekends.
>
> The mental state showed a rather tall and well-built young woman with short, streaked hair, dressed in clean but mis-

matched casual clothing. She had numerous expensive tattoos and half a dozen studs, including one in her tongue. She was agitated and talkative, weepy at times but given to brief, dismissive laughs. She was no longer suicidal but also had no plans beyond going out on the weekend to get away from her mother's drinking. She described pervasive performance and social anxiety associated with fairly high levels of general suspicion and mistrust of people. However, she was also sure she had "heaps" of friends and could easily get work and get back on her feet. There were no psychotic features and she was functioning in the bright-normal range of intellect.

She was started on a program of specific treatment for anxiety, including non-psychiatric medication and a form of brief cognitive therapy. At the first review a week later, she said she felt "heaps" better and the tablets were "magic" so she had started looking for work. At the second, she revealed she had used amphetamines on the weekend, had lost her tablets and had failed to attend a job interview so she wasn't feeling good. On the third appointment, she was more settled and said she was sure she would get a job but she missed the fourth appointment. Due to public holidays, she was rebooked for review in two weeks.

This time, five weeks after first being seen, she attended in a state of considerable excitement. Her job agency had referred her to a particular psychologist who had diagnosed major depression, dissociative identity disorder, and borderline personality disorder with bipolar tendencies. When reviewed two weeks later, she was excited and talkative. The psychologist had "broken through the resistance" and the patient now knew that all her problems were due to being sexually molested throughout her childhood. She was sure her father was involved somehow but mostly the offenders were men in the street and possibly some women, she wasn't sure. She was, however, sure there had been many hundreds of incidents, all of which she could recall in great detail except for the identities of the people involved. Mostly it took place in houses in their neighbourhood, by day or night, but often they would sneak into her house when her mother was asleep, or perhaps her father allowed them in.

At the next appointment, she said she intended to lodge "hundreds" of claims for compensation under victims of crimes legislation which would be worth "millions" (there was provision for only one claim for each class of crime) but she knew there were more bizarre incidents as the psychologist helped her uncover dozens more each visit except she couldn't talk about them yet as she was also "working on" the hidden personalities the psychologist was discovering. Meantime, she was feeling very much better and, as a victim and not a "mental patient," she didn't need to see a psychiatrist any longer but she would need a report for her application for victims' compensation to confirm the diagnoses the psychologist had made and that she was a victim of ritual sexual abuse by a cult she couldn't mention. She was not seen again.

Typically, the story grows and grows, becoming ever-more fantastic with each appointment. What started out as isolated episodes of sexual abuse spreads to hundreds of incidents involving dozens of people, known and unknown, famous and otherwise, who belong to a secret cult of satanic worshippers who steal children and even murder them. Others claim to have been abducted by aliens and taken in spaceships to the aliens' home planet where they are questioned and examined scientifically before being brought back to earth.

There is never a shred of evidence for any of this, and it merges with the medieval "blood libel," allegations of similar Jewish conspiracies, and with the cult of Q-Anon which has swept the US in recent years [11]. It is a combination of a moral panic, conspiratorial thinking and heretical religiosity which, in normal times, would be of little significance to psychiatrists—except these are not normal times. In the first place, psychiatrists are involved because some of the people who are convinced that all adult mental disorder is the result of grotesque childhood sexual abuse are psychiatrists who, keeping with Freud's tradition, force their views on their vulnerable clientele.

Second, it damages the people who are led to believe they have been sexually abused. The idea takes control of their lives, inducts them into a world of "true believers" similar to other cults, and cuts them off from their families and friends while debasing the experience of those who genuinely have suffered. Third, even the mere rumour of being a sexual predator can have a shattering effect on people's lives. Finally, it encourages psychiatrists to believe that all mentalism is of the same fantastic nature and should be dismissed out of hand. That is, because there is no demarcation criterion separating factual mental contents from fantasy, fabrication or delusion, then all mentalism is ridiculous and the search for the causes of mental disorder must be restricted to biology. So the unhappy people who were genuinely mistreated early in life are forced to take drugs but nobody wants to hear their stories.

3.5: Conclusion: observing the unobservable.

This brief but rather gloomy survey offers no answer to the demarcation problem. Even if we accept that humans have an inner mental life, there is no agreement in psychiatry on how that comes about or whether it is significant. We can't tell whether what a person perceives or remembers is factual so we can't prove that a particular event, past or present, has caused or contributed to a case of mental disorder. Yes, there are many studies that show a clear association between childhood abuse and neglect and adult psychosocial disorder, or between current psychological stressors and long-lasting mental disorder but, in the absence of a formal model of mental disorder, we reserve judgement as association isn't causation.

For orthodox psychiatrists today, the question remains: How much scientific weight can be placed on events which are in principle unobservable. Their answer? None. That's why psychiatry has lurched away from mentalism to embrace biological reductionism: it's easy to understand; it requires practically no intellectual or emotional effort from the psychiatrist; it sounds terribly medical with none of the arty nonsense about egos and ids; it's very good at stopping questions by uncooperative patients or aggressive lawyers; it puts a secure barrier between the psychiatrist and all those mental people; and it leads to all sorts of interesting research projects looking at genes and brain chemicals and other scientific things. Well, that plus the vast amounts of money flowing from pharmaceutical companies [1, 7].

References:

1. Scull A (2022) *Desperate Remedies: Psychiatry and the mysteries of mental illness*. London: Penguin.

2. Popper KR. (1974). *Unended Quest: An intellectual autobiography*. Glasgow: Collins/Fontana.

3. Popper KR (1972). *Conjectures and Refutations: the growth of scientific knowledge*. London: Routledge.

4. Masson JM (1984). *The Assault on Truth: Freud's suppression of the seduction theory*. New York: Simon and Schuster.

5. Masson JM (1990). *Final Analysis: The Making and Unmaking of A Psychoanalyst.* Addison-Wesley.

6. Crews F (1999). *Unauthorised Freud.* New York: Viking Penguin.

7. Harrington A (2020). *Mind Fixers: Psychiatry's Troubled Search for the Biology of Mental Illness.* New York: Norton.

8. Freud A (1936). *The ego and the mechanisms of defence.* Reissued: New York: IUP (1966).

9. Kahneman D (2011). *Thinking fast and slow.* New York: Allan Lane

10. Skinner BF (1978). Why I am not a cognitive psychologist. In: *Reflections of Behaviorism and Society.* New York: Prentice Hall.

11. Bloom M, Moskalenko S (2021). *Pastels and Pedophiles: Inside the Mind of QAnon.* Stanford, CA: Stanford U/Redwood Press.

4   Behaviorism: Not Sleeping, Just Dead

If we are uncritical we shall always find what we want: we shall look for, and find, confirmations, and we shall look away from, and not see, whatever might be dangerous to our pet theories. In this way it is only too easy to obtain what appears to be overwhelming evidence in favor of a theory which, if approached critically, would have been refuted.

Karl Popper (1902-1994), *The Poverty of Historicism*, (1957).

4.1: Behaviorism's origins.

When we try to locate the controlling mechanism in human behavior, there aren't many choices. Because we restrict ourselves to scientific principles, we exclude the world's most common approach, supernatural or magic control. We've already looked at two non-spiritual models, biological reductionism and mentalism, and concluded they aren't much help. Reductionism doesn't work, which means biological psychiatry is a project without a plan, while an unrestrained mentalism, such as psychoanalysis or a folkish cognitive psychology, will always want to float off into the sky. Unless it can be anchored to reality, mentalism can't be distinguished from mentalist fantasy and, at present, we have no anchor. In our search for a reliable model of mental disorder, things are not looking good. In fact, they haven't been looking good for the past hundred years, so we need to go back two hundred years, to the birth of Hermann Helmholtz in Potsdam in 1821 (d. 1894).

Helmholtz's father was a headmaster of a high school (gymnasium) who had studied philosophy and knew a number of influential philosophers, so young Hermann read widely in his father's books. He was interested in natural science but his father steered him into medicine although he practised only a few years before he moved into teaching anatomy and then physiology. Hermann was a restless spirit, committed to the idea of a natural explanation for the phenomena of life, and pioneered the application to living matter of what we would now call scientific methodology. There was very little that didn't interest him and he made major contributions to a number of fields, mostly directed at understanding the processes of life as natural events. His major impact was establishing physiology as a science to be investigated in the laboratory, not in an armchair. Helmholtz died in 1894, leaving the field of life sciences very different from when he embarked on his career.

One of Helmholtz's students was also a medical graduate with interests in philosophy. Soon after completing his medical training, Wilhelm Wundt (1832-1920) moved into physiology where he began applying his mentor's methods to matters of the mind. By the age of 32, Wundt had published the world's first book on psychological methods and, in 1874 at the age of 42, published *Principles of Physiological Psychology*, still regarded as one of the most important books in the history of psychology. He opened the world's first dedicated laboratory, in Leipzig in 1879, and was apparently the first person to refer to himself as a psychologist. Like Helmholtz, Wundt had wide-ranging interests. He published extensively in what he called Folk Psychology, the psychological beliefs and concepts of ordinary people. Part of this is the notion of the mind as a vivid thing in the head, which became a major part of his work. Wundt didn't see a clear division between matters of philosophy and matters that could be studied in the laboratory, so introspectionist studies remained a significant part of his work although he tried to put them on a formal footing.

Meanwhile, psychology was pioneering new fields, particularly the study of intellect, in the UK by Francis Galton (1822-1911), Charles Darwin's half-cousin, and in France by Alfred Binet (1857-1911). Possibly because of this success, it soon became clear that Wundt's introspectionist psychology wasn't going anywhere. As the years passed, it became a morass of conflicting claims and beliefs as there was no means of distinguishing fact from fantasy—no demarcation criterion, in Popper's terms. By the early part of the 20th Century, psychology's standing was suffering until in 1913, a self-appointed cavalry rode to the rescue. Delivering an address at Columbia University, John B Watson (1878-1958) made his position clear:

> I do not wish unduly to criticise psychology. It has failed signally,
> I believe, during the fifty-odd years of its existence as an experi-

mental discipline to make its place in the world as an undisputed natural science ... We have become so enmeshed in speculative questions concerning the elements of mind, the nature of conscious content that I, as an experimental student, feel that something is wrong with our premises and the types of problems which develop from them ... I can state my position here no better than by saying that I should like to bring my students up in the same ignorance of (the mind-body problem) as one finds among the students of other branches of science [1, 163,166].

In his lecture, titled *Psychology as the Behaviorist Views It*, Watson argued that all considerations of mind and mental contents, of consciousness and introspection "bound (psychology) hand and foot" so that it could not progress. Observable behavior was all that counted, he said; all talk of unobservable intervening variables, such as minds, was doomed to sterility. Very early, he adopted a rigid biologism: "The findings of psychology become the functional correlates of structure and lend themselves to explanation in physico-chemical terms." And the goal of all this was "...to learn general and particular methods by which I may control behavior." He believed it would be possible to write such a psychology in just a few years.

Watson had a confident style which, in the newly assertive scientific atmosphere after the First World War, and coupled with the confused results of fifty years of introspectionist psychology, had an immediate appeal. Introspectionist psychology soon collapsed, to be replaced by an aggressively objective, anti-mentalist "science of behavior." Psychologists saw themselves as flag-bearers in the continuing scientific revolution aimed at dragging Man from his special seat just a little below the angels. They were content to use the mind to investigate behavior but believed that mentalism and consciousness were red herrings, even a deadly trap, and swept away all mention of these archaic terms. In their place, they proposed that human behavior should be investigated only in terms of input, meaning the environmental stimuli, and output, meaning behavior. The trouble was, Watson had no suitable mechanism in mind, as it were. It's one thing to claim that the only reliable data are environmental stimuli and human behavior, but if a person reacts in a particular way to an event, how can we explain it if we can't talk of some intervening process that joins the stimulus to the behavioral response? Fortunately for his "behaviorist revolution," it wasn't long before Watson felt he had found such a mechanism, in a physiology laboratory half way around the world.

In short order, Watson built his behaviorist theory on the mechanism of conditioning, described by the Russian researcher, Ivan Pavlov (1849-1936). Every first year psychology student knows that Pavlov discovered the process of conditioning by observing dogs salivating in response to the dinner bell. At the time of his momentous discovery, Pavlov was studying digestion and had exteriorised the salivary flow in dogs so that their response to different stimuli could be precisely measured. He found that putting meat powder into their mouths caused a reflex flow of saliva but, before long, the dogs began to salivate almost as much when they heard the bell announcing lunch. That is, the dogs had acquired a new reflex. Pavlov's legendary formulation of this event was to regard the meat powder as the unconditioned stimulus and the salivary flow it stimulated as the unconditioned reflex response. During the process of conditioning, the lunch bell became the conditioned stimulus, and the secondary salivary flow the conditioned response.

Unlike Freud's almost bizarre concept of mental life, the principle behind conditioning is simple, biological and universal. Animals are born with certain innate or reflex responses to environmental stimuli. In turn, the environment reacts to the reflex behavior, either positively or negatively, to reinforce it. Positive reinforcers ("rewards") increase the likelihood that a behavior will be repeated; negative reinforcers ("punishment") reduce the chances of a repetition. A chance association of a behavior with a positive reinforcer will increase its incidence, while negative reinforcement will reduce it. Reinforcement is a biological concept, working at the level of the brain as a biological organ; traditional mentalist concepts, such as "likes" or "dislikes," play no role. Behaviorist psychology eliminates the fanciful "mind" as the unseen and unprovable causal mechanism in human behavior, replacing it with the reflex. The animal's behavioral repertoire expands as the limited number of innate reflexes is augmented by new learning. Psychologists investigated the conditions that affected the chances of a particular behavior being acquired or eliminated but there wasn't much more to the theory.

Seizing on this model of conditioning as the basic building block of human behavior, Watson extended the concept to cover all forms of human learning. In 1916, he announced his revolution in a paper in *Psychological Review* (which he had edited for five years) entitled *The place of the conditioned reflex in psychology* [2]. He expanded on the concept in his 1924 text *Behaviorism,* which met with rapturous reviews. One reviewer, quoted in McKenzie [3], said of it:

> Perhaps this is the most important book ever written. One stands for an instant blinded with a great hope... [3, xi]

Very soon, a new science of human behavior developed, championed in the US by Watson and his students and, in the UK by, among others, Sir Cyril Burt and his student, the German-born Hans J Eysenck (1916-1997). It influenced not just the management of mental disorder but, as the generic science of human behavior, it was applied in diverse fields such as normal parenting, education, criminology, industrial psychology, military training and in many others.

Needless to say, there wasn't a unified idea of behaviorism. In the US, the dominant model was Burrhus F Skinner's concept of operant conditioning (also known as Radical Behaviorism). Skinner believed that his theory could account for all human behavior, normal and abnormal, without relying on fairy-tale mentalist elements. His non-technical volume, *Beyond Freedom and Dignity* [4] published in 1972, created a sensation; everybody with any intellectual pretensions was expected to have read it. By the 1970s, as psychoanalysis and other mentalist theories began to retreat, behaviorism's fundamental learning theory seemed poised to achieve dominance. For example, in the introduction to his textbook, Yates [5] crowed over the impending collapse of psychoanalysis: "It will surely not be long before every Hollywood star has his or her behavior therapist" (for the benefit of the younger generation, behaviorist psychologists hated psychoanalysts who, in turn, regarded behaviorists as intellectual cockroaches).

This is written in all basic psychology textbooks; for decades, it was what all psychology students were taught. Such a pity then that like most legends, there's hardly a word of truth in it. We will start with Watson's concept of Pavlovian conditioning.

4.2. Pavlov and conditioning.

The first point is that Pavlov hadn't trained as a psychologist, didn't regard himself as a psychologist and disliked what psychologists were doing with the laboratory technique he had discovered. It is true that when he was investigating the process of digestion in dogs, he discovered something about saliva and lunch bells, but he never claimed to have discovered a general process called conditioning. As far as he was concerned, the concept of artificially-induced physiological responses was simply a means of laboratory investigation and probably nothing more. He never believed that it was the (or even a) basic element of human behavior, and he was antagonistic to the hope held by many psychologists of using it to build a universal psychology. In one of the last papers of his long career, which was also his first paper in the psychological literature, Pavlov attacked many of the concepts on which behaviorist psychology was based:

> The psychologist takes conditioning as the principle of learning, and accepting this principle as not subject to further analysis, not requiring ultimate investigation, he endeavours to apply it to everything and explains all the individual features of learning as one and the same process ... (the psychologist) takes one physiological fact and ... gives it a specific meaning in ... the learning process (but) does not seek an (empirical) confirmation of that meaning [6, 91].

Psychologists, he argued, were still too much influenced by their historical origins as philosophers to understand the scientific process. They were not empirical researchers but theorists who ignored scientific facts just as it suited them: "...a whole mass of concrete facts remain without the slightest attention on (the psychologist's) part" [6, p100]. Without putting too fine a point on it, Pavlov saw psychologists as scientific amateurs and didn't trust their profession. Despite their protestations of scientific determinism (which, in any case, he believed to be false), they simply "...disguised by various scientifically decent synonyms" the same "dualism and animism" in which ordinary people believed. He scorned the idea that a behavioral analysis will allow control and prediction of behavior: "The variety and number of these (cortical) stimuli are countless, even in an animal like a dog." All his research indicated that the cerebrum was more, not less, complex than anybody had previously thought. Simple reductionism in any form was anathema to him:

> I reject point blank and have a strong dislike for any theory which claims a complete inclusion of all that makes up our subjective world [6, 122; bear in mind that he also didn't take psychology's anti-mentalism seriously].

Physiology would eventually explain what reductionist psychology couldn't:

> … it is clear to me that many psychologists jealously … guard the behavior of animals and man from such physiological explanations, constantly ignoring (established physiological processes) and not attempting to apply any of them to any extent [6, p123].

This would seem to be a fairly clear and authoritative rejection of behaviorism's attempts to found a general psychology in the theories of Ivan Pavlov. On the other hand, it could be that the great man was wrong, that psychologists correctly saw more in his work than he did himself. This was not the case: Pavlov was right and the psychologists were wrong, because there is no *process* of conditioning. Without conditioning, there is no modern theory of learning, meaning psychology loses a large part of its claim to be a separate science.

The case against the notion of conditioning has been argued by different authors, including Karl Popper [7]. A paper by Efron [8] appeared at a time when behaviorists saw little standing between them and complete domination of the field of human psychology. In the title to his paper, Efron asserted that the concept of the conditioned reflex was meaningless. He pointed out that within psychology, different authors use the term 'conditioned reflex' in a variety of totally different ways. He cited a dispute between two authors, one of whom argued that worms can be 'conditioned' while the other insisted that the first didn't know the difference between 'true conditioning' and 'pseudo-conditioning.' Efron made a number of points:

a) that these types of disputes were due to 'epistemological chaos' rather that to disagreements over genuine scientific facts;

b) the chaos derives from the assumption that all human behavior can be explained by eliminative materialism, i.e. that all "concepts of consciousness, volition and the causal efficacy of mental processes" can and should be excluded from the field of science;

c) that in attempting to eliminate all mention of conscious mental processes, reductionist biologists (essentially psychologists) have progressively broadened the concept of the reflex to the extent that it has become entirely meaningless;

d) all attempts to salvage a meaning for conditioning, such as operationalism, are doomed to failure because they necessarily enter an infinite regress.

Efron showed that 150 years ago, the term 'reflex' had a very restricted meaning, essentially that of the automatic response to an external stimulus in an intact, functioning animal:

> The definition of 'reflex' action contains, therefore, by implication, reference to a class or classes of action which are non-reflexive... behavior which is automatic, innate, involuntary, and independent of consciousness (e.g. knee jerk, gag reflex etc.) needs to be isolated conceptually (i.e. defined) only because other behavior exists which is voluntary, learned and dependent on conscious activity... To attempt to use the concept 'reflex' while at the same time denying the validity of the concepts of 'consciousness' and of 'volition' is not logically permissible [8, p491].

But this is exactly what reductionist psychology and biology wanted to do: deny consciousness. Not explain it, not show it was necessarily irrelevant or an artefact, but to deny the mentalism of their own minds. The term 'reflex' was seized by late nineteenth century physiologists as part of a broad drive against the notions exemplified by Bergson's *elan vital*. Researchers were determined to get rid of the 'mysticism' inherent in such concepts as consciousness, intention, mentality, etc.. They therefore declared these notions to be non-scientific and wrote a new 'science' which did not depend on them. But they simply replaced one form of mysticism by another, all the more pernicious by being denied. The influential neurophysiologist Karl Lashley outlined the "reductionist's credo":

> Our common meeting ground is the faith to which we all subscribe ... I believe that the phenomena of behavior and mind are ultimately describable in the concepts of the mathematical and physical sciences (quoted in Efron [8], p500).

This particular form of mysticism is known as promissory materialism, which has been around a long time now without delivering on any of its major promises (that's why it's called 'promissory'). In order to eradicate mentalism, psychologists had to broaden the concept of the 'unthinking reflex' to the point where it was used to explain thought itself. Their campaign had to be managed this way. They couldn't eliminate consciousness by reducing it to matters of brain chemistry (i.e. neurophysiology), because that would also eliminate them as scientists. Therefore, they had to pursue the alternative approach, which was to squeeze consciousness out of existence by expanding the unconscious, automatic basis of behavior until it included everything that the concept of consciousness was meant to explain. In their mechanistic world, the basic element of behavior was the reflex (like a thought is the basic element in a mentalist world), but in order for it to subsume all that minds once did, it had to be redefined…

> …in such a fashion that it no longer rested upon the concept(s) of consciousness and volition … In sum, the mechanistic biologist (i.e. psychologist) retained the word 'reflex' because it enabled him to make implicit use of the old concept of the reflex (i.e. involuntary behavior independent of consciousness) without admitting that his 'new science of behavior' still logically rested upon the concepts of consciousness and volition. This epistemological procedure is known, in some scientific circles, as 'having your cake and eating it too' [8, p501].

Supported by lengthy quotes, Efron argued that Pavlov was one of those responsible for expanding the definition of 'reflex' to the point where it became facile. Using it, Pavlov could explain "every activity of man and beast" which, unfortunately, led directly to an infinite regress and even to self-contradiction:

> By virtue of (Pavlov's) definition, it is a reflex if a hungry dog salivates in response to a bell which has in the past signalled the appearance of food; it is a reflex if I purchase a painting today which I saw and enjoyed last year; and it is a reflex if a man tries to escape from his tormentors in a concentration camp [8, p506].

Of course, the researcher, the artist and the torturers would also be acting reflexly, although I read Pavlov's *Reply to the psychologists* of 1932 [6] as trying to rein in these wild applicatons of his technique. In any event, Efron's case against the conditioned reflex is unimpeachable yet it had remarkably little effect on behaviorist psychology. But it can be extended further. If we look at the term 'conditioned reflex' as it stands, it has no meaning. Reflex we understand (or we think we do); but conditioned? What does this mean? We think it has a meaning, but only because we have heard the term so often that we accept it as real. It is similar to the way American psychiatrists of the fifties and sixties thought they knew what they meant by the term schizophrenia: they appeared to agree only because none of them bothered to look at it closely.

The original meaning of Pavlov's term emerges through his writings but, due to his turgid style, not with any great clarity. It would appear that the salivating response his dogs showed to food was originally termed *unconditional*, meaning a reflex response which appeared without further conditions. The food was a *stimulus to an unconditional response* (shortened to *unconditional stimulus*) in that, without any conditions attached, it worked every time. So an *unconditional stimulus* (food) leads to an *unconditional reflex response* (salivation). The bell, however, has to be associated with the food before it can elicit any sort of response; its effect as a stimulus is *conditional* upon its relationship with the (unconditional) food stimulus. This is associationism; there is *no process of conditioning* to be found, but Pavlov's translators always used the term *conditioned reflex*, implying something quite different from *conditional reflex*. *Conditional* is an adjective, and its meaning is quite clear but, using the word *conditioned*, which has the form of a past participle, implies there is a verb *to condition*. Today, there is such a verb in English, but its meaning is exactly the same as *to associate*. Skinner himself admitted this as long ago as 1931: "If we remain at the level of our observations, we must recognise a reflex as a correlation" [quoted in 8, p498].

Pavlov was not much fussed which word people used to describe his concept of non-conscious automatism:

> Of course, the terms 'conditional' and 'unconditional' could be replaced by others of arguably equal merit ... We might retain the term 'inborn reflexes,' and call the new type 'acquired reflexes'; or call the former 'species reflexes' since they are characteristic of the species, and the latter 'individual reflexes' since they vary from animal to animal in a species, and even in the same animal at different times and under different conditions. Or again we might call the former 'conduction reflexes' and the latter 'connection reflexes' [11, p504].

Quite clearly, if he had used any of these other terms, then the concept would not have been reified so quickly or so thoroughly. And if psychology had not had the specious concept of conditioning as its basic building block, its history in the twentieth century would have been very different. So if there is no process of conditioning, and the conditioned reflex does not exist, how was academic psychology able to maintain these fictions for 75 years or more? As with many of the great theoretical movements of the twentieth century, we may never have a final answer but certain factors contributed.

Early in the last century, psychologists desperately needed an 'atomic element' on which to build their discipline. In the fifty years from its tentative, introspectionist beginnings, psychology made little or no real theoretical progress and was in grave danger of collapsing as a separate body of knowledge. Watson acknowledged this in his "call to arms" for behaviorism in 1913 [1]. Unless psychology got its act together, he saw no chance of progress in the next two hundred years (in 1915, shortly after slamming his colleagues' life-works, Watson was elected president of the American Psychological Association; nowadays, comments like those would probably sink a presidential hopeful's chances). Without the reflex theory of behavior, psychology was doomed to wander unprofitably on the edges of other, better-established disciplines such as philosophy or physiology, even to wither and die. Without "conditioning," there would be no modern learning theory, no behaviorist revolution and therefore no basis for psychologists to claim a separate existence. The need for psychology to find something, anything, was profound, as MacKenzie commented drily:

> Not for an instant, but for fifty years, psychologists were blinded with the great hope that they could make psychology a genuine and successful science ... [3, pxi]

Their need blinded them to the weaknesses of the 'reflex theory' of human behavior and condemned twentieth century psychology to a long and hugely expensive exercise in intellectual sterility.

Second point: at the time he proclaimed his behaviorist revolution, Watson knew practically nothing of Pavlov's work. He had never met the physiologist, never read any of his publications and had available to him only a few summaries:

> ...all of the researches have appeared in Russian and in periodicals which are not accessible at present to American students. At least, we have not been able to obtain access to a single research publication. The German and French translations ... give the method only in the barest outline. Bechterew's summary was the only guide we had in our work ... [2, p94].

Watson stormed the citadels of introspectionism, his mortal enemy, without realising his shells had no powder. Fortunately for him, the citadel was ready to collapse; its defenders vanished into the night without firing a shot. Almost certainly, this easy victory helped convince the early behaviorists they were on to something big.

Finally, Pavlov himself contributed to the widespread misunder-standing of his work. His writing was opaque and it is clear that his different translators had difficulty with his novel terminology. He was given to propounding "laws" on the basis of a few observations but even with the best efforts of his translators, their meaning was often obscure. For example, in his lecture *A Brief Outline of the Higher Nervous Activity* [9, pp48-50], he listed a series of 'laws' which today seem simply peculiar. Yet these were dutifully translated and closely studied for their essential meanings. So when Watson in particular was championing the concept of 'conditioning,' he did so with no exposure to the research on which the notion was based. The jump from a Russian experimental physiology to an American general psychology was blind. Even Watson himself leaves no doubt: he was motivated more by his wish to break with introspectionism than any certainty that the new 'science of behavior' could satisfy the needs psychologists were placing upon it [2, p105]. As an aside, the two volumes of Pavlov's *Conditioned Reflexes and Psychiatry* [9] are a major cause of much of the confusion. Without much effort, it is possible to find conflicting quotes on many topics. This was not limited to Pavlov. Hans Eysenck, Pavlov's most devoted supporter in the West, commented how the vague and fluid terminology of Russian researchers made it almost impossible to test their hypotheses [15, p247].

In simple terms, Watson's proselytising for his "truly scientific psychology" was largely based in his ambition of finding a means of thumping his many intellectual enemies. A forceful and convincing writer, it is perhaps not surprising that when he was forced to resign his chair for conduct unbecoming of a professor (in fact, only adultery), he moved to the world of advertising and died a wealthy man. Academ-ically, however, his early works leave no doubt that he had little idea of the foggy concepts with which his distant hero was grappling. Misled by fragmentary translations of complex gropings towards an inchoate science, and by his own ambition, Watson thought there was a law-like process connecting stimulus and response when all the experimental evidence suggested only a vague association. In his wake, generations of psychologists unquestioningly accepted the myth of conditioning. Would it be fair to say of them "They were conditioned to follow their leader"? No, it would not. They wanted to believe in him as a purely mentalist phenomenon. Biology had nothing to do with it.

4.3. Skinner's Operant Conditioning.

Despite Watson's crusade, the prize for the most far-reaching and thorough-going attempt to construct a non-mentalist human psychology goes to Burrhus Frederic Skinner's Radical behaviorism. Skinner (1904-1990) was an American psychologist raised in the 'Brave New World' of early twentieth century scientific psychology. He had an exceptionally long career, published profusely and was dismissive of anybody's efforts but his own. His theory generated an enormous secondary literature but his disdain for his opponents (and there were many) was so complete that he rarely if ever bothered to answer their objections. Eventually, late in his life, it started to become clear that he was incapable of considering that he may have been wrong. On the question of mind, you could say, his mind was closed.

Skinner wrote in a aggressively objective style, ostentatiously eliminating any and all mentalist references. He spoke of 'organisms' which 'emit behaviors' which are then 'reinforced' by their 'environmental consequences.' A behavior which acts or operates upon the environment is called an 'operant.' Operants can be reinforced so, depending on the reinforcers (rewards or punishment), they can be made to dominate the organism's behavior or eliminated. Since operants can be conditioned by their consequences, behaviorist psychology's ultimate goal of 'shaping and maintaining behavior' (i.e. controlling it, in Watson's blunt language) comes within reach.

In order to study the effects of reinforcement, Skinner developed a box where suitably hungry rats and pigeons could be forced to perform tricks for food rewards or punished with electric shocks. Armed with the Skinner box, psychologists tried to work out general laws governing the interaction of stimulus, response and reinforcers. Their goal was to reduce all behavior, human and otherwise, to a few simple rules that could be manipulated so that behavior could be controlled. This was such a big deal that, in the 1960s to 80s, it was quite common to see cartoons in magazines about Skinner boxes and reinforcement. The dystopian Kubrick film *A Clockwork Orange*, from 1971, was built around it.

To take a common example, a baby gurgles and grunts. By their happy responses, the doting parents encourage their infant to use closer and closer approximations of real words. Language is thus acquired without the aid of unseen and unknowable 'intervening variables' (minds), and correct use of language is maintained by, essentially, the fact that speaking properly gets us what we want (i.e. it is positively reinforcing). For a radical behaviorist, the reinforcing environment (the verbal community) shapes and maintains language by contingent reinforcement of the organism's verbal operants. A Skinnerian's account of learning to speak does not involve a mind.

Skinner's psychology was profoundly influential, especially in the United States. Generations of psychologists were trained in the theory and practice of radical behaviorism. An enormous research program developed, and Skinnerian methods of behavior management were widely applied, from education to industry, armies to prisons. However, and despite his vast output, there are problems pinning down his views as, in his successive publications, Skinner tended to supersede his work rather than to revise it. Thus, he could say at one stage that the mind was irrelevant, later that it existed but couldn't be studied, and later still that it was quite relevant but was nothing special anyway. However, not long before he retired as one of America's most distinguished scientists, he published several works which have to stand as the definitive statements of his position (because he never had the opportunity to revise them). In *Beyond Freedom and Dignity* [2], he wrote a popularised version of his otherwise fairly opaque theory, and in *About Behaviorism* [10], he outlined his philosophy of behaviorism.

From about the late 1950's onwards, his ideas were subjected to increasingly critical analysis. In 1957, Michael Scriven (1928-2023) dissected Skinner's assertion that a true account of human behavior must be essentially (or totally) atheoretical. This was the basis, Scriven argued, for Skinnner's intense hostility to Freudian psychoanalysis. Scriven concluded that Skinnerian radical behaviorism was itself definitely not atheoretical: "… Skinner has elevated the relatively atheoretical nature of his approach into a sterile purity that his (own) approach fortunately lacks" [11, 94]. An essential element in the Skinnerian program had failed. Radical behaviorism was therefore open to attack on theoretical grounds, which Skinner had previously denied (and which, typically, he continued to deny).

A broader critique of Skinner's *Verbal Behavior* by the psycho-linguist and philosopher, Noam Chomsky (b. 1928), was brief (about thirty pages to review Skinner's book of nearly 500 pages), precisely targeted—and devastating. In a series of carefully-marshalled points, Chomsky showed that all the basic premises of the radical behaviorist approach to language were devoid of scientific content. One by one, he took Skinner's major concepts, showing that:

> ... if we take his terms in their literal meaning, the description covers almost no aspect of verbal behavior, and if we take them metaphorically, the description offers no improvement over various traditional (folk) formulations [12, p54].

Chomsky argued that the scientific ethos in radical behaviorism was illusory, that terms such as stimulus, response, operant, reinforcement, control, etc., were hollow, merely "... the illusion of a rigorous scientific theory with a very broad scope ... Skinner's claim that his system ... permits the practical control of verbal behavior is quite false" [12, 30-32]. Skinner's every effort failed. He could not define stimulus with any precision; "stimulus control" lacked the sense he claimed for it; his law of reinforcement was tautological; "... the term reinforcement has a purely ritual function" (p38); genuine "behavioral analysis" was impossible, and so on. This led Chomsky to characterise the psychologist's work as "hopelessly premature" and "empty." He concluded: "If it were true in any deep sense that the basic processes in language are well-understood and free of species restrictions, it would be extremely odd that language is limited to man" [12, 30].

His critique was a small masterpiece; nobody improved on it because nobody needed to and nor, for that matter, did Skinner. He never revised his book to take account of Chomsky's objections. Since then and despite intense efforts, the Skinnerian research program on "verbal behavior" has faded from view. Towards the end of the 1970's, a number of critiques of radical behaviorism appeared, including those by a psychological methodologist, Brian MacKenzie, and by a philosopher, Daniel Dennett.

MacKenzie's work was another small wonder, a precisely detailed analysis of psychological epistemology. After an exhaustive and rather arcane review, he concluded that behaviorism had given us only "...some portion of the tools appropriate for building a science—but not the science itself..." [3, 170]. It would not be possible to summarise his work beyond this, his last sentence, but Skinnerian radical behaviorism was particularly criticised for its "systematic pretensions" (p163) and its total failure to deliver on any of its promises. After the intellectual edifices (of Skinner's psychology) had crumbled, all that was left was a set of skills which were not unique to radical behaviour-ism. Simply speaking, Skinnerians described and controlled animal behavior somewhat better than other psychologists and lion tamers, but not differently, and certainly not radically so.

Dennett's criticism of Skinnerian radical behaviorism [13] is articulate and equally incisive. In his opinion, Skinner made several substantial mistakes in his theory. Firstly, he mistakenly supposed that all mentalism is necessarily supernatural and thus no better than superstition. He (Skinner) therefore determined to sweep all mentalist explanations from his theory, but on this crucial first step, he failed. We cannot translate mentalist accounts of human behavior into non-mentalist statements. Skinner's work is in fact a good source of failed attempts to do this. Dennett was able to show that a non-magical account of that most mentalist of concepts, intelligence, was indeed possible, meaning that a major plank in the rationale for radical behaviorism collapsed.

Secondly, Dennett argued that Skinner made a mistake in generalising the results of his laboratory experiments on rats and pigeons to humans. It is one thing to place lower animals with limited means of dealing with the environment in a highly restricted environment, and then announce that their behavior is controlled by a few very simple principles. It is something else again to assume that those same principles necessarily govern all human behavior under all possible circumstances:

> Since all the explanations he has so far come up with have been of the unmasking variety (pigeons, it turns out, do not have either freedom or dignity), Skinner might be forgiven for supposing that all explanations in psychology, including all explanations of human behavior, must be similarly unmasking ... (but) Pigeons do not exhibit very interesting or novel behavior, but human beings do [13, p66-7].

Dennett's argument can be summarised as saying that genuinely intelligent creatures can always mimic the behavior of less-endowed animals. Therefore, the necessary first step for the Skinnerian program was to prove that humans don't have genuine intelligence, rather than simply assuming it to be the case. Anyway, as everybody who deals with animals knows, they're a lot smarter than people who don't deal with them think. This leads to a well-known contradiction for behaviorists, which is that if they argue that humans don't have intelligence, or creativity, or motives, then they must also believe it of themselves. The philosopher Alfred Ayer once said that to be a behaviorist is to pretend to be anaesthetised from the neck up. If, as Skinner argued, scientific creativity is just a matter of being in the right environment, why did he accept all his honours and awards? Kline [14] summarised this criticism pungently:

> If we only do what we have been reinforced to do, then presumably Skinner, also being subject to schedules of reinforcement, writes what he writes simply because he has been so reinforced. There is thus no reason to think that (Skinnerian psychology) is true, or ... that Skinner believes it to be true. Hence, why should we bother to examine it?

A genuinely non-mentalist theory of behavior cannot come to grips with such quintessentially mentalist concepts as truth and falsity. Only thinking creatures can appreciate errors—and falsehoods.

This leads to another of Dennett's criticisms, which is the notion of the 'undischarged homunculus' in Skinner's theory. Skinner claimed he had eradicated the need for mentalist explanations but, as a matter of logic, he had not. All he had done was shift them around, from an homunculus or 'little man' in the head to another man hidden in the environment. This led him to argue [4] that there was no such thing as a creative artist. What we think of as a creative artist, he insisted, is merely an artist skilled at arranging a 'creativity-inducing environment.' But who decides what constitutes a creativity-inducing environment? The artist, we assume, so Skinner merely shifted the problem from one of explaining creativity to one of explaining how people decide what environment will induce creativity (presumably a fairly creative exercise in its own right). There is an 'undischarged mentalist debt' or homunculus lurking in every one of Skinner's allegedly neutral environments.

As mentioned, Dennett is of the view that at the beginning of his career, Skinner made a profound and far-reaching mistake by equating mentalism with the supernatural. The psychologist was determined to eradicate from his "science of general psychology" all mentalist concepts, and therefore never looked seriously at whether mentalism is genuinely beyond analysis, i.e. the age-old questions of whether a non-mentalist psychology is possible. Thus, there was a great deal of circularity, even question-begging, in Skinner's psychology, meaning he frequently assumed the truth of that which required proof. For example, it is typical of humans that we 'plan ahead,' which means just what everybody thinks it means. But Skinner didn't allow any mentalist concepts, and planning ahead is entirely mentalist. Behavior is under the control of the environment, he believed, but since future events haven't yet happened, they can't control behavior. What appears to be a case of people planning ahead, he argued, is actually a matter of their past history of reinforcing contingencies controlling their behavior. Given a detailed account of everything that has happened to them in the past, we would be able to say just what compels them to act in a particular way right now such that, lo and behold, a few days or weeks down the track, they get whatever it is they said they wanted in the first place.

Unfortunately, in discarding mentalism as non-science, Skinner adopted another bit of non-science. As every psychologist knows, keeping track of the history of reinforcing contingencies of even a laboratory animal is difficult; working out what happened to a human years before, when no records were kept, is impossible. What he called a "proper behavioral analysis" is just *deus ex machina*. Skinner was led to this error by his major assumptions:

1. Mentalism is necessarily supernatural;

2. Therefore, behavior must be under environmental control;

3. But future events can't control behavior because they haven't yet happened;

4. Therefore, the controlling element must lie in the past history of environmental contingencies.

The real question here is whether we can derive a natural or non-question-begging means by which future events can control behavior (equivalent to the mentalist or folk explanation, "If you want to pass your exams, you'd better study now"). I believe we can, and an everyday example will demonstrate the point. I ride my bicycle to the university, locking it in the rack before attending a lecture. After the lecture, I decide to go to the library to find a book the lecturer has mentioned. However, for the life of me, I can't recall where I left my machine. I stand for a few moments, carefully retracing my movements since leaving home and then experience that flash of recollection which says: "Aha, it's outside the south door of the gymnasium."

Now it's true that I don't have any sort of real picture of all the university's bike racks in my head, nor is there a physical model of my pushbike rattling around in my head. In order to recall where I left my machine, I need to have a means of representing it in my head, and of coding that information in a system of memory. Since rats can easily recall how to get into a house after one attempt, and pigeons never forget where they have placed the first two sticks for a new nest, we can't argue that memory is not a natural mechanism. But if by manipulating the internal representation in my memory (whatever that is), I can successfully locate my bike even when I can't see it, then I would say that on first principles, the same or a similar mechanism should also be able to cope with organising to go the library to collect a book I have never seen. There is no substantive difference between my behavior being controlled by a bicycle I can't see and the book which I know exists but I have never seen. Both matters involve the manipulation of information coded in my head to produce a mental representation. If there is nothing supernatural about using this type of mechanism to explain the effect of past events on my behavior, then *ipso facto* there is nothing supernatural about using it to plan ahead.

Strictly speaking, of course, my wish to borrow the book was a past event as soon as I had formulated it and in that sense, Skinner couldn't object to it controlling my behavior. Collecting the book wasn't part of the wish, and that is true of all future events. I simply set up a behavioral program which, all things being equal, should have ended with my leaving the library with a particular book under my arm. If future events genuinely controlled human behavior, then we would never make mistakes. In his fanatical opposition to the notion of internal control of behavior, Skinner discarded the idea that future events could control behavior. 'Reflexly' rejecting that possibility led him to miss the point that current internal representations aren't in the future.

As it happened, the book didn't control my behavior as it was on loan. It was the (mental) expectation that I would find it that counted. But I tried.

Why didn't Skinner think of these obvious objections? The answer is that only a full-blown, anti-mentalist Skinnerian system requires the abolition of plans as mental events and, almost certainly, he didn't believe there was any chance of error in his system. What seeps through his later works in particular is a profound self-satisfaction with his ideas. Everything he described seemed to fit his notions remarkably well, and he devoted a lot of space in *Beyond Freedom and Dignity* to showing just this point. I suggest the reason human behavior fitted his flawed theories so very well was because he didn't offer an explanation of human behavior at all, just a redescription from a novel point of view, the environment, not the head. Explanations can easily be proven wrong but descriptions, even in a new language, can never be wrong. Intellectually, descriptions take no chances and Skinner fell straight into this trap.

For example, in our old, poetic ways, we say that a if slave driver wants a slave to work harder, he will give him a good whipping to teach him a lesson; in turn, the slave quickly works out that by appearing to be busy, he can avoid the lash. This is a fairly humdrum, mentalist 'explanation' which involves motives, hopes, fears and other unobservables. Skinner rewrote this to read:

> Thus, a slave driver induces a slave to work by whipping him when he stops; by resuming work, the slave escapes from the whipping (and incidentally reinforces the slave driver's behavior in using the whip) [4, p26].

All traces of mentalism have been removed; we are left with a bare, environmentalist account (well, not quite: I think the word 'induce' has a covert mentalist role), but the behaviorist account says no more than the mentalist acount it was designed to replace. It can't say more, as it's just another way of saying the same thing and, because it hides the mentalism in the environment, it doesn't say less. As an attempt to explain human behavior, *radical behaviorism is mere description masquerading as explanation.* It had to be description, it couldn't be anything else because Skinner himself booted the possibility of minds (and of generative mechanisms, and of media of implementation) out the door.

Skinner believed that he had found the non-mentalist key to controlling and predicting behavior, and argued that all human behavior fitted his concepts. Now this is true, all human behavior can indeed be made to fit his devastatingly simple concepts—just because it is description, *not* explanation. The real question is: why bother? The history of ideas is littered with failed theories where somebody tried to reduce all human activity to the outcome of one or two fundamental principles. Thus, Skinner needed to show why our understanding of ourselves would necessarily be improved by his particular stance, how his non-mentalist model was an improvement over the mentalist. For him, of course, there was a very simple answer: by eradicating superstition, our self-understanding would *ipso facto* be improved. Is this true? Or can there be a naturalistic account of mentalism? Behaviorists never addressed this question but, under the reigning positivist influence, simply assumed the answer to be in their favor. The fact that there had never been a rational theory of mentalism was enough to convince them that it could never happen, that rejecting mentalism was the only true path.

In *Beyond Freedom and Dignity*, Skinner did not argue this point but outlined his new way of looking at age-old questions. All behavior, he avers, can be seen as the outcome of a previous history of contingent reinforcement of essentially random actions or operants. Throughout this book, he shows that while we have long looked at human behavior through mentalist spectacles, we can also look at it from an environmentalist stance. To do this, he simply translates the mentalist concepts used in ordinary language, rewriting them so that humans appear to be no more than marionettes dangling from environmental threads. That isn't the case but his positivist ideology made him want to believe it.

Skinner never proved that his view was the only one available, nor did he show that it had greater predictive value or any of the other features that distinguish science from faith. He simply said: "We can look at all human behavior from this point of view," as though the reason for doing so was self-evident. As a good positivist, the goal of eliminating mentalism was indeed self-evident, but not to anybody else. Despite the unwavering conviction which sustained his research program for the better part of sixty years, he did not explain human behavior just because he failed to address the critical questions. He never wrote his technology of behavioral control, because he didn't have one. Skinner's Radical Behaviorism turned out to be just another jargon-laden description dressed up as explanation.

4.4. Conclusion: Whither antimentalism?

Until just recently, the overwhelming majority of people throughout history have accepted the reality of mental life. Our entire perception of ourselves is built around the concept that something vital takes place in the privacy of our heads, something we own, something that allows us to direct our lives, something ... that is *us*. Even our name, *Homo sapiens*, reflects this. Religions and systems of law were built on this idea, entire philosophies flourished, literatures flowered and everybody was happy, although it brought with it the vast conceit that we humans have something in our heads that no other creatures on earth have and therefore we can do with them as we please.

But then somebody invented Western science with its pedantic preoccupation with evidential precision: "Your religions and phil-

osophies and folk psychologies don't meet our concept of reliability,"
the scientists declared smugly. "Henceforth, we will banish them and
you must dance to the drone of our scientific pipes." So they tried. And
tried. For a hundred years, they tried to build a science of mind without
mentioning mind. And, as a few curmudgeons predicted, their huge and
hugely expensive project failed. As science, it has been an abject failure,
possibly without parallel, and all for reasons taught in Philosophy 101.

References:

1. Watson JB (1913). Psychology as the behaviorist views it.
Psychological Review, 20:158-177.

2. Watson JB (1916). The place of the conditioned reflex in psychology.
Psychological Review; 23: 89-116.

3. McKenzie BD (1977). *behaviorism and the Limits of Scientific
Method*. London: RKP.

4. Skinner BF (1972). *Beyond Freedom and Dignity*. New York: Knopf.

5. Yates AJ (1972). *The Theory and Practice of behavior Therapy*. New
York: Wiley.

6. Pavlov IP (1932). The reply of a physiologist to psychologists.
Psychological Review; 39:91-127.

7. Popper KR (1972). *Objective Knowledge: an Evolutionary
Approach*. Oxford: University Press.

8. Efron R. The conditioned reflex: a meaningless concept. Perspectives
in Biology and Medicine, 1966; 9: 488-514.

9. Pavlov IP (1941). Lectures on Conditioned Reflexes, Vol 2:
Conditioned Reflexes and Psychiatry. New York: International Publishers.

10. Skinner BF (1974) *About behaviorism*. New York: Knopf. Page
numbers refer to the Penguin edition, 1993.

11. Scriven M (1956). A study of radical behaviorism. *University of
Minnesota Studies in the Philosophy of Science*, Vol I.

12.Chomsky N (1959). Review of Skinner's 'Verbal behavior.'
Language; 35:26-58.

13. Dennett DC (1978). *Brainstorms: Philosophical Essays in Mind
and Psychology*. Hassocks, Sussex: Harvester Press.

14. Kline R (1987). *Psychology Exposed, or: The Emperor's New
Clothes*. London: RKP.

5 The Biopsychosocial Model: The Claytons model for psychiatry

The first and worst of all frauds is to cheat one's self. After that, all sin is easy.

Pearl Bailey.

5.1. Claytons, anyone?

Years ago, a soft drink called Claytons was launched in Australia and New Zealand. It was a non-alcoholic, non-carbonated drink coloured and bottled to resemble whiskey. The punchline to its advertisements was the irritating slogan: "Claytons. The drink you have when you're not having a drink." I never tried it and don't know if it's still for sale but its name lives on as it has come to mean sham or bogus. So a company may have a Claytons selection process for a position, meaning they've already made their decision and are just going through the motions; or two people are having a Claytons argument, meaning it's only for show; or a couple may be in a Claytons marriage; a government may conduct a Claytons investigation; or two political parties have a Claytons debate, meaning they don't actually disagree but they don't want to be seen to agree. And for the past forty five years, psychiatry has had a Claytons model of mental disorder.

5.2. A model for psychiatry.

In 1977, George Engel, a gastroenterologist from Rochester, NY, published a paper in the prestigious journal, *Science*. Under the title *The need for a new medical model: a challenge for biomedicine* [1], he outlined a case for a new orientation in medicine to counter the dominant, dehumanising biological ideal of mainstream medical practice. Instead of seeing the patient as a biological specimen to be prodded and dissected, he urged physicians to adopt an integrative approach incorporating the patient's psychological and sociological states. He presented several medical cases to demonstrate his idea and finished with a call for medicine to take up the challenge of building such a model, which he called a biopsychosocial (BPS) model.

Over the past 45 years, the numbers of papers referring to the BPS model has increased steadily, if not exponentially, as this table derived from the PubMed database shows. If nothing else, it indicates a growing dissatisfaction with the dominant reductionist model in psychiatry:

1977	1978	1980	1985	1990	1995	2000	2005	2010	2012	2014	2016	2018	2020	2022
3	3	22	26	69	66	113	167	274	357	422	573	660	897	1188

Table 4.1: numbers of citations of "Biopsychosocial" on PubMed.

As it transpired, it was initially psychiatry, not general medicine (and certainly not surgery) that was most influenced by Engel's work. More recently, the concept has spread to fields such as pain management, chronic disability including arthritis or diabetes, rehabilitation, sexual disorders, social work, child development, and so on. The idea of integrating the triad of mind, body and society appears to have broad appeal in health care. In psychiatry, it offers to bridge the (enormous) divide between those psychiatrists who see all mental disorder as the direct result of a physical disorder of the brain, and those who feel that psychiatry must give account of the humanity of the mentally-troubled. A recent paper praising the influence of the BPS model begins:

> Biological reductionism in psychiatry can be dehumanizing and/or demeaning. In many cases it exemplifies the faulty and simplistic logic that renders psychiatry liable to criticism; it can also be frankly unscientific [2].

British psychiatrist (and emeritus professor) David Kingdon was more to the point on the failures of the biological approach to psychiatry:

> Biological research has produced major advances in our understanding of our bodies and, where systems go wrong, is producing remedies to address these, but it has yet to do the same for the mind. This is because no causative biological evidence has been found for the major mental disorders in contrast to the wealth of psychosocial findings. This disparity in regard and resource needs to be addressed [3].

Historically, this division has always been a feature of psychiatry [4]. In the main, mental hospitals and public practice embraced the biological approach while private practice was strongly inclined to mentalist models, especially Freud's psychoanalytic model. This split was strongest in the US; in the remaining Anglophone world, practitioners preferred to avoid what they saw as extremes. Instead, they opted for a moderate stance, trying to fit the treatment to the patient in what they called an eclectic approach. That word comes from art, and means choosing the best from a range of sources to give a better result. There are also eclectic philosophers and eclectic architects, meaning they aren't tied to a particular school.

Similarly, an eclectic psychiatry wasn't bound to a dogmatic line but was able to choose from the various treatment options according to the patient's needs. A patient presenting in a psychotic state would be seen as suffering a biological illness and prescribed a range of medications or even ECT. An anxious patient would be seen as best suited to treatment within a learning or psychological model and would be managed using behaviourist techniques, while people with neurotic or personality disorders would be treated by insight-directed psychotherapy.

It all made good sense and seemed more caring and less procrustean than the alternatives but there was a problem: nobody could reliably define either the conditions being treated or the criteria used to allocate patients to different modes of treatment. The idea that there was an "eclectic" psychiatry turned out to be just a way of justifying "anything goes" [5], a high-sounding but empty trope bandied about by psychiatrists to forestall criticism (since the psychiatrists actually believed it themselves, it qualified as an urban myth). The word concealed the absence of anything approaching a scientific model for psychiatry; psychiatrists could pick and choose according to whim, and whimsy is not science. After that critique was published in 1996, "eclectic psychiatry" quickly fell into disuse but it was probably on the way out anyway, as Engel's BPS model gained traction.

As outlined in Chap. 2, for the last forty years or more, biological reductionism has dominated psychiatry to the extent that very few psychiatrists now use an exclusively psychological model. However, many more would be happy to say they practice a biopsychosocial psychiatry, or are guided by that model in their practice, their teaching and their research. In fact, this would be the only real alternative to what has been called the biomedical model (even though in reality, no such model exists, see Chap. 2). In the rest of this section, we will look at the current status of the BPS model in psychiatry.

Starting in 1960, Engel published a series of papers arguing for a wider understanding of health and illness [6-10]. The most influential was his 1977 article in *Science* [1] which is taken as the source of his BPS model. By the time of his death in 1999, there was widespread support for the model, especially in the UK, Canada, Australia and New Zealand. In a series of commemorative papers commissioned by the *Australian and New Zealand Journal of Psychiatry* in 2002, Singh, who knew Engel well enough to visit him at home, opined that Engel saw himself as a "medical Darwin" who was "driven by a narcissistic belief in his own 'specialness'." Notwithstanding, Singh was in no doubt: "What no one can deny is that he did leave a towering edifice, the BPS approach ..." [11, p. 471].

In the same issue, Smith and Strain took a broad view:

> Medicine in Australia became biopsychosocial without knowing it... A generation of Australian medical students and psychiatry trainees have been taught (the BPS method) (p458) ... The integration of biology, psychology, social issues and behavior, and the interaction among them, is the hallmark of the biopsychosocial model of disease... Engel's biopsychosocial model stands as one of the most influential ideas in Medicine in the 20th Century" [12, p459].

The tributes have continued to the present. Philosopher Bradley Lewis asked whether Engel was a pragmatist:

> George Engel's BPS model has achieved worldwide recognition as one of the most influential developments psychiatry and medicine. Unveiled in 1977 as a comprehensive and integrative alternative to the dominant but highly restrictive biomedical model, the BPS model has become a beacon for a balanced and humanistic approach to clinical encounters. Indeed, it has become a beacon for the soul of medicine and psychiatry in the twenty-first century [13, p299].

In 2014, Allen Frances, former chairman of the DSM-IV committee, offered his support:

> ... (Engel's) BPS model of mental illness and mental health care created a conceptual underpinning that unified psychiatric practice ... Psychiatry places a bad bet for itself and for its

patients if it expects quick biological breakthroughs, and tamely accepts a restricted role as a pill prescriber. The BPS model can't by itself cure the mental health mess or rejuvenate the clinical practice of psychiatry, but it is a useful and perhaps necessary starting point [14].

Earlier, psychologist and sociologist David Pilgrim had seen the BPS model as a humanist pole fighting a losing battle against the hegemony of bioreductionist psychiatry [15]. By 2015, he was more sanguine, concluding: "The BPS model has been of considerable utility to those researching health and illness" [16]. Soon after, Seawright entitled a review article *The Biopsychosocial Model: 'Reports of My Death Have Been Greatly Exaggerated'* [17]. While aware of some of the complaints levelled against it, he urged further work on the model:

> ... the BPS has been refined and reshaped. While more work needs to be done, the result will hopefully be a more theoretically rigorous, clinically relevant, and empirically testable integration of the multiple factors determining health and illness.

In an extensive editorial in the *British Journal of Psychiatry*, philosophers Will Davies and Rebecca Roache examined the BPS "paradigm" and found it had an "elusive influence" in psychiatry:

> Psychiatry uncomfortably spans biological and psychosocial perspectives on mental illness, an idea central to Engel's BPS paradigm. This paradigm was extremely ambitious, proposing new foundations for clinical practice as well as a non-reductive metaphysics for mental illness ... Engel did not provide details as to how biological, psychological, and social factors should be combined in diagnosing, describing, explaining, and treating mental illness. And yet the conception of psychiatry as a BPS discipline remains influential ... The BPS paradigm is, in a sense, everywhere and yet nowhere [18].

Note, however, that they referred to it not as an articulated model but as a paradigm, presumably in the Kuhnian sense. As a result, they suggested it should be further developed to expand its "continued relevance." Subsequently, Davies reverted to identifying it as a model but, in case there was any doubt, reiterated his point about its elusive nature: "For half a century, the BPS model has beguiled and frustrated researchers and clinicians across psychiatry ... In clinical practice, BPS is, in a sense, everywhere and yet nowhere" [19]. The BPS model persisted, he suggested, because of the emphasis it placed on social factors. Outlining the social approach, he argued that a purely reductive biologism could never give a full account of mental disorder. While Davies wondered where the BPS model may be, well-known psychiatrist and commentator Ronald Pies entertained no doubt:

> ... academic psychiatry—for at least the past 30 years—has advocated a "bio-psycho-social" model of mental illness, as originally proposed by Dr George Engel ... This position has been quite consistent ... (Affective) disorders are best understood using a bio-psycho-sociocultural model, which has been the mainstay of academic psychiatry for over 30 years [20].

This has to be seen in the context of an earlier paper when he had asked: "Can we salvage the BPS model?" By this, he meant it didn't reach criteria for a formal scientific model and perhaps should be seen as a paradigm, as defined by Thomas Kuhn. He correctly saw paradigms as higher level explanations than models:

> As I interpret Kuhn, a paradigm is essentially a *world-view*—a way of seeing things—that guides the practices within a given discipline. Paradigms often generate ("provide") very specific models but are themselves both broader and more heterogeneous than models [21].

Either way, he saw psychosocial factors as important in mental disorder. In 2018, British psychiatrist Linda Gask penned a heartfelt and personal corrective, *In defence of the BPS model*, concluding "...the BPS model is, and remains, a model for the whole of medicine—not just psychiatry" [22]. The next year, psychologist Derek Bolton and ethicist Grant Gillett published a volume providing strong support for the notion of the generality of the BPS model, albeit with some reservations:

> The (BPS) model is popular and much invoked in clinical and health education settings and has claim to be the overarching framework for contemporary healthcare ... It is not straightforward to find the right metaphor for the relation between the biological, the psychological and the social [23, 33].

Psychiatrist Richard Porter also saw problems, suggesting the concept should be seen as a "BPS spectrum," with separate conditions located at different points on the spectrum according to the aetiological factors that contribute to them [24]. Unfortunately, that doesn't work. As every first year maths student knows, it is not possible to chart three parameters on a single axis. Separate factors can only be graphed on separate axes, meaning three in this case. In any event, while it may have some descriptive value, a spectrum, or continuum as it used to be known, is wholly descriptive and explains nothing. Despite Porter's apparent misunderstanding of the nature of axes [25], psychiatrist William Lugg evinced no concern over this point:

> The BPS model remains the predominant theoretical framework underpinning contemporary psychiatric training and practice ... An aetiological model for mental disorders that involves psychological, biological and sociocultural factors has existed since at least the 1940s [2].

Support for the BPS model within psychiatry is not restricted to a few grumblers who are unhappy with the reductive biological approach. Writing as president of the Royal Australian and New Zealand College of Psychiatrists (RANZCP), Janice Wilson said:

> The BPS model is fundamental to our profession, as is written in our position statement *What is a psychiatrist and what does a psychiatrist do?* This underpins every aspect of our training, and should underpin our day to day thinking and action within our own clinical practice ... Fundamentally, we must remember our underpinning principle: we bring a BPS integration into our daily therapeutic work with patients [26].

It was RANZCP Position Statement No. 39 of 1998 that asked *What is psychiatry? What does a psychiatrist do?* and answered with these definitions:

> 1.1: Psychiatry is a branch of medicine specialising in the prevention and treatment of mental disorder, and the promotion of mental health in the community.

> 2.1: Psychiatrists are medical practitioners with a recognised specialist qualification in psychiatry. By virtue of their specialist training they bring a comprehensive and integrated BPS approach to the diagnosis, assessment, treatment and prevention of psychiatric disorder and mental health problems [27].

In October 1998, a similar statement was placed on the official RANZCP website where it remained for five years. In 2013, the

RANZCP issued a revised Position Statement which reads: "This 'bio-psycho-social' model is a holistic approach that recognises the impact of social adversity and physical health on mental well-being" [27a]. In 2023, the RANZCP put a submission to a Senate enquiry into mental disorder which stated: "Psychiatrists' unique and comprehensive understanding of the bio-psycho-social assessment and treatment ..." etc. Meanwhile, in the UK, support for the BPS remains strong. In reviewing Bolton and Gillett's volume, Leslie Frazier said:

> (... this book could ...) challenge a new generation of scholars and scientists to demonstrate that the BPS model is more relevant than ever ... theory, research, and practice focused on health, disability, illness, and wellness should remain grounded in the BPS model [28].

In Britain today, it would be fair to say that the idea of psychiatry as a self-contained specialty hangs on this model to the extent that, without it, psychiatrists may start to lose their reason for existing [29]. Since general practitioners are trained in biological medicine to manage chronic disorders such as diabetes, arthritis, asthma, etc., and given that mental disorder has strong biological features and is mostly chronic, it follows that GPs are equally qualified to manage mental disorders. If psychiatrists embrace a wholly biological model of mental disorder, they could easily be without a job. Thus, their *raison d'être is* their unique conceptual grasp on the psychological and sociological aspects of medicine afforded by the BPS model. In the US, psychiatrists Glen Gabbard and Jerald Kay had made this quite clear:

> Almost all psychiatrists, and certainly those who are leaders in our field, endorse the notion that psychiatrists are distinct from all other mental health professionals in that their training and expertise allow them to be the ultimate integrators of the biological and psychosocial perspectives underlying diagnostic understanding and treatment. However, the BPS model made famous by Engel has been relegated to political lip service in our managed care era [30].

To bring us up to date, two commentaries in the *British Journal of Psychiatry Bulletin* from 2022 set out somewhat differing views. In an opinion piece, *Looking forward to a decade of the biopsychosocial model*, philosopher and psychologist Derek Bolton said:

> The topic of this article is the biopsychosocial model. My main contention is that—notwithstanding doubts as to what exactly it is, or indeed whether it is anything—there is a coherent account of it, in terms of both applications to particular health conditions and mechanisms with wide application ... There is accumulating evidence from recent decades that psychosocial as well as biological factors are implicated in the aetiology and treatment of a large range of physical as well as mental health conditions... the biopsychosocial model has to do with many or all types of health conditions, professions and specialties, and so we should hardly expect it to be *simple* [31, p228; his emphasis].

He argued that because we have "... major new explanatory theories that integrate biopsychosocial factors across very wide ranges of health conditions ..." (p229), and because of the dearth of any indicators of biological causes of mental disorder [32], we should devote the coming decade to studying the role of psychosocial factors, not just in causing and prolonging mental disorder, but also their role throughout the field of general medicine. However, he pointed to the general lack of formal models in the entire field, by asking: "But ... what exactly is the biomedical model?" that Engel had criticised. As shown in Chap. 2, this is, of course, a very worthy question as there is no such model.

In a further commentary, academic psychiatrist Simon Williamson agreed that the term "paradigm" may be more appropriate as Engel's concept sits higher on the ontological ladder than a mere model. While people talk about using the BPS approach or whatever, in practice, it is largely ignored in favour of simply making a diagnosis, as that is what determines treatment, and treatment is all. He suggested we look at the different levels of complexity of the human organism, from basic biology and genetics, to psychological systems and thence to social systems:

> Although higher levels regulate lower ones, each new level's proper functioning is entirely dependent on the lower levels from which it has risen. With such a framework, interactions between BPS factors can be theorised coherently, as existing in the same ontological space ... The BPS model is valid and useful, but it can be of no use to our patients if we fail to implement it ... a concerted effort is required to revive it in practice ... The BPS model will always be of significance to the history of psychiatry [33].

As this brief survey shows, any fair-minded person can conclude that, championed by influential psychiatrists and philosophers around the world, Engel's BPS model enjoys broad and deep support at the highest institutional and academic levels. This is also true of many medical schools and psychiatric training programs [11, 17, 27]. At the same time, there is practically no critical commentary published so it seems journal editors are also strongly supportive of the BPS model. Clearly, this model carries a great deal of cultural and intellectual weight, to the extent that, in some parts of the world, it is taken as defining psychiatry. So where's the problem? The problem, in five words, is this: Engel's biopsychosocial model doesn't exist. It doesn't exist as a model, approach, paradigm or spectrum and, due to psychiatry's profound misconception of what constitutes a science, it never can.

5.3. The status of the BPS model.

Given this fulsome praise, we need to look closely at the status of the model. The primary source is Engel's 1977 paper in *Science* entitled *The need for a new medical model: a challenge for biomedicine* [1]. Surprisingly, authors often cite the BPS model without providing a reference, as though it were axiomatic [e.g. 24]. Nobody would get away with that in general medicine or any other scientific field, so we can't take any of the claims above at face value. It's also important to remember that Engel was a physician talking about ordinary medical illnesses.

Given the title of his paper, Engel's definition of a model is crucial. On p130, he talks about "the existing medical model of disease," and soon specifies it as a reductionist or biomedical model, "... with molecular biology as its basic scientific discipline... " which explains behavioral aberrations...

> ... on the basis of disordered somatic (biochemical or neuro-physiological) processes ... the language of chemistry and physics will ultimately suffice to explain biological phenomena ... the only conceptual tools available to characterise and experimental tools to study biological systems are physical in nature (p130)

However, he then says the reductionist biomedical model is *also* a dualist model but says nothing further about the dualist element. Instead, he leaves the reader to infer that it is a natural dualist model and that the ordinary methods of physical science would account for it.

By this means, he throws a net over psychogical and social factors in human behaviour and pulls them into the orbit of conventional medicine. This is unprecedented. I'm not even sure that the expression "natural dualism" had been coined in 1977 as it is closely associated with the work of philosopher David Chalmers [34]. In any event, given the fact that it is not further explained, and in view of the complexities of Chalmers' case for a natural dualism, I conclude that Engel had no inkling of these matters.

He then defines a model as "... nothing more than a belief system offered to explain natural phenomena, to make sense out of what is puzzling or disturbing (p130)." His definition is further qualified to yield a class of scientific models which "... involved a shared set of assumptions and rules of conduct based on the scientific method and constituted a blueprint for research (p130)."

Now this is all a bit garbled and appears to have misled generations of psychiatrists and philosophers. A model is *not* a "set of beliefs": a model is the instantiation or actualisation of a set of beliefs in a form that yields viable predictions, *and* aids in testing those predictions [29]. All Engel did was classify psychological and social factors in such a way that they came under the umbrella of "things medical people ought to take into account." The mainstream of medicine, of course, follows the positivist ethos by excluding unobservables such as mind and society. That it may produce a shallow, dehumanised practice doesn't concern them. By adhering strictly to the reductionist program, they aren't saying "These things don't count," they are saying only "We don't know how to account for them in our approach so we're not going to bother." Given their reductionist approach, that's fully justifiable but it didn't suit Dr Engel's concept of good medicine.

Next, Engel outlined what he saw as the deficiencies of the biomedical model, none of which were new and would not surprise most physicians. This segues into his account of "The requirements of a new medical model" (p131). At this point, his attempt at a model actually collapses into a matter of his opinion but that's almost incidental, because now we come to the central problem: there is no model. Suddenly (p132), he jumps to talking about "a biopsychosocial model" in the context of various conditions such as diabetes and grief, after which he stated:

> The development of a biopsychosocial model is posed as a challenge for both medicine and psychiatry ... (Physicians) are

now ready for a medical model which could take psychosocial factors into account (p134).

Subsequently, he suggested the General Systems Theory (GST) of Ludwig von Bertalanffy [30] could provide an intellectual framework for his proposal:

> ... systems theory provides a conceptual approach suitable not only for the proposed biopsychosocial concept of disease ... If and when a general-systems approach becomes part of the basic scientific and philosophic education of future physicians and medical scientists, a greater readiness to encompass a BPS perspective of disease may be anticipated (p133-34).

Before finishing, he fired a number of parting shots at his nemesis, reductionist biomedicine, summarising his position as:

> The dominant model of disease today is biomedical, and it leaves no room within its framework for the social, psychological and behavioral dimensions of illness. A BPS model is proposed that provides a blueprint for research, a framework for teaching, and a design for action in the real world of health care.

So where's the problem? It's here: as he makes crystal clear, his model doesn't exist. There is no such thing as a "biopsychosocial model" just because he didn't write it, and he didn't write it because he didn't intend to. He left it to somebody else. From the title to the summary, his case is written in the future conditional tense, not past. It is entirely a matter of what could be, not what is. The title does not claim, nor at any point in the paper did he state anything like: "Here is a new medical model." In the last sentence, he states "*A* BPS model is proposed..." not "*The* BPS model" or "*My* BPS model." Nothing in Engel's title or the paper itself can be taken as a statement that his "model" has been articulated as a series of explanatory propositions with testable predictive power, i.e. as a scientific model [35]. All he ever said was "We need an integrative model of mind, body and society to challenge the biomedical model." This small point appears to have eluded several generations of psychiatrists. Certainly, Singh's "towering edifice" has no more substance than a shimmering mirage.

The case against GST is quite simple. Von Bertalanffy's singular approach hung upon a critical point, which he termed the matter-energy transfer functions. If, in any complex system (and the human brain and mind are surely complex), these cannot be isolated, identified and formalised as mathematical functions, then GST cannot address that system. In the 75 years since von Bertalanffy's work first gained psychiatric attention, nobody has ever offered anything that would amount even to an attempt to resolve this issue, let alone a solution. There is certainly nothing in von Bertalanffy's book [36] or in any of the other works Engel cited that would amount to an analysis of mind-body interaction in terms of matter-energy transfer functions. Here, absence of proof can be taken as proof of absence: it doesn't exist because it can't be done. Even if somebody had tried, it would be a hopeless task because however the human brain/mind complex functions, it is not as a manipulator of energy *per se*. Instead, everything we know about the brain says it is an information processor, which GST does not address. This probably explains why GST has faded from view in psychiatry over the past forty years.

None of this is new, it was spelled out in detail a quarter of a century ago. After a detailed analysis of the nature and status of scientific models, that paper concluded:

> In its present form, (Engel's BPS model) is so seriously flawed that its continued use in psychiatry is not justified… (I)t is not a theory… not revolutionary… not a model in any interesting sense of the word… just a case of wishful thinking [35].

If anybody were to publish an article entitled "The need for a bridge to Tasmania: a challenge for transport," concluding with the sentence: "A bridge from mainland Australia to Tasmania is proposed that provides a blueprint for building, a framework for study, and a design for action in the real world of transport," nobody would be so foolish as to drive to the coast near Melbourne looking for the access ramp.

Moreover, using his definitions, Engel's project starts badly. Given certain "puzzling or disturbing natural phenomena" (observations), the theorist builds an explanatory hypothesis linking those observations via some unseen mechanism. Nobody working with models would accept that a set of beliefs constitutes a model, as beliefs and models are of different orders of epistemological significance [35]. A model is the *instantiation* of the proposed explanatory mechanism, it renders those ideas in real form suitable for testing. A model is not merely an ontological opinion, hunch or intuition of the form "Biological, psychological and sociological factors are involved in the aetiology of mental disorder." Mere description is not a model as it has neither explanatory nor predictive power.

There is nothing in Engel's 1977 paper or any of his other papers cited above that amounts to a scientific model of any type. Beyond giving a name to a pious hope, there is not even the *beginnings* of a model, only a space on a library shelf where an integrative model could go. There is no statement of his ontology: we are left to presume he was committed to a natural dualism of some sort but he gave no indication of its form and there was no attempt at a methodology. Compounding these serious objections, apart from implying "everything that biomedicine doesn't do," Engel gave no indication what his model actually does. He never claimed it was a model of mind, and it certainly wasn't. He started with the fact that physical and mental illness are real, not social constructs, but it wasn't a model of illness *per se*, either physical or mental. He did not explain mental disorder nor give any clues as to how his approach improved on the prevailing psychiatric model. It was definitely not a model of personality and therefore had nothing to say about personality disorder. It said nothing new or interesting about mind-body interaction (but absent a model or theory of mind, that would have been impossible anyway). No treatment programs followed from it, either psychological or physical; it did not justify involuntary treatment; and it did not generate a novel research program.

As far as scientific models go, there aren't any more tests to fail. And the *coup de grâce*: it wasn't about psychiatry anyway.

Did Engel believe his model would emerge ostensively, i.e. by the clinical examples he offered in this and later papers? Not on the information available to us: his clinical examples were mundane, with no suggestion that he was offering a novel understanding of illness. Assuming he had a natural dualism in mind (and that's just surmise, he never addressed this point), it won't work as the concept of mind is metaphysical and can't be defined empirically. I have set out the case for a natural dualist model of mind [37]; this leads to its own explanation of mental disorder, one which immediately takes psychological and social factors into account.

To summarise this section, in 1977, a specialist physician published a paper on general medicine in a general scientific journal. Since then, psychiatrists have adopted it as a guiding intellectual principle for the profession. However, it has never been further developed and says not one word more today than it did 45 years ago. In particular, psychiatrists have added nothing conceptually new to Engel's unremarkable idea that psychosocial factors contribute to mental disorder. Note that none of the authors cited above includes a quote from Engel's 1977 paper demonstrating the precise nature or mechanism of his "model." No other authors have ever done so either which, in the context of scientific publishing, must be without precedent.

My case, first published a quarter of a century ago [35], is that there cannot be quotes, or development, just because there is no model. All Engel offered was his workaday intuition that psychosocial factors influence diagnosable disorders, essentially a description with no explanatory scope, aka a motherhood statement. In Davies' words [19], the BPS model is "… beguil(ing) and frustrat(ing)… everywhere and yet nowhere." In academic circles, this is a polite way of saying the whole thing is just a wish-fulfilling and self-deceiving mirage. To make matters worse, ignoring repeated warnings that it doesn't exist as a formal model is a betrayal of the scientific ethos.

After nearly half a century, anybody who still wants to claim that George Engel wrote a viable model of mind-body integration must produce a copy of it. In this era of "evidence-based psychiatry," his many supporters must produce evidence that it actually exists in the form of a scientific model although they should be mindful that, by his own words [10], it doesn't exist in that form. Until we actually see it, all claims about the reality, scope, practicality, etc. of the BPS model remain false claims. Scientific truth is not established by dint of repetition of a falsehood.

5.4. The illogicality of the BPS model.

Knowing that the model doesn't exist, it is perhaps overkill to point out that actually, there are further errors. By all accounts, Engel genuinely believed he had made a major contribution to medical science. While his "disciples" saw him as "one of the leading figures in medicine and psychiatry of our time" [11, p471], it seems he firmly agreed with their opinion. If so, how could he have made such an egregious mistake as to believe that simply by providing a name for a model, and leaving it to others to fill in the blanks, he had done humanity a great service? I suggest he fell into two elementary but common mistakes in logic.

The first is from the field known as logical semantics, specifically the relationship between the three words, *The Biopsychosocial Model*, and what those words can conceivably signify. In grammatical terms, the expression is a noun phrase comprised of the definite article *the*, the adjective *biopsychosocial*, and the noun *model*. The problem lies in the noun, because a model exists only insofar as it models a demonstrable entity. Thus, the point of a model is that it models. Conceptually, this is not demanding:

> A singer *sings*.
> A robber *robs*.
> A sailor *sails*.
> A cook *cooks*.
> A timer *times*.
> A writer *writes*.

These examples differ from the noun phrase *The Biopsychosocial Model*, in that they are complete sentences consisting of an article, a subject and a verb. In Kantian terms, each of them is an analytic truth, specifically a proposition whose predicate concept is immanent in its subject concept. Their definitions depend on their actions and could not be otherwise. It would be an absurdity worthy of Monty Python to claim that the subjects don't act as defined:

> "Oh look, there's that wonderful singer."
> "How exciting. What does she sing?"
> "Nothing. She doesn't sing at all. She hates music."

We could expand the sentences listed above by giving each one an adjective, thus:

> A *famous* singer sings.
> A *shifty* robber robs.
> A *brave* sailor sails.
> An *adventurous* cook cooks.
> A *careful* timer times.
> A *creative* writer writes.

While these are still sentences, they feel incomplete: what do the subjects sing, rob, sail, cook and so on? In each case, the verb is both transitive and intransitive, i.e. the meaning of the action can either stay with the subject (as in the terse examples above) or it can pass from the subject to some other thing, known as the object of the sentence: Article, subject, verb, object. These constitute complete sentences. Sentences with transitive verbs but no object are incomplete:

> A famous singer sings *a lovely song*.
> A shifty robber robs the mysteriously-darkened house.

> A brave sailor sails his tiny cockleshell over the towering crests.
> An adventurous cook cooks a delicious meal fit for a king.
> A careful timer times *the oft-delayed race.*
> A creative writer writes a combative paper that says everybody else is wrong.

If nothing else, it feels right to insert an object for the subject to act upon. Now we see the semantic deficiency in Engel's concept. Start with the bare noun: model. What does a model do? A model models. Here you see how the action of the subject must pass to an object to make sense. Even if we add an adjective, giving " The biopsychosocial model," we still need to know more, as in:

> The biopsychosocial model models.... What?

What does it model? Here, we run into a problem, because Engel never specified what his model would actually do. He left it as the bare noun phrase. Look at each of the examples again: if we parse each of the complete sentences above to their primary noun phrases (the subject of the sentence), we are left with:

> A famous singer.
> A shifty robber.
> A brave sailor.
> An adventurous cook.
> A careful timer.
> A creative writer.

Correctly, anybody reading that list would ask "Which famous singer, which shifty robber or brave sailor?" That is because the noun phrases refer to the sets of famous singers, or shifty robbers, or brave sailors, etc., but without specifying any particular member of that set. So the noun phrase *The Biopsychosocial Model* can only refer to the set of biopsychosocial models. However, as was shown as far back as last century, the ugly fact remains that there is no member of that particular set. Certainly, George Engel never wrote one, and nobody else has ever claimed to have done so since. The set of biopsychosocial models is an empty set. We can refer to it as a set but, until it has at least one member, it is a hollow and useless concept, a name tag on an empty library shelf.

However, for the purpose of discussion, let's assume that Engel did write a model. Next question: A model of what? Look at some other examples. A model aircraft models the concept of heavier than air flight. An animal model of a disease uses a simplified form of the disease to explore its physical consequences. A computer model of climate is a mathematical formula that, after a certain number of iterations, can predict the weather on a particular day. By listing probable outcomes, an algorithmic model of an epidemic does much the same thing. In science, a model instantiates or renders in real form an idea, usually called a theory, although it may be simply an hypothesis or even a hunch. But what did Engel's model model? To this day, we don't know. It wasn't offered as a model of mind, so we can dispense with that general possibility. Was it a model of disease? No, he used different diseases or illnesses as examples but his model couldn't say anything about a particular sickness or about sickness in general. Was it a model of, say, chronic illness? Again, no; he mentioned it but didn't nominate it. Was it a management model? In a way it was, but more along the lines of how to approach *assessment* of a patient, the correct attitude or disposition in the interviewer but not a model *per se*. Was it a model of treatment? No, definitely not. Finally, was it a model of mental disorder? No, most emphatically not, he had practically nothing to say about it.

Thus, we can only assume that Engel thought he had written a model of something when, in fact, he hadn't. So we arrive at the second objection to his spurious model: How could he have made such a grievous mistake as to think he had written a model when it didn't exist? I suggest he fell into one of the most basic errors of philosophy of language: he thought that by naming his model, he had also defined it. That's not possible: you cannot nominate something and, in the same illocutionary act, define it separately from its name, as in this everyday example:

> "Who's that?"
> "That's Bill Smith."
> "No, I mean *who* is he?"

Bill Smith, the name which nominates him as a distinct human entity, exists as a separate category of discourse or acquits a different language function from whatever role he occupies that defines the person *Bill Smith* as a social entity. These categories are not one and the same thing: the act of acquitting one language function, by naming something, does not simultaneously acquit the other, of defining it through its role. Same goes for the three word 'biopsychosocial model':

"This is my biopsychosocial model."
"What's a biopsychosocial model?"
"This is."

Engel believed he had found an intellectual/humanitarian gap in medicine (not in psychiatry; he was not a psychiatrist and didn't think much of psychiatrists or their trade [11]); he decided that if we had an integrative model of mind, body and society, we could do better for our patients. But that's all he did, and even that was hardly news. What he *didn't* do was give some sort of intellectual framework for his model, as distinct from the name he gave it. Epistemologically, naming a model and defining it are different acts.

Finally, what led him to this error? Most likely, it was, as his student and friend, Bruce Singh, suggested, his "narcissistic belief in his own 'specialness'" and his vision of himself as a "medical Darwin." Simply, he wanted to believe he had created "a towering edifice," "one of the most influential ideas in Medicine in the 20th Century," so he convinced himself he had. Moreover, a generation of psychiatrists desperately needed to believe it and he was so taken with the adulation that nobody bothered to look at the details.

4.4. Psychiatry and the emperor's new clothes.

In Hans Christian Andersen's version of the fable, the swindlers told the emperor and his courtiers that his lovely new suit was only visible to clever and competent people. Rather than run the risk of being called foolish, everybody pretended to be able to see the clothes. So for psychiatry, the real question is this: How can so many people have been so completely misled by this mirage? Answer: Their common sense was overwhelmed by their desperate need to show that psychiatry's unique intellectual basis means it must be taken seriously: *Mundus vult decipi.* The world wants to be deceived, just because the alternative is so painful that people can't confront it. Imagine any of the authors quoted above saying: "I don't like biological reductionism but I have no alternative. I have no scientific model to guide my psychiatric practice, my teaching and research, although I want to retain my status, my power and my income as a specialist." Imagine the RANZCP submission to the Senate stating: "We don't actually have a model of mental disorder and our treatment is pure serendipity but we think you should only listen to our views." Just imagine. The renowned astrophysicist Carl Sagan noted this years ago:

> One of the saddest lessons of history is this: if we've been bamboozled long enough, we tend to reject any evidence of the bamboozle. We're no longer interested in finding out the truth. The bamboozle has captured us. It's simply too painful to acknowledge, even to ourselves, that we've been taken [38, p230].

Upton Sinclair pointed to a more elementary reason why psychiatrists refuse to admit they've been eager dupes: "It's difficult to get a man to understand something when his salary depends on his not understanding it." There is no *a priori* reason to presume that, as humans, psychiatrists are immune to the normal human cognitive biases [39], particularly the illusory truth effect (people are more likely to believe false material if they have heard it before), confirmation bias (people selectively notice and recall information that confirms their pre-existing opinions, regardless of its validity) and *argumentum ad verecundiam* (people are swayed by opinions coming from authorities, regardless of whether the authority is an expert on the topic, or is even right).

All this was set out in the 1998 paper which showed that all Engel did was write a heartfelt plea for more humanity in medicine. He hardly talked about psychiatry and certainly didn't see himself as a psychiatrist [11]. These points have been reiterated a number of times since [40, 41] but the hermetic world of psychiatry is determined to maintain the falsehood that they have a unique integrative model of mind and body which gives them a particular advantage in dealing with the mentally-troubled.

Most publications on the BPS model does not refer to the 1998 paper; those authors who do so pointedly omit to mention its central point, that Engel never wrote a valid model of mind-body integration. This does not say that the concept of mind-body integration is wrong, or that it can't be done [37], only that Engel didn't do it. Psychiatry has actively convinced itself, the general public, governments and funding agencies, as well as our patients, medical students and trainee psychiatrists that he did, that psychiatry has thereby a solid and unique intellectual foundation when every psychiatrist knows, or ought to know, that it doesn't. This is a very serious matter, but it is hardly new. In his critique of medical practice from 1976, Holman argued that ven as American health care was facing a major crisis, it was common practice for medical institutions to label themselves as "centres of excellence." Holman deplored this development:

> In the aggregate, medical institutions and practices are not excellent. The self-acclaimed excellence is, in practice, a myth … the medical establishment is not primarily engaged in the disinterested pursuit of knowledge and the translation of that knowledge into medical practice; rather, in significant part, it is engaged in special interest advocacy, pursuing and preserving social power. The concept of excellence is a component of the ideological justification of that role [42, p11].

If we insert 'psychiatric' in place of 'medical,' and 'biopsychosocial model' in place of 'excellence,' this observation appears custom-made for modern psychiatry's function as a self-protective guild [43]. As an aside, the biopsychosocial model was first called a myth in 2006 [44].

The question then arises: Is this apparent self-deception deliberate or is it just intellectual laziness? First, those who claim Engel's BPS model exists must explain exactly what they are endorsing, and why they have ignored repeated warnings that there is something seriously wrong with Engel's proposal *as they claim to understand it. A fortiori*, this applies to editors, not just to authors and academics. Second, does it matter? Yes, it does: deception is as deception does, including self-deception. Science is about eliminating error and self-deception. It is inexcusable to perpetuate an error over nearly half a century, convincing a "… generation of … medical students and psychiatry trainees…" [12] that psychiatry has an integrative aetiological model of mental disorder when none of their teachers can produce it. That implies a refusal to consider error, a wilful blindness or conceit that goes far beyond self-satisfied carelessness. In a profession such as medicine, that's dangerous. Writing on the contribution of the physiologist, Claude Bernard, to the development of positivist science, the Polish philosopher and historian, Leszek Kolakowski noted:

> It is too easy to gain cheap satisfaction by labelling a phenomenon and assigning it a subdivision in a rank order. It is not correct classification that matters, but *understanding the mechanism* governing the phenomenon [44, p94-5, emphasis added].

On the crucial question of the mechanism by which body, psyche and society are to be integrated, Engel was entirely silent, not least because he didn't have a theory of mind from which to derive a model of mental disorder: a theory of mind necessarily comes before a theory of disordered mind. That's also true of every other author quoted above. The next question, the process by which his followers simply slipped into the same mistake, is more complex. While creative people are often quick to proclaim the wonder of their own works, it is something else again for educated people to accept their claims without demur. This phenomenon has attracted the attention of a political scientist with an interest in the increasing medicalisation of society. In a rather dense but carefully-argued paper, Alex Roberts dissected the model as Engel proposed it, concluding:

> What the BPSM is, then, is essentially the *general proposition* that illness involves biological, psychological, and social factors... The model is thus vague, all-inclusive, and lacks meaningful scientific content. Essentially the BPSM states a truism about illness (p3) ... the BPSM can appropriately be called a "conceptual framework," but it is not a scientific model or an explanatory model of disease. There is nothing in the model itself that would allow us to distinguish disease from non-disease, define specific diseases, or separate genuine cause-effect relationships from spurious correlations [45, p4, emphasis in original].

How, then, has it attracted such a wide and loyal following among psychiatry's "key opinion leaders"? Roberts has proposed a number of steps by which psychiatrists have led themselves to believe they are dealing with an authentic scientific model, producing what he terms "wayward BPSM discourse," which is the thrust of his argument. These steps include:

> 1. Concept shifting. ... researchers will sometimes inappropriately blur the conceptual distinction between disease and illness (or syndrome).

> 2. Question begging. ... (using premises that contain, or presuppose the truth of, one's conclusion).

> 3. Appeals to authority. ... many arguments ... boil down to the following: D is a disease caused by factors X, Y, and Z because the BPSM says so.

This leads him to a reappraisal of the status of the BPSM, concluding:

> It is not a model that can produce scientific explanations of phenomena. Rather, it is a general perspective one can take to

> research and treatment.... The empirical data "fit" the BPSM *because* it is all-inclusive and unfalsifiable; they do not demonstrate that the BPSM is a valid scientific model... [45, p5].

After considering a number of conditions in the text and in the accompanying supplement, Roberts outlines the ways in which "wayward BPSM discourse" adversely affects the practice of psychiatry. These include introducing "dysfunctional disease constructs" by creating difficulties in revising research constructs and producing "... unstable illness constructs that place research on a fundamentally chaotic path, especially over the longer term..." However, his main concern is the ability of this flawed reasoning to extend the reach of medicine to fields that should not be seen as subject to medical intervention:

> Wayward BPSM discourse is also a potent and potentially dangerous vehicle of medicalization. In particular, it has the capacity to [1] prematurely represent ambiguous states of suffering as organic problems falling under medicine's purview, and [2] expand the domain of "disease" in ways that unjustifiably increase the power of medicine and the state [45, p13].

Since psychiatry is granted essentially unassailable civil powers to detain and inflict involuntary treatment on people who have broken no laws, this conclusion is far from trivial. In detaining a person and inflicting treatment against the person's will, psychiatrists are under the gravest moral duty to be *certain* that they know *precisely* what they are doing. This means they must have a formal and publically-available, *explanatory* model (a scientific model) of mental disorder, articulated to the point where they *could not be wrong*. They have nothing of the sort. Moreover, it is now established to the level of *certainty* that Engel's "biopsychosocial model" is not, and never could be, such a model.

Sondern trägt der Kaiser keine Kleider.

The emperors of psychiatry are wearing no clothes.

5.5. The law on fraud.

This raises the possibility that this long-standing deception is neither accidental nor reckless, but is an act deliberately undertaken with the intention to deceive, i.e. it may be of fraudulent intent. The dictionary definition is:

> Fraud: *n* 1. deliberate deception, trickery or cheating intended to
> gain an advantage. 2. an act of such deception. 3. something false
> or spurious. 4. *Inf.* a person who acts in a false or deceitful way.

At the least, Definition 3 (something false or spurious) seems to
apply in this case. The Queensland Criminal Code at S.408C states
inter alia:

> (1) A person who dishonestly ... (d) gains a benefit or advantage,
> pecuniary or otherwise, for any person; ... commits the crime of
> fraud [47].

Presumably, psychiatrists benefit from claiming the BPS model is
real, otherwise they wouldn't do it. The benefit need not be financial as
S.408C (3)(a) specifies broadly "... any benefit or advantage, anything
evidencing a right to ... receive a benefit ..." Maintenance of one's
status as a specialist with extraordinary civil powers, and insulation
from criticism (i.e. "special interest advocacy, pursuing and preserving
social power") would be one such advantage.

S.408C (2A) of the Code lists aggravating factors, including: "... (b)
the offender carries on the business of committing the offence." The
fact that it has been carried on for 25 years since the first warning
constitutes an aggravation, as does the fact that psychiatrists routinely
misrepresent the nature of the warning. However, criminal codes
normally provide a defence relating to ignorance of the facts, thus:

> S.24. Mistake of fact.
> (1) A person who does or omits to do an act under an honest and
> reasonable but mistaken belief in the existence of any state of
> things is not criminally responsible for the act or omission to any
> greater extent than if the real state of things had been such as the
> person believed to exist [47].

Was Engel guilty of fraud? I don't believe so. I have argued that he
made a common-enough mistake [34] but, because of his "narcissistic
belief in his own 'specialness'" [10], and amplified by the obsequious
and uncritical adulation showered on him, he really thought he had
achieved something of historical significance. Perhaps he genuinely did
believe he was a "medical Darwin" but that doesn't excuse his
followers. The whole point of a university education is to learn how to
analyse material and criticise the received wisdom, not to parrot it.

Is the defence of "Mistake of Fact" available to professors who have
chosen to ignore repeated warnings that their preferred model doesn't

exist? I don't believe so. If the engineers engaged to design the "proposed bridge to Tasmania" ignored warnings that it lacked adequate support, they would be in serious trouble. Psychiatry's lavish support for a non-existent model is neither honest nor reasonable as it ceased being a mistake in 1998. If accused of fraud, the only defence available to the hordes of Engel's palpitating followers is to plead self-serving stupidity (see end note).

5.6. BPS Model: A name with no horse.

When psychiatrists claim that Engel's BPS model is "fundamental to our profession," "the mainstay of academic psychiatry for over 30 years," "a towering edifice" and "one of the most influential ideas in Medicine in the 20th Century" which "has achieved worldwide recognition as one of the most influential developments psychiatry and medicine" and now, given its role as the "overarching framework for contemporary healthcare" due to being "the predominant theoretical framework underpinning contemporary psychiatric training and practice," stands as "a beacon for the soul of medicine and psychiatry in the twenty-first century," it becomes burdensome for even compulsive naysayers to resist the temptation to throw aside their vexatious quibbles and join the happy throng of "ultimate integrators of the biological and psychosocial perspectives underlying diagnostic understanding and treatment." True. I agree. In fact, after half a lifetime of being practically the only skeptic at the BPS party, I am ready to throw in the towel. First, however, I would like to sort out some objections received from reviewers.

The first objection to my assertion that a scientific model for psychiatry should meet the general criteria for scientific models is that Engel didn't really mean "model," he meant "approach," or "perspective" or possibly "paradigm" or even "spectrum." This may be the case although he never said that. Moreover, it would be most unlikely that he would have invoked General Systems Theory if all he had in mind was such vague and amorphous notions. He said model, he offered his definition of model, so we are forced to accept that is precisely what he meant. In any event, we can dismiss this objection as "approaches" and "spectra" have no basis in science, while the idea he meant paradigm in the modern sense is completely wrong. Psychiatrists who prefer a "BPS approach" or whatever are only saying they don't like the prevailing reductionist or biological ontology. They are using it as a rallying call for anybody who wants to retain a place for mentality in mental disorders, i.e. adopting a dualist position but without the "thought crime" of overt dualism (another example of having your cake and eating it too). In my view, this is the most likely motivation for psychiatry's reluctance to accept that it is operating without warrant.

Next objection: "What counts for a model 'to exist' would depend on the nature of the model, be it physical, mathematical, statistical, etc.." This is a spurious objection. The criteria for scientific models are general and are independent of the specific field under study. They were set out in a form suitable for psychiatry many years ago [29] but those who support the BPSM much prefer to ignore them.

Continuing, one reviewer took an uncompromising view: "The reasoning is leaping in reaching claims of deception and fraud. Even if your premises were true, the conclusion is not a necessity (that is, the inference is not valid logically)." Firstly, the premises of the argument are factually true. All quotes from psychiatric authorities were referenced, and quotes from the Qld Criminal Code are readily available online. Implying they were not true is verging on dishonest. Second, since when does science operate on a standard of "logical necessity"? Reductionist science is and always has been empirical, that is, based in evidence derived from the senses, meaning subject to interpretation, and always open to refutation by further evidence. Suddenly claiming that your opponent (and not your own side) must adhere to an impossible standard of proof is definitely less than honest. Third, the decision whether psychiatry is actively or passively misleading itself and the general public is a matter for investigation. My duty as an author, and as a citizen, is to report what I believe to be institutional-level wrong-doing. I am the complainant, not the jury. That duty rests with the larger scientific community, and with the general community (who double as tax-payers).

Some psychiatrist, however, argue that all debate over models is beside the point, on the basis that psychiatry is evidence-based rather than being a captive of one theory or another. The problem with this objection is that what is taken as evidence is *itself* theory-driven. By virtue of their unacknowledged views, two people looking at the same event can ascribe to it different or even contradictory significance, as Kolakowski pointed out:

> ... the data of experience always leave scope for more than one explanatory hypothesis, and which one is to be chosen cannot be determined by experience. Rival hypotheses accounting for a

given aggregate of facts may be equally sound from a logical point of view, and hence our actual choices are accounted for by non-empirical considerations ... the conception of science as descriptive 'generalisation' from 'brute' facts, as a one-way movement of thought from 'facts' to 'laws,' is naive and superficial [45].

In practice, as Roberts has emphasised [46], the process of "evidence-basing" becomes self-reinforcing: from all possible observations, some are selected because they fit the theory but are subsequently used to justify the choice of the theory. The idea that collecting evidence frees us of the need for an articulated world view is pure laziness: we cannot free ourselves of our prejudices, the model does that for us. And because psychiatrists deal with people's lives, their prejudices count; if they think they don't have any, their prejudices are all the more pernicious.

Now to one final quibble mentioned by Davies and Roach: "Engel did not provide details as to how biological, psychological, and social factors should be combined in diagnosing, describing, explaining, and treating mental illness [18]." Bolton and Gillett also alluded to the same point: "It is not straightforward to find the right metaphor for the relation between the biological, the psychological and the social" [23].[2] Later, Bolton mentioned the same point *en passant*: "My main contention is that—notwithstanding doubts as to what exactly it is, or indeed whether it is anything—there is a coherent account of it ..." [31, p228].

And it is on this thorn that the balloon of the BPS model, or paradigm, or approach, or spectrum, or perspective, so assiduously inflated over the past half century by so many eminent psychiatrists and philosophers, arrives at its *Hindenburg* moment: an integrative model of mind, body and society that has no "details as to how biological, psychological, and social factors should be combined," one that may even be nothing at all, is not a model, it is a mirage. A model is not a metaphor and vice versa [23]: if you need a metaphor to explain what your model was supposed to demonstrate, then you don't have a model at all. The idea that there could be a "coherent account" of something that doesn't exist is absurd.

None of this has anything to do with the question of whether psychological and social factors are of significance in physical illness

---

2   This is academese for "We haven't the faintest clue."

and mental disorder, a point which appears to have eluded Prof. Bolton: "There is accumulating evidence from recent decades that psychosocial as well as biological factors are implicated in the aetiology and treatment of a large range of physical as well as mental health conditions... " Yes, there is, heaps of evidence, although it goes back to time immemorial. Bolton seems to think that evidence for mind-body interaction is somehow evidence for Engel's model, which it isn't. Mind-body interaction is an empirical fact; all we need is a formal, integrative model, for which the *sine qua non* is a model of mind, which psychiatry most certainly doesn't have, and which Engel didn't write. Ronald Pies, however, dismisses this as a bagatelle:

> The BPS paradigm imposes no need to solve the ancient "mind-body" conundrum that has bedeviled philosophy for millennia (eg, "What is the mind? Is it distinct from brain? How does mind interact with the brain?"). Those issues, though philosophically important, are at a different epistemic level than that of the BPS paradigm [21].

That is, he believes that a scientific model of mind-body interaction does not require us to provide a mechanism or means of mind-body interaction. But his "bio-psycho-social paradigm" can only exist when the ontology says that mind and body are different; without that, you have to say they are one and the same thing, which is biological psychiatry by another name. By this reality-bending move, Pies puts his finger on a point we will revisit in the final chapter: the reflex inability of psychiatry to accept that the mind is a real, causally-effective thing. This is part of the positivist legacy which we will explore in more detail in Part II of this work.

5.7. Conclusion and a challenge.

I conclude that Engel's phantom BPS model is an illusion created and maintained as an important part of psychiatry's covert program of "special interest advocacy, pursuing and preserving social power." Psychiatry's vaunted biopsychosocial model is a Claytons model, the model you have when you don't have a model. I don't necessarily blame Dr Engel. He tried, but he got it wrong, which is more than can be said for all the panting professors and salivating sages in his cheer squad. They *did* it wrong, which is an inexcusable breach of the most basic principle of higher education.

These are strong words so I will offer my many opponents a face-saving escape: produce something, anything, written by George L Engel, late gastroenterologist of Rochester, NY, that meets the criteria for an integrative scientific model of mind, body and society, and all will be well. But if nobody produces it, say by the fiftieth anniversary of the publication of his paper, April 8th 2027 (and I have been issuing this challenge for years, so I think that's generous), then psychiatry stands exposed to allegations of major scientific misconduct ranging from intellectual neglect via reckless egotistical conceit up to and including actual scientific fraud.

Having ignored repeated warnings over the past twenty-five years, psychiatry cannot claim the defence of "an honest and reasonable but mistaken belief in the existence" of a biopsychosocial model.

All they have to do is produce it.

Note: Many of the authors quoted in this chapter were contacted to provide precise details of where Engel's model is set out as a series of axiomatic propositions. Not one replied. The original paper for this chapter was submitted to, and rejected by, four journals. There were six reviewer opinions from the first three journals, all completely different and not addressing the central points: that George Engel's BPS model does not exist; that psychiatrists know this; and they are attempting to conceal this point. The fourth journal's editorial manager said "This paper will not be approved by our reviewers so I will not be sending it out." At least it was honest about their lack of integrity.

References:

1. Engel GL (1977). The need for a new medical model: a challenge for biomedicine. *Science* 196:129-136.

2. Lugg W. (2021). The biopsychosocial model—history, controversy and Engel. *Australasian Psychiatry.* On line publication

.doi.org/10.1177/10398562211037333

3.Kingdon D (2020). Why hasn't neuroscience delivered for psychiatry? *British Journal of Psychiatry Bulletin,* 44: 107–109, doi:10.1192/bjb.2019.87

4. Scull A (2022) *Desperate Remedies: Psychiatry and the mysteries of mental illness*. London: Penguin.

5. McLaren N (1996). The myth of eclecticism. *Australasian Psychiatry*; 4: 260-61.

6. Engel GL (1960). A unified concept of health and disease. *Perspectives in Biology and Medicine*; 3:459-485.

7. Engel GL (1977). The care of the patient: art or science? *Johns Hopkins Medical Journal.* 140:222-232.

8. Engel GL (1978). The biopsychosocial model and the education of health professionals. *Annals of the New York Academy of Sciences.* 310:169-181.

9. Engel GL (1980). The clinical application of the biopychosocial model. *American Journal of Psychiatry.* 137:535-544.

10. Engel GL (1997). From Biomedical to Biopsychosocial: Being Scientific in the Human Domain. *Psychosomatics.* 38:521-528.

11. Singh BS (2002). George Engel: a personal reminiscence. *Australian and New Zealand Journal of Psychiatry,* 36: 467-471 (note that for at least ten years, this paper was missing from the *ANZJP* archive).

12. Smith GC, Strain JJ (2002). George Engel's contribution to clinical psychiatry. *Australian and New Zealand Journal of Psychiatry,* 36: 458-466 (note that for at least ten years, this paper was missing from the *ANZJP* archive).

13. Lewis B (2007). The Biopsychosocial Model and Philosophic Pragmatism. Is George Engel a Pragmatist? *Philosophy, Psychology and Psychiatry,* 14: 299-310.

14. Frances A (2014). Resuscitating the biopsychosocial model. *Lancet Psychiatry.* 1: 496-97.

15. Pilgrim D (2002). The biopsychosocial model in Anglo-American psychiatry: Past, present and future? *Journal of Mental Health.* 11: 585–594 .

16. Pilgrim D (2015). The Biopsychosocial Model in Health Research: Its Strengths and Limitations for Critical Realists. *Journal of Critical Realism.* 14:164-180.

17. Seawright HR (2016). The Biopsychosocial Model: "Reports of My Death Have Been Greatly Exaggerated." *Culture, Medicine and Psychiatry.* 40: 289-98.

18. Davies W, Roache R (2017). Reassessing biopsychosocial psychiatry. *British Journal of Psychiatry.* 210: 3-5.

19. Davies W (2017). Social explanation in psychiatry. https://19c76db5-af9a-45c4-84d9-

2efc3f98d570.filesusr.com/ugd/ea0e11_178b0921f8814894b95c63c523ad
c691.pdf

20. Pies RW (2019). Debunking the two chemical imbalance myths, again. *Psychiatric Times*. At:

https://www.psychiatrictimes.com/view/debunking-two-chemical-imbalance-myths-again

21. Pies RW. (2020) Can we salvage the biopsychosocial model? Psychiatric Times, at:

https://www.psychiatrictimes.com/view/can-we-salvage-biopsychosocial-modelde

22. Gask L (2018). In defence of the biopsychosocial model. Essay, *Lancet Psychiatry*. 5: 548-549.

23. Bolton G, Gillett G (2019). *The Biopsychosocial Model of Health and Disease: New philosophical and scientific developments*. Cham, Switzerland: Palgrave McMillan/Springer Nature. Open Access

24. Porter RJ (2020). The biopsychosocial model in mental health. *Australian and New Zealand Journal of Psychiatry*.. 54:773–774.

25. McLaren N (2021). Debate: The Biopsychosocial Model: Reality Check. *Australian and New Zealand Journal of Psychiatry*. 55: 644-645.

26. Wilson J (1998). President's Letter. *Australasian Psychiatry*. 6:83-84.

27. Royal Australian and New Zealand College of Psychiatrists (1998). Position Statement No. 39: 'What is a psychiatrist, and what does a psychiatrist do?' Archived; available from RANZCP, Melbourne. https://www.ranzcp.org/home.

27a. Royal Australian and New Zealand College of Psychiatrists (2013). Position Statement No. 80:b Available from RANZCP, Melbourne. https://www.ranzcp.org/home.

28. Frazier L (2020). The past, present, and future of the biopsychosocial model: A review of *The Biopsychosocial Model of Health and Disease: New philosophical and scientific developments* by Derek Bolton and Grant Gillett. *New Ideas in Psychology*. 57: 100755. https://doi.org/10.1016/j.newideapsych.2019.100755

29. Holmes J (2000). Fitting the biopsychosocial jigsaw together (editorial). *British Journal of Psychiatry*. 177; 93-94.

30. Gabbard GO, Kay J (2001). The Fate of Integrated Treatment: Whatever Happened to the Biopsychosocial Psychiatrist? *American Journal of Psychiatry.* 158: 1958-1963.

31. Bolton D (2022). Looking forward to a decade of the biopsychosocial model. *British Journal of Psychiatry Bulletin,* 46: 228–232, doi:10.1192/bjb.2022.34

32. Kingdon D (2020). Why hasn't neuroscience delivered for psychiatry? *British Journal of Psychiatry Bulletin,* 44: 107–109, doi:10.1192/bjb.2019.87

33. Williamson S (2022) The biopsychosocial model: not dead, but in need of revival. *British Journal of Psychiatry Bulletin,* doi:10.1192/bjb.2022.29

34. Chalmers DJ (1996). *The Conscious Mind: in search of a fundamental theory.* Oxford: University Press.

29. McLaren N (1998). A critical review of the biopsychosocial model. *Australian and New Zealand Journal of Psychiatry.* 32; 86-92.

36. Bertalanffy L v (1968-1969). *General Systems Theory.* New York: Braziller/Penguin. 1968-1969

37. McLaren N (2021). *Natural Dualism and Mental Disorder: The biocognitive model for psychiatry.* London: Routledge.

38. Sagan C (1997). *The Demon-Haunted World: Science as a candle in the dark.* New York: Random House.

39. Kahneman D (2011). *Thinking fast and slow.* New York: Farrar, Straus and Giroux.

40. McLaren N (2020). The Biopsychosocial Model: the end of a reign of error. *Ethical Human Psychology and Psychiatry,* 22:71-82.

41. McLaren N (2023). The Biopsychosocial Model and Scientific Deception. *Ethical Human Psychology and Psychiatry,* 25: 106-118.

42. Holman HR (1976). The 'Excellence' Deception in Medicine. *Hospital Practice* 11:11. (April, 1976).

43. Whitaker R, Cosgrove L (2015). *Psychiatry Under the Influence: Institutional Corruption, Social Injury, and Prescriptions for Reform.* New York: Palgrave MacMillan.

44. McLaren N (2006). The myth of the biopsychosocial model. Letter: *Australian and New Zealand Journal of Psychiatry;* 40:277.

45. Kolakowski, L. (1968). *Positivist Philosophy: From Hume to the Vienna Circle*. New York: Doubleday. Page numbers refer to Penguin Edition, 1972.

46. Roberts, A. (2023). The biopsychosocial model: Its use and abuse. *Medicine, Health Care and Philosophy*. https://doi.org/10.1007/s11019-023-10150-2. ePublication April 17th, 2023.

47. Queensland Criminal Code 1899-2021. Available at: https://www.legislation.qld.gov.au/view/pdf/inforce/current/act-1899-009 . Accessed February 22nd 2022.

6   Thomas Szasz and Antipsychiatry: the myth of the myth

In all of history, we have found just one cure for error—a partial antidote against making and repeating grand, foolish mistakes, a remedy against self-deception. That antidote is criticism.

David Brin.

6.1. To eliminate mental disorder.

So far, we have looked at a number of different options in explaining mental disorder, with little success. Since biological reduction doesn't work, mentalism merges into irrationality, behaviorism is dead in the water and the biopsychosocial model is a pseudo-model, what's left? One recurring theme that was strong in the 1970s and 80s is the notion that there is no such thing as mental illness, only persecution/ misunderstanding/ malingering/ bad behaviour/ lack of love etc. This slogan points to quite a different position from the approaches above, namely that they're all wrong because nobody is actually mentally ill or disordered or whatever or, if they are, it's somebody else's fault and can be fixed with less persecution, more understanding, getting a grip, less drugs, following the rules, more love etc.

These ideas are generally lumped together under the heading "antipsychiatry," which is (wrongly) lumped together with branches who believe that mental disorder is indeed real but modern psychiatry is entirely on the wrong track and is a destructive folly and/or racket and/or power trip etc. For most people, the term "antipsychiatry" is indelibly associated with the writings of Thomas Szasz (1920-2012), a Hungarian-born psychiatrist from Syracuse, NY, but the ideas long predate him. Why are they so persistent? Because the institution of psychiatry has never articulated a model of mental disorder to guide its practice, its teaching and its research, and thus lumbers blindly from one crisis to the next, thereby providing lots of ammunition for its opponents. The history of "antipsychiatry" is too big to cover here, so we will focus on Szasz's work because, like it or not, he was the face of antipsychiatry for over half a century.

Thomas Szasz was a prolific author, publishing some 35 books over about fifty years, including no less than seventeen books in the last twenty years of his long life, as well as hundreds of articles, papers, commentaries, lectures etc. He travelled extensively and must have given thousands of lectures and talks on his theme. All of this has stimulated an enormous secondary literature of many thousands of books and papers, not least because Szasz was a provocative and even deliberately inflammatory polemicist who delighted in his role as torturer-in-chief of the psychiatric establishment. Trouble is, psychiatry hardly noticed him while he was alive and, as I had predicted, his name has rapidly faded since his death. In the 1970s, practically every university student knew of him and what he was about. Now, hardly any have heard of him.

Szasz did not publish a complete autobiography, only a single chapter. This introduced a volume edited by Jeffrey Schaler, a close associate, entitled *Szasz Under Fire: the psychiatric abolitionist faces his critics* [1]. The book consists of twelve chapters by critics with commentaries by Szasz. His introduction shows he was born into a secure, upper middle-class Jewish family in Budapest, shortly after Hungarian independence. His father, who had trained as a lawyer, was a successful businessman while his mother, whom he described as "beautiful" in every respect, was devoted to her family and home. He felt his parents had a warm marriage and his mother appeared to have doted on him, not least because he was the younger of her two sons and was "sickly" as a child. His uncle was a renowned mathematician who moved to the US and was later able to sponsor the family to migrate before the Second World War engulfed Hungary's large and intellectually influential Jewish community.

While still in high school, and against his father's wishes, Thomas decided he wanted to study medicine, but for his own reasons: "I wanted to go to medical school not because I wanted to practice medicine but because I wanted to know medicine" [1, p9]. He arrived in the US in late 1938 and, after a few years, was able to study medicine. Subsequently, he began training in psychiatry in Chicago which, at the time, essentially meant psychoanalysis. In the early 1950s, he served a "comfortable" two year term in the US Navy, based in USN

Medical Center, Bethesda, Maryland. From there, he moved to Syracuse as he wanted a quiet, rural setting where he could read and write.

The most striking feature of his brief autobiography is that he had a charmed life, indulged at every turn by practically everybody who met him. To my mind, this is significant in the opinions he embraced throughout his long career. The other thing to remember about him is that his disciples, because that is what they are, react badly to the merest hint of criticism of any word he wrote, on which point they are following their master's lead.

6.2. Szasz the polemicist.

Some years ago, while writing two chapters on Szasz's contribution to 20th Century psychiatry [2], I read about a dozen of his best-known books, starting where it all began in 1961. His five most important works appear to be:

> *The Myth of Mental Illness: Foundations of a Theory of Personal Conduct* (1961; my copy is the revised edition, 1974) [3]

> *The Manufacture of Madness: a Comparative Study of the Inquisition and the Mental Health Movement* (1970; my copy 1977) [4]

> *The Theology of Medicine: the Political-Philosophical Foundations of Medical Ethics* (1977) [5]

> *The Myth of Psychotherapy* (1979) [6]

> *Insanity: the Idea and its Consequences* (1987) [7]

Some 3,000 pages later, his major points can be summarised:

> 6.2.1: Mental illness is a myth. So-called mental illnesses are either problems of living, including moral dilemmas, none of which should be medicalised, or physical illness of the brain, which physicians (real doctors) should treat.

> 6.2.2: So-called mentally-disordered people are deceivers. Their so-called mental illness is a game of deception.

> 6.2.3: Psychiatrists are willing partners in a conspiracy to defraud.

> 6.2.4: Psychiatrists in public practice are agents of the repressive society.

6.2.5: Treatment in psychiatry must be a voluntary, pecuniary contract between coequal adults.

A quick reading of any of his works will give dozens, if not hundreds, of quotes to support each of these points:

6.2.1.1: "...mental illness is a non-existent or fictitious condition" [7, p107]. That is, there is no objective physical basis to the types of behaviours termed psychiatric diseases: "...mental illnesses are not *bona fide* diseases... they are personal problems in living... I simply prefer not to place deviance in the category of disease" [7, p162]. All of what is now called mental illness, disease or disorder is simply problems of living compounded by frank deceit and should be dealt with accordingly. Crime must not be attributed to or excused by mental disorder because that is the worst form of dishonesty. Soldiers with "so-called war neuroses" are simply acting crazy or sick to escape their duty [6, p90-91].

6.2.2.1: People who claim to be mentally ill or whose actions attract the label are acting fraudulently and with full conscious intent to deceive: "...Mesmer's practice, like that of all psychotherapists before and since him, was devoted exclusively to persons who pretended to be ill" [6, p49]. There are dozens of points throughout this book where he explicitly states that patients are only pretending: "...their patients who pretend to be ill... persons with pretended illnesses..." [6, p55]; "...both had hysterical—that is, pretended—illnesses..." "What was wrong with these 'nervous patients'? ...the patients pretended they were ill, because they malingered or faked illness" [6, p96]. "I have described elsewhere the pretences of neurotics and psychotics claiming to be patients..." [6, p196]. "...patients with ...most so-called mental illnesses do not make 'appropriate efforts' to get well. Indeed, they usually make no such efforts at all, and try, instead, to be authenticated as 'sick'..." [6, p197]. He repeats this claim hundreds of times in his other works.

6.2.3.1: Psychiatrists who diagnose or treat people as mentally ill are party to a conspiracy to defraud. There are so many supportive references that one can almost open any of his books at any page and find comments to this effect. For example: "All this (psychiatry) is fakery and pretence whose purpose it to 'medicalise' certain aspects of the study and control of human behaviour" [3, p4]. Except for a very restricted form of psychotherapy, all psychiatric treatment is either a money-grubbing sham or state-sanctioned brutalisation of society's scapegoats: "…doctors have invented two different kinds of such non-existent diseases, bodily and mental… mythical disorders of the uterus and ovaries… mythical ailments of the liver… examples of the (mental) are all of the mental diseases… the various anxiety and stress disorders today… as the medical profession and the public have redefined the rules of the medical game, (telling the truth) has ceased to be an option altogether" [7, p36].

6.2.4.1: Psychiatrists in public practice are complicit agents of the repressive consumerist society, deceitfully classifying people as deviants in order to free society of nuisances and keep themselves in jobs. They are the modern equivalent of the medieval witch hunters who eliminated marginalised and unwanted individuals so everybody else could have a better life.

6.2.5.1: All psychiatric treatment other than the "autonomous psychotherapy" of fee-paying adults is fraudulent and brutalising. Treatment of mental problems should be by voluntary pecuniary contract between coequal adults with absolutely no coercion whatsoever. Third party (insurance) payments are not permissible: "…in autonomous psychotherapy, the relationship between the therapist and the patient is like that between an architect and the workmen who actually build a house" [5, p61].

All of this is delivered in a supremely confident manner with no attempt at a balanced view of the various questions – or an awareness that there may even be two sides to the argument. All psychiatrists except Thomas Szasz are cheats and liars; all patients are cheats and liars; governments are full of cheats and liars; total personal freedom is the only moral imperative needed in order to build a perfect society; anything less is anathema.

6.3. Unpicking Szasz's legacy.

Where to start? Probably the easiest place is his opening shots: There is no such thing as mental illness as illness is physical and nobody has ever shown a physical disturbance of the brain that would justify calling a mental state an illness. He appears to have come to this opinion some time in the early 1930s, while he was still at school and knew nothing about mental disorder—and, given his privileged life, most likely had never seen a mentally disturbed person. He appears to have had no knowledge of modern neurosciences, there is no analysis of his position and he very rarely referred to the current psychiatric literature, so his position was pure ideology. In fact, he was probably right but that was luck, not science. In any event, even if psychotic conditions are found to have a physical basis, who will look after them? Neurologists? Not likely, the last thing they want on their wards are deluded psychiatric patients.

Next: psychiatrists occupy the same role as medieval witch hunters. Here, it gets a bit confusing as he makes it perfectly clear that he believes all psychiatrists are frauds. But he could never claim that witch hunters didn't believe in what they were doing. They did, they were totally committed to the idea that witches exist and must be found and destroyed. Whatever else, they were not frauds, so Szasz's parallel immediately fails. Moreover, the people accused of witchcraft or sorcery were not acting like witches to defraud the society. With very good cause, they were terrified of being labelled whereas Szasz believes mental patients are actively pretending to be crazy in order to get a free lunch. In both cases, the hunters and the hunted, the roles were actually the reverse of what he claimed, so Szasz's claim of an historical homology breaks down completely, taking a large part of his corpus with it.

Next is one of Szasz's major points: mentally-disturbed people are only pretending. He said they are playing a game but didn't explain why they opted for such a self-destructive game in life. As was so often the case, his "explanation" wasn't so much to enlighten as to stop further discussion. For myself, I can't understand how anybody could arrive at that conclusion. Sorry, I can: anybody who has decided beforehand that all mental patients are frauds would not be able to see their distress as genuine, any more than medieval witch hunters were moved by their victims' protests of innocence. His conviction appears to have two historical bases. He relied heavily on the psychoanalytic and historical concepts of "hysteria," but this has long since been discredited, a case of bad evidence producing bad conclusions [2]. The other was more pernicious. As he makes perfectly clear in his chapter in Schaler [1], young Thomas Szasz was a remarkably deceitful child. He pretended to be sick to get what he wanted and his anxiously indulgent mother fell for it every time:

> I intensely disliked going to elementary school ... I learned to malinger... I had a powerful motive to malinger ... I learned not only how to lie about feeling ill, but how to cough, how to vomit, and how to have a fever, by surreptitiously placing the thermometer close to a lighted light bulb. I was well aware of the difference between being ill and occupying the sick role... [1, p4].

As a result, he assumed everybody else is playing the same game, but generalising to the whole human population from research based on a series of one case (himself) is bad science and even worse philosophy.

We move on: Addictions, deviance and so on are just problems of living or moral problems and can be sorted out without invoking notions of "chemical imbalances of the brain." In fact, he was probably on fairly strong ground here but he didn't have an argument to support his view, just an opinion. Which leads to his next point, that psychiatrists who "treat" people with problems of addiction, deviance, compulsive behaviour and so on are part of a conspiracy, pulling nuisances of the streets and pretending they are ill just to keep themselves in a job. Again, close but not quite right. He was correct in saying that psychiatrists are party to a serious misrepresentation but it wasn't the one he thought it was. Psychiatrists put it around that they have models of mental disorder (see previous chapters) when in fact they don't [8].

On the issue of post-traumatic states, Szasz simply ignored the question. In the five books listed above, there are no references to concentration camp syndrome and only one to post-traumatic stress disorder, in Insanity: the idea [7], which reads: "PTSD, simulation of, 205-206." It refers to a convicted robber who claimed to have "Vietnam Stress Syndrome" when he had never served in Vietnam. In that book, however, there are seven references to "Factitious Illnesses," twenty to "Malingering" and twenty-two to "Imitation of Insanity." In Schaler's volume [1], there is a chapter entitled Bombing the Cradles: The Disordering Mental Effects of Off-the-Chart Life Experiences, by Margaret Hagen, which describes the effects of massive psychological trauma on children. This is a twenty page essay, well-written and supported by several dozen references. Szasz's considered reply was a dismissive and evasive page-and-a-half that essentially said "If you can't prove physical damage, then they don't have an illness. They may be spiritually crippled (his words) but that's not mental illness" [1, p276].

Similarly, while talking of treatment of "so-called war neurosis" in World War I, he stated "In this vignette, we can thus see war neurosis unconcealed as malingering..." [6, p95]. His opinion seems to be completely unsupported by any objective evidence but, as his dismissal of Hagen's view shows, he didn't need evidence to support him. He believed that anybody who wanted to could see he was right; people who didn't agree with him were either dupes or part of the conspiracy because, in his world, there were no other categories. You're either with Szasz or you're against him, but as Szasz is invariably right/incapable of being wrong, everybody who isn't on his side is wrong and should be silenced.

However, the bizarre point to all this is that Szasz need not have made this hostile and irrefutable claim. He could have said something like: "These soldiers have a severe, permanent disturbance to mental life, call it spiritual crippling if you will, but they don't have brain damage so there is no mental *illness* present." Problem solved, but he couldn't bring himself to say it because he had already said that there are only three categories: problems of living, or moral problems, or malingering. If the stressor has been removed (the war ended, the soldier was discharged), then, by Szasz's estimate, he should have got better. Of course, as the appalling history of World War I showed, they didn't get better. Oh well, says Szasz, that just proves they *didn't want to get better,* they wanted a pension for nothing. Perhaps it was proof for Szasz, but not for any decent human being.

When it comes to treatment we see his ideological bias shining through the clouds of obfuscation: patients have to pay out of their own pockets. They can't even have the foresight to have insurance to cover their costs (throughout his career, Szasz's medical insurance was paid by the university). This is pure ideology, unsupported by any conceivable argument, and, to my mind, exposes him as part of the heartless and repressive consumerist society. Szasz was what is called a libertarian, which translates as "Every man for himself, the devil take the hindmost because that's what they deserve." It's possible that one could make a case that the problems of the wealthy (Szasz came from a wealthy background and was wealthy in his own right), the problems of wealth are minor issues of self-indulgence seasoned by a few problems of life ("Husband has run off, has he? Sue him for his back teeth and find another one") but the poor are in a different boat. Even if their problems are moral and social, they can't sort them out themselves otherwise they would do so. They don't need globe-trotting professors to tell them to get a grip; their answer is there is nothing left to grip:

> "Sue him, doctor? You don't understand, I have children to support. I can't work because my ex-husband broke my elbow. I can't pay the rent or the school fees or my medical bills, so where will I find money for lawyers?"

> "Suck it up lady, you can't fight reality. Suicide? Sure, if that's what you want, go ahead. Next please."

In simple terms (and I've set the argument out in more detail in [2]), Szasz's "autonomous psychotherapy" was just a licence to shift responsibility onto the unfortunate and then charge them heavily for "help" in getting out of the mess. In other words, it authorised psychiatrists to be even more heartless than they already are. Was Thomas Szasz heartless? He made it perfectly clear that he studied medicine and then psychiatry not from any wish to help people, because he didn't believe they needed help, but to understand them. But I don't think he understood anything. All he did was try to generalise his own peculiar personality into a general philosophy of mind and then justify punishing people who didn't measure up to his standards. What were his standards? They were the standards of a self-centred person who had had everything served up on a plate.

I don't believe Thomas Szasz made a real or lasting contribution to psychiatry or to the relentlessly miserable lot of the mentally-disturbed. By coincidence, another Jewish Hungarian refugee from the Nazis set out the case against libertarianism. Economic historian and social philosophyer Karl Polanyi (1886-1964) came from a similar background in Budapest. However, he concluded that the free market so avidly embraced by Szasz could only result in destruction of the natural environment and all that we hold important, everything that separates human society from an ant colony. In his carefully argued and documented treatise, The Great Transformation (1944) [9], Polanyi sets out the brutal and inevitable consequences of a radical free market.

By his many, historically inaccurate and one-sided polemics, Thomas Szasz shows exactly what happens when the free market is applied to mental distress: the heartless destruction of all that we hold important, of everything that separates human society from an ant colony.

6.4. Conclusion: moving beyond Szasz.

Putting this aside, what effect did Thomas Szasz have on mainstream psychiatry? Again, that's a separate topic but at the time, he provoked initial astonishment followed rapidly by intense hostility. He gave psychiatrists another excuse to circle the wagons and shoot at critics. As a group, psychiatrists are offensively defensive, they react badly to criticism and quickly start attacking the messenger. As individuals, they are easily reduced to resentful muttering by any questions targeting their lack of intellectual grounding. As I know too well, during the 1970s and '80s, merely mentioning Szasz's name during a meeting or lecture provoked such aggression that they sometimes had to be abandoned. By the late 1980s, he wasn't mentioned. The consensus was that Szasz was a destructive and publicity-hungry narcissist who had nothing interesting or constructive to say about psychiatry. For a critic, that's the kiss of death.

Is there any mileage in the notion that mental disorder is "just" persecution, or deprivation, or misunderstanding, etc? For anybody who holds to a rigid biological determinism of mental disorder, the answer is an emphatic No. If mental disorder is genetically determined, then life experiences are irrelevant. Fortunately, there would be very few people so sure of themselves as to deny the obvious: perfectly ordinary, healthy, educated and well-adjusted people can be turned into life-long nervous wrecks purely as a result of psychological stressors. Most biological psychiatrists would accept that adverse life events can have an adverse effect on the mental state. The problem for them is to explain how this comes about, for which a resolution of the mind-body problem is an essential first step. However, they sidestep the problem with the smug rejoinder: "Well, regardless how it came about, it's all biological now so take your tablets and come back in a month."

Objectively, of course, there is overwhelming evidence to show that adverse life experiences in childhood and as adults are associated with poor mental outcomes in the short and long term; if genetics has any part to play, it's trifling [10]. All that is missing is a model to show how mental damage is effected, and a willingness among influential psychiatrists to take the matter seriously. Szasz appeared aware of this but didn't elaborate on it. As high priest of the "antipsychiatry" movement, he took psychiatry's lack of a model as irrefutable proof that all people complaining of mental symptoms are malingering, otherwise known as "blaming the victim." However, we have to take him at face value: Can it be said that all mentally-disturbed people are frauds who must be exposed? Yes, but only in the sense that it can be said witches exist and must be tortured to death and their vile bodies burned.

References

1. Schaler, JA (2004) *Szasz Under Fire: The Psychiatric Abolitionist Faces His Critics*. Chicago: Open Court.

2. McLaren N (2012). *The Mind-Body Problem Explained: The Biocognitive Model for Psychiatry*. Ann Arbor, MI: Future Psychiatry Press.

3. Szasz, T.S. (1961). *The Myth of Mental Illness: Foundations of a Theory of Personal Conduct*. Revised Edition. New York: Harper and Row (Perennial Library). Page numbers refer to the revised edition (1974).

4. Szasz, T.S. (1970). *The Manufacture of Madness: a Comparative Study of the Inquisition and the Mental Health Movement*. New York: Harper and Row (Harper Colophon Books). Page numbers refer to the reprint, 1977)

5. Szasz, T.S. (1977). *The Theology of Medicine: the Political-Philosophical Foundations of Medical Ethics*. Baton Rouge: Louisiana State University Press.

6. Szasz, T.S. (1979), *The Myth of Psychotherapy*. New York: Anchor Press/Doubleday.

7. Szasz, T.S. (1987). *Insanity: the Idea and its Consequences*. New York: Wiley.

8. McLaren N (2013). Psychiatry as Ideology. *Ethical Human Psychology and Psychiatry* 15: 7-18.

9. Polanyi K (1944). *The Great Transformation: The political and economic origins of our time*. Boston: Beacon Press.

10. Joseph J (2006). *The Missing Gene: Psychiatry, heredity, and the fruitless search for genes*. New York: Algora Publishing.

Part II:
Philosophical contributions.

7 # Chomsky's cognitive model:
decline and fall

IT IS THE RESPONSIBILITY of intellectuals to speak the truth and to expose lies.

Noam Chomsky, 1967.

7.1. Why linguistics?

The American linguist, philosopher and public intellectual, Noam Chomsky (b.1928), has often been acclaimed as one of the most influential thinkers of the past century. He is a singularly prolific author, with something like 150 books to his credit, as well as innumerable scientific and philosophical papers, articles, critiques, commentaries, videos and lectures. Even today, aged 95, he still gives regular lengthy interviews. As an author, he has been central to what has been called the cognitive revolution, the movement to analyse and understand human mental function in rational terms, but he has not contributed to our understanding of the irrational, either mental disorder or violence [3].

His work as a linguist established his credentials as an original thinker, particularly his 1957 text, *Syntactic Structures*, and his 1959 critique of *Verbal Behavior* (1957) by the behaviorist Burrhus Skinner (1904-1990; see Chap. 4). His critique is a small masterpiece, lucid and precisely on target. It signalled the beginning of the end of behaviorism in general and Skinner's model of operant conditioning in particular. While over the past thirty years or so there has been increasing criticism of Chomsky's cognitive mode, it continues to exert an influence in the theory of language, especially formal languages such as

---

3   Chomsky's supporters will object to my saying he has not made a significant contribution to our understanding of violence. "He talks about it all the time," they will say. Yes, he does, but he doesn't explain it.

programming languages, automata theory and other somewhat arcane disciplines.

His political work looks critically at totalitarianism and its roots in different societies. He is mainly concerned with US, Western and Israeli policies, particularly what he sees as their rapacious, race-based capitalism, but not so much with other regimes such as USSR/Russia, China, North Korea or Cambodia, not least because they aren't listening anyway. Over the last half century, he has used his background in linguistics to argue forcefully that Western countries are pursuing a brutal policy of domination of any and all countries for the purpose of using them as sources of wealth and power for themselves. Regardless of whatever governments tell their populations, anybody can look beneath the surface of their propaganda to see the real truth of their actions. At times, this has put him at risk, e.g. when he was put on Richard Nixon's list of enemies. However, it has never discouraged him and he remains a major figure, beatified by the left and reviled by the right.

Readers may wonder why a politically-minded linguist is included in a work on psychiatric theories, particularly as he doesn't talk about mental disorder. Language is, of course, of central importance in the concept of mind and thence of mental disorder and its treatment, but I will argue that Chomsky's approach to mind demonstrates a particular and widespread conceptual error. Any project to assemble a working model of mind which shows the same fault cannot be completed. Nonetheless, the error is ideological and is thus readily avoidable.

Now I appreciate that a psychiatrist opening a section on philosophy of mind with frank *lèse-majesté* is inviting scorn so a few digressions will be necessary to establish the case. I don't intend to review Chomsky's vast output; only the most committed devotees would try that but it isn't necessary. We will look at two influential volumes, *New Horizons in the Study of Language and Mind* [1], a collection of essays from 2000, and *Why Only Us. Language and Evolution* [2] from 2016, coauthored with his long-term colleague, Robert Berwick. *New Horizons* was published to the most effusive accolades. Gilbert Harman of Princeton University said "These essays represent the most significant work that has been done in the general area of philosophy of language and philosophy of mind." The latter work comes near the end of his career and should stand as a definitive statement. They set a fairly high bar so I will take time to develop my case.

7.2. Chomsky's position.

Today, when talk of a mental life is so often equated with the supernatural, authors and researchers often go to great lengths to show they are not contaminated by "wrong thinking." Hence the many attempts at non-mentalist theories of the mind over the past century, but the questions Descartes tried to answer nearly 400 years ago haven't gone away. I know from firsthand experience that there is something going on in my head that seems to be significant, so every attempt to explain human behaviour without taking it into account uses only half the available data. I decide to correct a word in this script and my hand reaches for the mouse. That isn't coincidence. I look outside to see the clear blue of the sparkling winter sky yet there is nothing blue in my head. In some crucial but so-far-undefined sense, these things are real.

At first glance, if the research program starts with a blanket refusal to admit the reality of mental events, it seems impossible to assemble a plausible theory of human mental life. It would be a bit like trying to explain human reproduction and population growth without ever mentioning sex, or writing about capitalism without mentioning greed[4]. And this is the basis of the error that I claim is pervasive in modern western thought: that we all want to talk about the mind and make sense of it, but we don't want to admit it exists in the form Descartes recognised: insubstantial, unlocalised and yet causally-effective. Under positivism's stern gaze, every sensible person agrees that minds are indistinguishable from souls, spirits and so on, crude magical wrong-thinking that we abandoned a hundred years ago. Therefore, in order to tame the mind, modern authors have to wrestle reality into bold new shapes. The quickest and easiest way of doing this is simply to amputate half the mind, to leave it out of any discussion.

These days, people say "All this talk of mental events doesn't meet our standards of scientific purity." Possibly so, and there's always the option of changing the concept of science but, for people who were suckled on the notion that mentality and mysticism are one and the same primitive thing, that's too threatening. So they press on, trying to account for human behaviour while leaving out the bit that seems to do a very large part of the work, the mental life. In the rest of this chapter, I will show that this is exactly what happened to Chomsky's program.

Without much trouble, we can extract Chomsky's basic position

---

4   In his acclaimed work, *The Road to Serfdom*, Friedrich Hayek managed this astounding feat.

regarding his field of study, language. In what follows, all emphasis is in the original. Where a quote includes a quote, the primary source is shown in single quotes for clarity:

- 7.2.1: Language is exclusively a capacity of *Homo sapiens*. While other creatures can "communicate," none of them has anything like the linguistic capacity of human beings. At birth, all healthy modern humans have the same immanent capacity for language regardless of their origin or status.

- 7.2.2: Language emerged in a small group of *H sapiens* in southern Africa between 200,000 and 60,000 years ago, most likely about 80,000 years ago [2, pp50, 54, 66, 92, 149, 157, etc]: "Roughly 200,000 years ago... there were no languages" [2, p54] and "... there is no room in this picture for any precursors to language... " [2, p72].

- 7.2.3: Language arose in *H sapiens* alone due to a fortuitous genetic mutation "... presumably involving some slight rewiring of the brain..." [2, p67, 107] and quickly spread through the species. Since then, it has not evolved further [2, p92].

- 7.2.4: No healthy humans lose the skill of language because it is a genetically-determined biological "organ of the body" "... on a par with the visual or digestive or immune systems... a cognitive organ, like the systems of planning, interpretation, reflection..." etc. [2, p56]. This organ acquits the "faculty of language" as its "... basic character is an expression of the genes" [1, p4] and it thus qualifies as a natural object [1, p119]. As a biological function, language is, however, a "... curious mental organ..." [2, p57] because, as observed over 150 years ago by Alfred Wallace, co-discoverer of evolution by natural selection, there is no biological demand which can't be managed without it [2, p3].

- 7.2.5: Cognitive organs fall among "... those aspects of the world loosely 'termed mental' which *reduce somehow* to the (organic structure of the brain)" [2, p56; emphasis added].

- 7.2.6: "We can think of language as a mental organ, where the term *mental* simply refers to certain aspects of the world, to be studied in the same way as chemical, optical, electrical and other aspects..." [1, p106, 134; 2, p56]. His program "... undertakes to study a real object in the natural world—the brain, its states and its functions—and thus to move the study of the mind towards eventual integration with the biological sciences" [1, p6]. "… the study of language is again much like that of other organs" [1, p17], to be pursued by "naturalistic inquiry," meaning the principles and methods of the natural sciences. "That may leave untouched many other questions, but it remains to be shown these are real questions, not pseudo-questions…" [1, p45]. For example, "If 'cognitive science' is taken to be concerned with intentional attribution, it may turn out to be an interesting pursuit (as literature is), but it is unlikely to provide an explanatory theory or to be integrated into the natural sciences" [1, p23].

- 7.2.7: The goal of a "naturalistic approach to linguistic and mental aspects of the world … (is) eventual unification with the 'core' natural sciences: unification, not necessarily reduction" [1, p106; 2, p56]. "… no one should ask whether the study of linguistic expressions and their properties belongs to linguistics, psychology, or the brain sciences". He opposes "some form of dualism, an insistence that we must not treat the domain of the mental, or at least the linguistic, as we do other aspects of the world" [1, p140], a persistent "…dualism that … is prevalent and pernicious" [1, p78]. There is, however, "… a matrix of human actions, interests, and intent in respects that lie far outside the potential range of naturalistic inquiry," but they will probably fade away with the progress of natural science "… to whatever extent the 'mental'-'physical' distinction is intelligible" [1, p21]. Here, he states he has no theory or model of mental life because a *science* of linguistics, the mechanisms by which we acquire language and *how* we speak, doesn't involve itself with *what* we speak. He is both vague about and dismissive of " … mental aspects of the world."

So far, we have learned that language is a recent and uniquely human biological function, mediated by a part or parts of the brain we can study using the standard methodology of ordinary science. That will tell us everything interesting about language; if it doesn't tell us, it isn't worth knowing. Dualist talk, that there is something about language that laboratory science can't investigate, is silly and will eventually disappear as the scientific program expands. Although he freely uses terms like 'mind,' 'imagination,' 'idea,' 'thoughts,' 'meaning,' and so on, Chomsky doesn't resolve the nature and significance of these and other mental phenomena, but nor does he say there isn't such a thing as the mind. His program is correctly classed as eliminative materialism, i.e. the belief that with the progress of science, these questions will be shown to be mistaken or irrelevant. Compare this with the statement of positivism by Moritz Schlick (Chap. 1),

We are now in a position to specify the nature of his proposed language "organ" or "faculty."

- 7.2.8: The whole of the human capacity for language is the "faculty of language" which has a number of subsections. The internal part is the higher functions such as thought, planning, intention and so on, which are natural properties of the brain: "... brains provide the mechanisms of thought ... thought and language are properties of organised matter—in this case, mostly the brain..." [1, p113, 115; it is not clear why he said "mostly" the brain]. It exists at "... an abstract level, in terms of mentally-represented rule systems... all of this is standard natural science" [1, p56].

- 7.2.9: In the externalising side of language, we find there are two subsystems involved, the first being the receptive or auditory side of speech, and the other being the expressive part of the sensorimotor system by which speech is physically articulated. There are thus two "interfaces" involved, namely that between thought and language organ, and the other between language organ and the sensorimotor system (note that this is actually two systems, the sensory side and the motor side). Consistent with his critique of Skinner from nearly 65 years ago, Chomsky dismisses any hints of a behaviorist rejection of the role of thought. He devotes a large part of Chapter 3 in *New Horizons* to establishing this point. At the same time, he does not accept the dualist argument that systems of language are of a nature that "natural science" cannot investigate (see S.7.2.7 above, re "pernicious dualism").

- 7.2.10: He is not much concerned with thought, sensation and other higher mental processes which can be left to philosophers if they want it [1, p81-2] (see S7.6); the interaction of systems of the body is biological. What counts for him is what happens once these rather ephemeral mental processes reach the language organ. Once received, they must be translated into an ordered sequence of instructions to be delivered to the articulatory side of the sensorimotor system, a central role of the language organ.

- 7.2.11: Each child is born with a naive language organ in an "initial state" (this expression recurs throughout both texts) and acquires a spoken language by means of a "Language Acquisition Device" or LAD [1, p81]. This is " ... not about the mind, about psychological mechanisms" [1, p94]: "Inquiry into the initial state of the language faculty ... is an attempt to discover the 'principles or notions implanted in the mind' that are a 'direct gift' of nature, that is, our biological endowment ... the theory of the initial state is sometimes called 'Universal Grammar' (UG)..." [1, p81]. (LAD is not referenced in [2]).

- 7.2.12: By exposure to a very limited range of the possible sentences and constructions in the native tongue, each child gains the ability to generate and to understand an infinite range of grammatically-correct sentences. This is just because the language organ is perfectly adapted to its function. Part of it consists of features of the mind that "... enter into naturalistic inquiry; call them the 'science-forming faculty' (SFF). Equipped with SFF, people confront 'problem situations,' consisting of certain cognitive states (of belief, understanding, or misunderstanding) ... Like other biological systems ..." SFF can deal with some things (problems) but not with others (mysteries). Some questions, e.g. consciousness, may forever lie outside its scope and remain mysteries, suitable only for philosophers and novelists [1, p82-83].

- 7.2.13: Overall, language is a biological function; it is a mistake to believe its function is communication [2, p63]. "... (T)he overwhelming use of language is internal—for thought" [2, p64, 111] which "...suggest(s) that language evolved as an instrument of internal thought, with externalisation as a secondary process" [2, p74]. There is convincing evidence that the human vocal tract was capable of the full range of sounds of articulate speech for half a million years before there is any evidence of the emergence of speech as we know it (i.e. artwork, funeral rituals etc). The origin of language lies in a chance mutation that allowed pre-existing brain and somatic structures suddenly to come together and produce a remarkable property "... largely unique in the organic world" [2, p64].

- 7.2.14: It is legitimate science to posit unobservable forces or entities to explain observations and test results. For his proposed language organ, investigation of its nature and inner workings are matters of ordinary laboratory science. Granted, its workings are currently beyond our technology but rational enquiry within the framework of natural science is producing results where elimination (as in behaviorism) and armchair philosophising did not.

We can pause to note two points. First, his position has changed dramatically over the years, which makes it difficult to be clear on the details of his account of language acquisition and generation. This is legitimate; science grows and never stands still but, rather than growing, the complexity of his original transformational grammar has shrunk to a few operations [1, p13]. Confounding this, his recent publications are long on opinion and worryingly short on actual results. Like, next to none. The second point is that he says remarkably little about language perception. It hardly rates a mention in *New Horizons* and is not indexed in *Why Only Us*. Even though he insists language is *not* about communication, this is a bit shocking because, without an audience, there's no language. The unclear implication is that auditory perception is entirely biological, and the path from ear to imagination is simply the expressive path in reverse. We now look briefly at the core of his current position, named Minimalism, before summarising the matter.

- 7.2.15: The critical cognitive operations in the language faculty are the ability to associate one item with another, which he has named Merge, and another called Move: "The operation Merge takes two distinct objects X and Y and attaches Y to X. The operation Move takes a single object X and an object Y that is part of X and merges Y to X" [1, p13]. These operations largely or entirely replace the arcane rules and processes of the original versions of his generative/transformational grammar, dramatically simplifying the process of language generation. Note, however, that later in that section he conceded: "There is a fair amount of hand-waving [5] in this brief description" [1, p15].

- 7.2.16: The advantage of Merge is that "… narrowly focusing the phenotype in this way greatly eases the explanatory burden for evolutionary theory…" [2, p11]. "… the evolution of language will reduce to the emergence of Merge … the lexicon, the linkage to conceptual systems, and the mode of externalisation." Shortly, he warns: "Note that there is no room

---

5   For those who aren't familiar, "hand-waving" is a dismissive expression used to indicate that the relevant details aren't known, as in "He dismissed the questions with a wave of his hand."

in this picture for any precursors to language... no direct evidence for such 'protolanguages'..." [2, p71-2].

- 7.2.17: Merge "... may have arisen from something as straight-forward as a slight rewiring of the brain..." [2, p79] but the survival of this mutation in the gene population is problematic as "communicative needs" would not have produced sufficient selection pressure to produce such a complex system as language [2, p81]. He warns: "... any approach to the 'evolution of language' that focuses on communication... may be seriously misguided" [2, p84].

In summary, Chomsky's position is that language is essentially an internal and wholly biological function which, by our good luck, allows us (and only us) to communicate. He dismisses the notion that control of language can be located in the external environment (Skinner's model), arguing instead that the crucial elements are of a biological nature and are under genetic control. He expects that with progress in the various fields of science relating to language, it will be shown that language control reduces to a biological function. Any remaining "mentalist" factors will be of no significance beyond the ephemeral.

While grouped as a "language faculty," the performance elements of language separate functionally into internal and external systems. The internal factors are thoughts, which hardly concern scientists, and a "language organ," which takes thoughts, converts them into a set of instructions and despatches them to the motor centres of the brain. This organ is entirely a biological function, genetically-determined and preset to encompass any conceivable human language. In language perception, the process works in reverse.

In the rest of this chapter, I will show that Chomsky's scientific program is at once...

- 7.2.18: incomplete,

- 7.2.19: internally incoherent and ...

- 7.2.20: irrefutable, and thus ...

- 7.2.21: cannot ever reach its goal of an empirical, naturalistic account of the full richness and complexity of human language.

Worse still, by his singular insistence on the abrupt appearance of language about 80,000 years ago, effected by a single genetic mutation several hundred thousand years after early modern humans first appeared, he has distracted research and intellectual attention from the far more likely picture that language as communication is hardly unique to humans; that it appeared much earlier and slowly developed; that it is dualist in nature; that it is the primary means of human communication and persists by virtue of this fact; and that we need to give an account of mind before we can deal with how minds communicate. All of this depends on a single erroneous assumption resulting in a flawed program which, unfortunately, is widespread in those fields dealing with facets of mind.

7.3. *Caveat lector.* Let the reader beware.

The first point to mention is that, in contrast to his political writings, Chomsky's scientific/technical material is dense to the point of opacity, discursive, unfocussed and repetitious. He repeatedly drops hints, fails to expand on them then later acts as though they were established fact. The reader is constantly asking "Did I miss something? Where did he prove that?" As a result, I believe there will always be "spirited discussion" on what he actually meant, meaning people will tend to interpret his vast oeuvre to suit themselves. And that leads to another point to note: "scare quotes." Chomsky makes liberal use of this literary device, of introducing a contentious topic with this little warning as to how it should be taken. It is legitimate to bring the venacular into a technical work by means of quotation marks, as we read on page 1 of *New Horizons*:

> It is also worth remembering that lack of understanding of "mind/brain interaction" is not the only respect with which progress has been limited since the origin of the modern scientific revolutions.

The proper use of quote marks is to introduce a topic from lay usage then define it technically. However, the next time we see "mind/brain," a few lines down the page, it is naked, as though the entire concept has been fully explained. This particular pairing is sprinkled throughout both books but we are not provided with an explanation of what mind is, how it arises, how it interacts with the brain, if at all, and why they should be conjoined. The reader is covertly invited to understand that they are in some vital sense one and the same thing, and that any disputes over the meaning of the term have been resolved, even though that is most emphatically not the case. An uncommitted reader will reach the end of the volume and still not know what it means. Most readers, however, will either assume it has been defined and they didn't quite see it but they assume the error is theirs, or they will attach their own meaning to it and press on, comforted by the notion that the author agrees with them. So in this sense, what are commonly known as "scare quotes" are better characterised as "smuggler's quotes," they allow the author to smuggle something in that sounds impressive but carries hidden or unstated meanings. Daniel Dennett does this (see Chap. 8) but the worst offender was surely Thomas Szasz (Chap. 5). The reader either accepts the inferred content or puts the book back on the shelf.

Science begins with definition. Anybody writing on the concept of mind needs to state at the outset what the word means, just because everybody has a private meaning. It's like the concept of schizophrenia in American psychiatry. In the early 1960s, a study showed that while psychiatrists in major centres across the US were comfortable applying the diagnosis and talking about it at conferences or in their research and academic papers, there was less than 20% concordance among psychiatrists on what they actually meant. Speakers assumed that the audience agreed with them while members of the audience were thinking the speaker was using the word in the way they did. For decades, they were happily talking past each other. In the context of works on language and mind, the expression "mind/brain" has set the same trap. It is of critical importance to Chomsky's project yet it can't be defined and is thus meaningless: anybody who doesn't realise this will be led astray.

"Mind/brain" is a good example of what Dennett calls an "intuition pump" [6, p399-400]. This handy bit of jargon means that a first or superficial reading of a text leads to a conclusion which is not actually carried by its literal meaning. It "pumps" an intuitive meaning into the reader and is thus misleading. "Mind/brain" is not defined meaningfully just because it cannot be. It has become a shibboleth, identifying people who want to reduce the tricky bits of mind to brain, who need to believe that the hard philosophical work has been done and they can embrace the author's conclusions as their own. In the same way as the devout pore over their religious texts, mining them for hidden meaning, committed reductionists can comfortably divine widely differing pictures of Chomsky's work, which raises further serious questions as to its scientific nature.

7.4: The biology of language.

Chomsky's basic stance is clear: he is opposed to behaviorism in its various forms [1, p46-60], especially as his reputation as an innovative thinker was greatly enhanced by his acute critique of Skinner's 1957 500 page tome, *Verbal Behaviour*. In thirty pages, Chomsky took aim at Skinner's "scientific pretensions," concluding:

> If it were true in any deep sense that the basic processes in language are well-understood and free of species restrictions, it would be extremely odd that language is limited to man [7, p30]. ... if we take (Skinner's) terms in their literal meaning, the description covers almost no aspect of verbal behaviour, and if we take them metaphorically, the description offers no improvement over various traditional (folk) formulations [7, p54].

That is, Skinner's attempt to separate language from some sort of rule-governed internal processes was doomed to failure. Chomsky's "faculty of language" is his attempt to provide a natural rule-governed internal process. However, he is also firmly opposed to any suggestion that the critical elements of language are not firmly in the physicalist camp, as in S7.2.5 above:

> ... a cognitive organ ... falls among those aspects of the world loosely "termed mental" which reduce somehow to the "organical structure of the brain" ... We can think of language as a mental organ, where the term *mental* simply refers to certain aspects of the world, to be studied in the same way as chemical, optical, electrical, and other aspects, with the hope for eventual unification ... [2, p56].

The critical point in this claim is the loaded expression "reduce somehow." Reduce somehow. Let's think about that expression: What does it mean? What does he mean by "a cognitive organ"? What's cognition if not mental? What other mental aspects of the world are there hidden in his verbiage, and how can the mental be given a biological explanation? How do "thoughts" get from mind to the tongue (see S.7.3.9)? He glosses over these points but they are exactly, precisely the questions that drove Descartes to frustration. Chomsky gives no explanation of any of this because, of course, he doesn't have an explanation. What he offers instead is industrial grade promissory materialism with a forest of hands waving in the general direction of the hills where, one fine day, the scientific cavalry are expected to appear. Four centuries of scientific progress and all he can do is rehash Descartes' *Meditations*. The reader either accepts his assurances and reads on, or gives up, i.e. readers sort themselves into true believers in the Chomskyan miracle, and infidels.

Moving on, Chomsky defines a cognitive organ as a biological system of the body but the immediate objection is that an organ is not a system. An organ is a discrete collection of tissue performing a particular function. The lung is an organ; the respiratory system is everything that works with the lung to allow respiration but it is a *system*, not an organ *per se*. The eye is an organ; the visual *system* is not. The thymus is an organ; the immune *system* is not. Each muscle, each bone or each nerve is an organ, the musculo-skeletal *system* is not. It is not clear why his editors allowed this howler through. What he has done is take a collection of largely unknown and unlocalised brain functions, lump them together with an unspecified range of rule-based mental abilities and deem the resultant jumble a biological unity amenable to routine scientific investigation. This is apparently based in the intuition that thoughts are fluffy but rules are hard; therefore if it is rule-based, it must be biological. This led him to postulate a large number of rules of formation of language, akin to the way, in the 1930s and 40s, Clark L Hull tried to reduce psychology to psychobiological rules. Hull's idiosyncratic and mechanistic psychology died with him [8, p145] (see S.7.7).

As Chomsky reveals at numerous points in these texts, his 26 "highly detailed rules for a fragment of English" [2, p6] have been drastically modified and reduced over the years, leaving only two "operations," Merge and Move, described in Ss.7.3.15-17 above. The main impetus behind this regular pruning has been the steadily accumulating evidence that all the major proposals in his innate grammar have been falsified empirically [e.g. 9, 10]. His original work tried to incorporate all rules relating to language production. As associationism rewritten as biology, the latest version, known as the Minimalist Program [2, p94] will have to be final because there's nothing left to discard. However, when we look for the details of the biology he relies on, perhaps something to match the spectacular advances in immunology or in genomics, there aren't any. There is nothing to indicate where this linguistic activity takes place, how it is implemented, how it is switched on or off, etc. That is, all the Minimalist Program does is take two apparently cognitive (i.e. mental) operations and relabel them as biological, accompanied by what, even by academic standards, amounts to a degree of hand-waving more suited to a North Korean parade saluting the Dear Leader. At what must be the terminal stage of his career, Chomsky's remnant program to explain language in *biological* terms has been pared down to just a pious hope.[6]

At this point, we can step back a little and ask: "What does folk

---

6   I use the term "pious" advisedly, as "a hope held on faith by a true believer."

psychology have to say about language?" I suggest the proverbial woman in the local shops would say something like "Well, it starts with what you want to say in your mind. Then there's what you've learned at home and at school about how to talk, like grammar and so on, and if you've got a healthy brain—and your tongue and teeth, of course— then somehow it all comes together." That is, folk psychology sees two elements, the mental plan, consisting of current intentions and learned material, and the physical machinery by which the wish is implemented. Immediately, there remains the problem of how the mental plan gets across to the biological machinery for it to effect the intent to speak, aka Descartes' 400 year old mind-body problem.

Now we see the point behind Chomsky's use of the conflated term, "mind/brain": it discards the mind-body problem as something for philosophers and novelists to amuse themselves with but nothing to bother real scientists. By fiat, the rules governing speech are biological while the effector sensorimotor "machinery" of the brain is also biological, albeit "… not part of the core faculty of human language" [2, p79], as he explains:

> We can now… carve the difficult evolutionary problem of "language" into three parts…:
>
> (1) an internal computational system that builds hierarchically structured expressions with systematic interpretations at the interfaces with two other internal systems, namely…
>
> (2) a sensorimotor system for externalisation as production or parsing and …
>
> (3) a conceptual system for inference, interpretations, planning , and the organisation of action—what is informally called "thought" [2, p11].

His interest lies in the genetically-determined "internal computational system," which is why he placed it first; as the smuggler's quotes in pt (3) indicate, "thought" lies outside the realm of natural science, fit only for poets and the odd philosopher. The sensorimotor system isn't "core" and can be left to the physiologists, allowing linguists to race ahead with analysing the rules of language. However, this ploy raises two questions, the problem of what he called the "interface" between mental elements and the language organ, and that between the language organ and the motor areas of the brain. In Chomsky's schema, the latter problem is, of course, artificial: both parts of the system are deemed to be biological so their interface is just a matter of neurophysiology. At the same time, the critical question of how rules are written into the brain's microstructure is nowhere addressed; in due course, neurophysiology will take care of that.

Meanwhile, the question of how "thoughts" jump the apparent barrier from the mental realm to the physical remains unresolved. By decree, Chomsky deems this not an issue for the natural sciences. He has nothing interesting to say on how "thoughts" can give rise to speech, nor about thoughts themselves. Thus, he leaves us at exactly the position in which Descartes found himself: Plus ça change, plus c'est la même chose, except the Frenchman made an honest effort to resolve the quandary. Applying his extensive empirical knowledge of neuro-anatomy within the mechanistic ontological framework of the day, Descartes offered an interesting but ultimately unsuccessful resolution of the mind-body problem.

So what is the "single erroneous assumption resulting in a flawed program ... in those fields dealing with facets of mind"? (see end of S.7.3). It is the same as drove Skinner into a dead-end: the wholly spurious positivist notion that dualism means magic. Anybody following the positivist program must write mind out of the equation; conversely, we know immediately that anybody who tries to assemble a non-mentalist account of mental functions already believes that mentalism = dualism = magic. But that is an ideological position, not scientific, so what seems to be a scientific argument will always be shown to be specious.

Anybody who wants to explain the mind has to start somewhere, and the obvious starting point is the immediate experience of something happening in the head, the seeing, hearing, feeling, tasting, laughing, hurting, regretting, planning, plotting and forgetting that goes on and on between waking and dozing off. We can either accept that as the raw given of mental life and proceed forward, as Chomsky does, or turn and try to explain all that noise between the ears. But, and this is a very big BUT, the explanation must not involve magic. THEREFORE, all the messy bits, like sensation and emotion, are EITHER amputated, as Chomsky does, OR simply moved across into the biological basket so that there is none of this nonsense about a "mind-body problem," thank you. We will see this play out repeatedly in the remaining chapters, but meantime, back to Bro. Chomsky.

7.5. Evolution of language.

For Chomsky, language is part of the human biological heritage so, as biology, it must be explicable in evolutionary terms. Axiomatically, if the behaviour or feature exists, it must confer an advantage on the species, or at least no disadvantage. He mentions the conundrum first put forward by Alfred Wallace, who independently developed the theory of evolution by natural selection, who " ... could perceive no biological function (of language) that could not already be met by a species without language " [2, p3]. As mentioned above, Chomsky is convinced language is a very recent development. For millions of years, he believes, the various species of Homo did not have language, then suddenly and very recently, H sapiens did, and the rest is history. This ability arose from a minor genetic mutation which somehow changed human neurology, allowing the explosive flowering of language as we know it, with no changes since. This view is widespread: Daniel Dennett speaks of Neanderthal language as "caveman grunts and howls" [11, p264].

Chomsky proposes that a minor mutation allowed the brain to implement the operation of associating one entity with another, which he calls Merge. He goes to considerable lengths in Why Only Us to show that minor genomic mutations with dramatic phenotypic effects are well-known in nature. That is, he is conceding that there is no actual "language organ" because the entire system of language did not spring into being overnight (meaning with the birth of a particularly fecund child). This makes perfect sense: teeth existed long before protohumans were able to speak, and ears, and mouths and so on, and they exist on lots of animals that don't speak to us. We can only assume he is opting for the moderate emergent position that...

> **Practically the whole of the language apparatus existed in its modern form before humans could speak in complex sentences; a tiny mutation provided a "key" that allowed the whole to function as a linguistic system.**

The importance of this view, which I believe is heading in the right direction, cannot be understated. It suggests language is the fortuitous outcome of a minor change which bridged, as it were, a number of other features and functions with established survival value. It says that human language is a free lunch that conferred enormous benefits on the lucky few.

As an example, consider swimming. It is the case that humans, like practically all terrestrial animals, can swim (elephants, rats and snakes are all good swimmers, much better than we are). In the case of humans, we are able to swim because we have a fairly long tubular body with a specific gravity of about 0.98 and paddles on each corner of the trunk. If our SG were even 1.01 (say from heavier bones), we would have great difficulty swimming. Despite this ability, we do not have a swimming faculty or swimming organ. Similarly, it would be foolish to talk about the "evolution of swimming." Nobody would argue that it is essential for survival or represents a breeding advantage. While practically all Australian- and New Zealand-born children can swim, it was (possibly still is) the case that most English-born children could not. Apart from the generally superior stock of Antipodean children, there is no genetic basis to this. Swimming did not arise as a result of a single minor mutation a short while ago. The parameters were always there, all that was needed to activate them was a pool of water with fish swimming around, a long stick and a hungry Neanderthal creeping over slippery rocks.

The same goes for dancing, although there probably is a genetic basis for our sense of rhythm and timing. Sport is also very much part of human behaviour but, apart from the competitive urge, there is no genetic basis to it. As for evolution of a "sporting faculty," some would argue that modern sports are evidence that evolution can run backwards. Similarly, all higher animals play to some extent or other just because the options are available. It is like people dyeing their hair blue. Hair exists; blue dye exists; somebody, somewhere, will put the two together without there being a genetic basis for a "blue hair organ."

It would be facile to talk of a "swimming faculty" produced by a sudden mutation of motor function when the reality is that complex behaviors emerge when all the necessities are in place and a reason pops up. The same applies to mental functions: we should speak of the evolution of the whole cognitive capacity, of which language is an integral part, but not of the evolution of disparate elements of human cognitive ability. If anybody needs a memorable term for that, call it "stochastic evolution of complex behavioral performances" (I prefer not to).

In each case, the behaviour develops just because it can, not because it is suddenly enabled by a mutation. With language, which requires vastly more fine motor control and cerebral computational power than paddling around in a creek or kicking a ball, the prerequisites for speech as we know it are at least:

> small regular teeth (it is difficult to pronounce unvoiced TH around fangs);
>
> a highly mobile, pointed tongue;
>
> fine mobile lips which can be pursed;
>
> a mobile larynx with full motor control able to produce a wide range of distinct sounds;

an expansive motor system capable of minute control of the dozens of muscles involved;

a highly developed auditory system able to detect and discern sound at a wide range of frequencies and volumes;

a highly-developed auditory pattern-detecting apparatus coupled with a vocal pattern-generating apparatus;

capacious and rapidly responsive lexical memory coupled with sensory and motor memory systems (these are actually separate systems), and...

finely-coordinated sensory feedback which tells us precisely where each and every physical element is in space and what is happening to it (otherwise we would bite our lips and tongues all the time).

Manifestly, these did not all evolve in a single mating somewhere near the (modern) Blombos Cave in southern Africa about 80,000 years ago. Each and every part of the linguistic apparatus listed above was essentially intact half a million years before Chomsky's chosen date, which he does not dispute. What happened, he believes, is that a small and harmless mutation allowed all these elements to be united in a single, novel function whose spectacular evolutionary advantage lay not in communication but in allowing "internal thought." He suggests that the generative procedure which is the core of his "language organ" is the cognitive operation he calls Merge, and that this "... emerged suddenly as the result of a minor mutation" [2, p70] which led to "a slight rewiring of the brain" [2, p79].

In my view, the whole of this positivist fable is so unlikely (read: stupid) as not to be worth considering: the ability to associate X with Y is fundamental to the most rudimentary cognitive capacities in the animal world. As Charles Darwin demonstrated, even earthworms can do it. In order to see why, we need to consider two other elements essential to speech which are less developed in other animals and which appear to be under genetic control.

First, there is the minute respiratory control underlying prosody, the inherent natural rhymicity of speech. The breath has to be released slowly and irregularly, otherwise words sound strange and the speaker will run out of breath in the middle of a sentence: try saying "He hit his head hard on the hefty haft of his hired hoe" while exhaling in a steady stream. Impossible.[7] If you can't control exhalation, you will never be able to speak fluently. Impairment of this particular function is seen in cerebellar damage and in the group of conditions known as cerebral palsy, in which intellectual function is generally preserved but motor control is seriously affected. It is feasible that this level of motor control arose quite recently and allowed the rapid expansion of what had previously been restricted speech (but vastly more than grunts and howls). However, the cheerfully raucous calls of kookaburras, which are common in my area, also demonstrate remarkable breath control, as do many other animals such as gibbons, so this is probably not a candidate.

The second possibility is the capacity to mimic sounds. Children who are just learning to speak can copy vowel sounds and most consonants with little or even a single exposure. They quickly learn to say "mama" and "dada" and can generally copy the salient words in an utterance with ease. They may use the word incorrectly but they can copy it and, without the ability to mimic, without the hard-wired connection between the brainstem auditory processors and the fine cerebellar control of the vocal musculature (which are physically close and closely related anyway), there will never be speech.

Either of these possibilities is far more likely than some undefined, undefinable notion like a single cognitive operation reduced to a brain structure. Do I think either of these possibilities is likely? I do not. My view is that the notion that early modern humans and our close hominin relatives couldn't speak beyond "grunts and howls" is akin to the European attitude that, for example, Australian Aboriginal people weren't really human because they didn't have imposing buildings for worshipping gods or kings, or written language, or cultivated farmland, or elegantly-gowned courtiers and so on, and could thus be pushed to extinction without transgressing the Fifth Commandment (not that Europeans have ever taken the slightest notice of that). The implication that Neanderthals couldn't think or communicate better than chimps is latter-day racism with a pseudoscientific gloss [9, 10]. Moreover, there is recent, firm palaentological evidence against Chomsky's peculiar views (see Chap. 16).

As an aside, and overlooking the small point that there is no such thing as "external thought," Chomsky's proposal that language arose as an aid to "internal thought" (S7.2.13) leads to a range of problems. First, the suggestion is irrefutable, not as technology but as

---

7   Australians have mastered it: "'E 'it 'is 'ead 'ard on the 'efty 'aft of 'is 'oired 'oe."

metaphysics. Second, if perchance that's what happened, and by some bizarre stroke of luck, everybody in the tribe developed the same inner language (it's private so why should they?), anybody who believes it must begin by explaining thought, the very feature that language arose to assist. Chomsky makes no attempt. Third, if there is "internal language," then it must have some generative mechanism and a medium for its implementation, but what are they but mind itself? And something must listen to these thoughts, so now we have mind split three ways in an infinite regress, which is not an improvement.

Explaining thought first requires an explanation of mind and of mind-body interaction, whereas the whole thrust of Chomsky's work has been to redefine language as biological/non-mental, in order to escape the "siren song of dualism" and its immanent mind-body problem. If you only talk about the mind/body, as Chomsky does, then you don't need to address the mind-body problem. But the entire concept of thought as symbol manipulation is dualist, and necessarily precedes language (children can think before they can talk), so his project has been self-defeating. Finally, if language developed for thought and not for communication, that would leave only gesture for those unfortunates who, born before the general rewiring of the brain 80,000 years ago, wished to tell each other "Save a bit of the mammoth for me." But that's communication which, as Chomsky often indicates, is not a function of language except for one crucial but widely-overlooked point: If language arose as a minor mutation in one person, that mutation has spread in 80,000 years or 3,000 generations to 8billion people with no trace of the former genome, which suggests it is highly advantageous. I say that's impossible but even if it did occur, the only conceivable advantage would be communication.

The least-problematic explanation of language is that it *created* a niche that allows each of us to communicate our mental states to our neighbours, and thus to understand each other. Language allows the audience to recreate in the privacy of their minds a facsimile of part of the speaker's mental state, of the speaker's intent. From this, they can coordinate their activities, share jokes or continue arguments, and so on. But such an explanation will never occur to theorists who scorn mentalism or, if it does, they will immediately blot it out as heretical to the paradigm. But it occurred to me when, decades ago, I first heard Chomsky's suggestion because I don't think in words and never have. I think in impressions and images, coupled in vague and amorphous relationships which I may struggle to define. If I can't verbalise what is on my mind, as happens in writing a text like this, I speak aloud what I want to say and then copy it. But the images *precede* and generally don't *need* speech. And on the occasions I actually do have mental speech rattling around in my head, it never has anything to do with what I'm doing, which annoys my wife.

I don't believe that people "think in words" because we think very much faster than mere words. I don't issue inner instructions to myself: "Reach for cup with right hand, place index finger through handle, steady cup with other fingers, raise cup 42.4cm and 48° to lips, open mouth 6mm and purse lips, inhale slightly to test temperature of beverage..." If I'm looking for something and come across it, I don't say aloud "Aha, there it is," nor do I "say" in mental speech "Aha, there it is." If I can say or "say" that, I already know where it is and don't need a reminder. In daily life, nobody uses internal speech except as an exception. The mere existence of the expression "internal speech" reminds us that there is a great deal of mental activity that isn't in the form of speech. Hunter-gatherers, as were *H erectus, H naledi* and *H neandertalis* (and *H sapiens* until just recently), most certainly don't waste time on internal chatter otherwise they would have been the hunted and the gathered. The suggestion that "... language evolved as an instrument of internal thought, with externalisation as a secondary process" [2, p74] is patently absurd.

Since plenty of humans actually do think in images, the corollary is that animals also think, which goes back at least to David Hume's *Treatise of Human Nature* (1740), in which he argued that "beasts are endowed with thought and reason as well as men." There is no remotely interesting case to suggest they aren't.

That still leaves two important questions about the evolution of speech. First: Why is it so important to talk about evolution of speech? We don't talk about evolution of sport or entertainment, or even of warfare (which we should but don't, but see [13]). The answer is that for people who want to believe that language is biological, it follows that they must show that, like all things biological, language follows the laws of evolution. If it doesn't, then it's probably not biological, meaning it would have to be emergent and thus dualist, which is anathema. *Hysteron proteron*: the conclusion precedes and determines the argument.

The second is: Why did it survive? What was the survival advantage? For all the possibilities Chomsky listed [2, p80-81], like winning suitors, coordinating hunting, improving tool-making or for telling better jokes or lies, it seems to me he has missed the most obvious: language created its *own* survival value by allowing humans to indulge more creatively and effectively in their favourite hobby, slaughtering their neighbours. Language dovetailed neatly with our insatiable urge to be dominant at all times, by any means and for no reason other than dominance itself [12, Ch. 9; 13; 14, p250-254]. That is, the emergence of complex language drastically altered the evolutionary calculus, toward the group that could plan and coordinate stealthy attacks on its somewhat less-gifted neighbours. This may help explain why Neanderthals and perhaps *H floriensis* and others didn't long survive contact with modern humans although, hidden in the victorious *sapiens'* genomes, their genes did.

7.6. Language as an emergent phenomenon.

Set out this way, these are fairly elementary oversights and they require some explanation. In S7.1, I suggested Chomsky's program suffers from a widespread error but it is cultural, a matter of ideology, not of formal science. Behaviorist psychology, both Pavlovian and Skinnerian, was born in and part of positivism's early, aggressively anti-mentalist phase (we're still stuck in it, of course). In particular, Skinner's operant conditioning, outlined in S4.3, was devoid of any hint of internal control of the "organism's" behaviour. The very language he used, such as organism for humans (which Chomsky does occasionally) meant there was nothing separating *H sapiens* from all other animals. Our vaunted "minds," Skinner insisted, had no role to play in our conduct.

But Skinner wasn't playing to the gallery, he was part of the positivist movement in what are now known as human sciences trying to write the dualist mind/soul/spirit out of the equation. As described in Chap. 1, positivist science is only about observables; the mind is in principle unobservable; therefore the mind is not science. For 20th Century scientists, the entire concept of mind was an abomination. This ethos was very powerful and, coupled with the normal adolescent urge to overthrow one's teachers, it meant that anything mental or spiritual had to be exorcised. Starting in 1945, aged just 16yrs, Chomsky's tertiary education took place in this "brave new world" atmosphere.

In trying to write the mind out of the human equation, Chomsky the linguist didn't go as far as Skinner the behaviourist. As described, Skinner tried to locate the controlling element in human behaviour in the environment; the brain was simply the physical switching device that took its instructions from the surroundings and sent them to the different organs to be implemented. It was all very mechanical but it was doomed, and Chomsky exacted great pleasure in despatching Skinnerian psychology to the history books. But if the locus of control of language didn't reside outside the individual, where was it? It couldn't be in "The Mind," because every young rationalist of the day knew the concept was puerile magical thinking.

Thus, Chomsky split his concept of mind in two. Half of it he deemed "thoughts" and thus non-scientific, fit only for philosophers, novelists, poets and other fabulists, while the rest, the rules-based part (the "easy problem of consciousness," see Chap. 10) is biological and therefore a legitimate subject for scientists to study in the laboratory. This part he tried to shoehorn into a computational approach but its first iteration became a case study of rules gone mad [2, p6], of rules strangling themselves in their complexity. Since then, he has "carved" his idea (his expression) to the point where there are only two operations, Merge and Move, even though at a functional level (see S.7.2.15) theirs is a distinction without a difference. And still it goes nowhere. The reason is self-evident, as he explicitly states of his remnant program:

> ... the evolution of language will reduce to the emergence of Merge, the evolution of conceptual atoms of the lexicon, the linkage to conceptual systems, and the mode of externalisation. Any residue of principles of language not reducible to Merge and optimal computation will have to be accounted for by some other evolutionary process—one that we are unlikely to learn much about ... [2, p71-72].

I submit this amounts to nothing more than:

> "The evolution of language will reduce to the evolution of language except for the mentalist bits we can't understand."

That is, seventy years of academic effort has explained exactly nothing. His program depends totally on the concept of emergence, which Chomsky has not specified, leaving himself open to allegations that he is using it as *deus ex machina*, a free pass allowing him to claim the benefits while avoiding the hard work of showing how all this originates and how it fits together. Philosopher Paul Humphreys proposed six *characteristics of emergence [15]*:

> 1. Novelty: "A previously uninstantiated property comes to have an instance."

> 2. Qualitative difference: "Emergent properties (are) qualitatively different from the properties from which they emerge."

> 3. Absence at lower levels: "An emergent property is one that could not be possessed at a lower level—it is logically or nomologically impossible for this to occur."

4. Law difference: "Different laws apply to emergent features than to the features from which they emerge."

5. Interactivity: "Emergent properties... result from an essential interaction between their constituent properties."

6. Holism: "Emergent properties are holistic in the sense of being properties of the entire system rather than local properties of its constituents."

More recently, after detailed explication, Humphreys has proposed that just four criteria capture the essence of emergentism: emergence is relational (i.e. emergent entities must result from something else); and it shows novelty, autonomy and holism [16]. My view is that his Pt (4) above, Law Difference, is critical because an emergent phenonomen does not follow the laws of the system that generated it. I prefer to include it, even if it serves only as a reminder that *emergent phenomena are not physical phenomena.* We do not call the eggs that emerge from chickens emergent phenomena.

And it is on this point that Chomsky's attempt to assemble a non-mentalist account of language sunders: as he himself admits at a thousand points, language *just is* emergent. It arises from the entire body and functions according to rules or laws which are *not* those of the physical systems that generated it:

> The rules and laws of syntax which govern language are not related at any conceptual points to the rules and laws governing physical neuronal function.

Language, *as Chomsky understands it,* is the very exemplar of the dualist notion, that there are "two incommensurable orders of being" to the human experience, the physical and the irreducibly non-physical. Moreover, he quotes Brentano who said "intentionality won't be reduced and won't go away" [1, p22] (intensionality, as it is usually spelled, relates to the directedness of mental contents, that they are *about* something). As noted in S7.2.6 above, he commented:

> If 'cognitive science' is taken to be concerned with intentional attribution, it may turn out to be an interesting pursuit (as literature is), but it is unlikely to provide an explanatory theory or to be integrated into the natural sciences [1, p23].

That is to say, "If our science can't account for the directedness of mental states, we will simply declare them out of bounds and leave them to poets and dreamers. We will not talk about meaning, only the vehicles that carry it." Nonetheless, by invoking *the criteria of emergence*, he has admitted that the non-physical just won't go away. It isn't possible to build a monist model of mind simply by verbally excluding dualism: an antidualist model is always incomplete. At the end of the day, the reductionists surreptitiously leave the door open for a spirit to jump in and drive their elegantly-contrived but mindless machine.

7.7. Conclusion: Whither antidualism?

In 1945, when Chomsky started university, behaviorist psychologist Clark L Hull (1884-1952) was at the peak of his career. Hull attempted to construct a non-mentalist "mathematico-deductive" model of behaviour which became increasingly idiosyncratic. He didn't formally dismiss the idea of consciousness, he just made it so difficult that nobody would attempt to bring it into a science of behaviour. For example, in his 1937 presidential address to the APA , he stated:

> The task of those who would have consciousness a central factor in adaptive behavior and in moral action is accordingly quite clear. They should apply themselves to the long and grinding labor of the logical derivation of a truly scientific system (quoted in [8, p110]).

This was more or less the end of the matter; most of his audience understood that it wouldn't happen. Even though a survey in 2002 rated Hull as the "21st most cited psychologist of the 20th century," his work quickly faded from view following his death. Burrhus Skinner, the frequent and deserving target of Chomsky's ire, tried to do better. His goal was explicit: by locating the controlling element in human behavior in the environment, he hoped to write a psychology with no mention of mind or consciousness. Skinner was hugely influential—his methods were widely applied and were even made into a film (Kubrick's *A Clockwork Orange*, 1971, from the novel by Anthony Burgess). The same survey rated him as the most influential psychologist of the century, yet his work has had little lasting impact. The same thing happened to the combative Hans Jurgen Eysenck, the German-born professor of psychology at London University's Institute of Psychiatry, who championed Pavlovian psychology. His enormous output and profound influence hardly survived his passing. By the ends of their respective careers, their work was largely kept alive by the influence of their personalities (none of them qualified as "retiring"), the numbers of their students holding key academic positions, and the potboilers they kept churning out.

In each of these cases, and there were many more, theorists had a major impact during their lifetimes but, following their demise, they soon slipped from professional and public attention until only history books refer to them. Why did this happen? I submit that, from the outset, their work was fatally flawed as it is not possible to write a non-mentalist account of human mental function. Why did they try? Because they were all infected by the doctrinaire antidualism expressed so forcefully by the first true behaviorist, John B Watson, and by the Vienna Circle of positivists. In his address to Columbia University in 1913, Watson denounced the idea of the mind-body problem and the dualism from which it arose. That theme echoed throughout the century, leading philosopher David Oderberg to complain that anybody who upheld a dualist account of human mentality was regarded as soft-headed, if not frankly loopy [17]. We will come back to this point in the remaining chapters of this book.

I propose that it is now well past time to say that dualist explanations of human behaviour should be given the most serious attention (and not just "equal time"). Anti-dualism has been promoted to the level of a cult and, as Chomsky's work shows convincingly, it has failed spectacularly. By trying to evade what Chalmers has called the "hard problem of consciousness," Chomsky ended up, not with a model of mind but with a model of half the mind, the mechanical and unexciting half. Even then, in the end, he had to call on dualism to save his model. I suggest his work will not long survive his passing and will eventually be seen as part of the death rattle of antidualism. However, we must not underestimate the tenacity of cultists: they never give up, which led Max Planck to opine:

> A new scientific truth does not triumph by convincing its opponents and making them see the light, but rather because its opponents eventually die, and a new generation grows up that is familiar with it (paraphrased to: Science progresses, one funeral at a time).

References

1. Chomsky N (2000). *New Horizons in the Study of Language and Mind*

2. Berwick RC, Chomsky N (2016). *Why Only US. Language and Evolution* (page references are to the MIT Press paperback edition of 2017).

3. Descartes R (1637) *A Discourse on the Method*. Trans. MacLean I (2006). Oxford: University Press.

4. Descartes R (1641) *Meditations on First Philosophy*. Revised Weinberg D (2007). Hawthorne, CA: BN Publishing.

5. Descartes R (1649). *The Passions of the Soul*. Published in English 1650, Unknown translator. Available online: TheVirtualLibrary.org.

6. Dennett DC 1991. *Consciousness Explained*. London: Penguin Books (1993).

7. Chomsky N (1959). Review of Skinner's 'Verbal Behavior.' *Language*, 35:26-58.

8. McKenzie BD. *Behaviourism and the Limits of Scientific Method*. London: RKP, 1977.

9. Evans, V. (2014). *The Language Myth: Why language is not an instinct*. Cambridge: University Press.

10. Everett, D.L. (2017). *How Language Began: The story of humanity's greatest invention*. New York: Liveright/Norton.

11. Dennett DC (2017). *From Bacteria to Bach and Back: the evolution of minds*. London: Allen Lane. Page numbers refer to the Penguin edition (2018).

12. McLaren N (2021): *Natural Dualism and Mental Disorder: The biocognitive model for psychiatry*. London, Routledge.

13. McLaren N (2023). *Narcisso-Fascism: the psychopathology of right wing extremism*. Ann Arbor, MI: Future Psychiatry Press.

14. Spindler K (1994). *The Man in the Ice: the preserved body of a Neolithic man reveals the secrets of the Stone Age*. London: Weidenfeld and Nicholson. See: Chap. V.10.

15. Humphreys P (1997). Emergence, not Supervenience. *Philosophy of Science*. 64: S337-S345

16. Humphreys P (2016). *Emergence: a philosophical account*. New York: Oxford UP.

17. Oderberg DS (2005). *Hylemorphic Dualism*, in Paul EF, Miller FD, Paul J: *Personal Identity*. Cambridge: University Press.

8   Dennett's dysfunctional Functionalism

The whole history of science, right up to the present, is a story of refusal to accept fundamental new ideas; of determined adherence to the *status quo*; of the invention of acceptable explanations, however ridiculous, for uncomfortable facts; of older people of scientific eminence dying in confirmed possession of their life-long beliefs; and of painful readjustment of younger people to new concepts.

Robert Youngson.

8.1. Toward an objective psychology.

At the risk of sounding repetitious, one of the dominant themes in twentieth century philosophy was to write a theory of mind that avoided the mortal sin of substance dualism. This is the notion, formalised in about 1640 by the French polymath, René Descartes, that the universe is composed of two distinct substances, each of which requires nothing other than itself to exist (actually, he said three, including divine substance). The physical world is composed of material substance which obeys the laws of physics, while the mind is composed of a completely different substance whose only property is thought. As Descartes himself recognised, this immediately creates the intractable problem of how mind and body interact. There is also the secondary problem of how we can turn subjective mental events into the sort of objective data we need to build a rational (non-magical, non-circular) theory of mind.

In order to avoid these problems, many philosophers decided to eliminate the mind-body disjunction by recasting mental events as brain events. Given this move, mental life can be investigated by the normal methods of laboratory science until, one fine day, we will see that what seems like the ineffable mentality of mental events is illusory. The task for such a monist philosophy of mind is showing that in some crucial respect, mental events just are brain events and are thus able to influence the body without magical intervention. In Chapter 3, we looked at behaviorism, particularly Skinner's operant conditioning, which took it to its limit by arguing that the controlling element in all behaviour, human and animal, is located in the external environment. The relationship between an environmental stimulus and the subject's response gives a full understanding of all behavior, leading to a science that can "predict and control" behavior. As history showed, that doctrine went nowhere so modern theories have tried to give account of mental events in terms of brain events, as these are the only other objective data available.

One of the most influential schools today is known as function-alism, the idea that mental states can be characterised by their role in the total behaviour or function of the individual. We don't need to waste time debating the *nature* of mental events, what counts is the *part they play* in the cognitive system. Thus, the mental event we call pain is seen as the state intervening between bodily injury and the behavior of wincing and pulling away. Any subjective qualities to pain add nothing to the explanation of its role so are beside the objective point.

Like most branches of philosophy, functionalism is a house divided. Very few people outside philosophy will have heard of any of its branches except that espoused by Daniel Dennett, of Tufts University, in Boston. This is because, even by philosophical standards, functionalism is arcane and thus largely a closed book to outsiders, whereas Dennett writes for outsiders. His most recent volume, *From Bacteria to Bach and Back: the evolution of minds* (2017) [1] could well be the last of a very long career in philosophy (some 60 years) and stands as the definitive statement of his philosophy. Other works providing essential background are:

- *Consciousness Explained* (1993) [2]

- *Kinds of Minds: Towards an understanding of conscious-ness* (1996) [3]

- *Freedom Evolves* (2003) [4].

Two earlier works, *Brainstorms: philosophical essays on mind and psychology* (1979) [5] and *The Intentional Stance* (1989) [6], outline the basis of his approach. In this chapter, I will try to distill well over 2,000 pages of text into a balanced critique but two words of warning are necessary. Firstly, Dennett has not offered an account of mental disorder and almost never mentions it so our interest is restricted to the question: Can his model be developed to the point of providing a framework for mental disorder? If it can't, then he should join Henri Bergson, Sigmund Freud, Burrhus Skinner and all the others in the history section of the library.

Second, Dennett has high verbal facility and is unashamedly partisan in his views. He uses this to write popular philosophy for non-philosophers; much less does he write technical philosophy for other philosophers to ponder and debate, possibly because he doesn't see much left to debate. Very few other philosophers express such strong opinions as he does, both positive opinions of his own work and negative of everybody else's. He uses a lot of witticisms and joking asides and while this may add to his appeal to keen undergraduates in philosophy and biology, it is a distraction for the serious reader. For example, the section on binary digits [1, p108-9]: anybody who needs binary logic explained won't be able to judge the validity of his arguments, while those of us who don't need it are irked by his glib condescension and tend to skim those sections. However, these are often the places he slips in contentious matters as though they were settled. In discussing language, he says:

> We don't yet know how to identify brain-tokens of words by their physical properties—*brain "reading"* hasn't been figured out yet, though we're getting closer ... [1, p183].

He means "getting closer" in the sense that a man who wants to go to the moon who climbs to the top of a tall building is "getting closer." Otherwise, there is no truth whatsoever to this biological claim but professional philosophers and undergraduates in any field are unlikely to know this. We will touch on these points as we look at his two major themes: Antidualism and biologism.

8.2. Dualism as "the ectoplasm that oozes."

> Those new to the study of Descartes should engage his own works in some detail prior to developing a view of his legacy (Gary Hatfield, 2014).

Dennett's interest goes back to his first year in college, when he read Descartes' *Meditations* from 1641 and was "...hooked on the mind-body problem" [2, xi]. The classic Cartesian formulation was that the mind is a real thing which interacts with the brain to control the body.

Unlike the body, the mind has no shape, no form, size or colour, nor even a location inside the skull. Nobody has ever seen a mind, spirit or soul yet, from direct experience, everybody knows that there must be something "in there" that does the thinking and experiencing. To Descartes, it had to be a special kind of real thing, made not of bone and meat stuff but of spirit stuff, a stuff we humans have but which animals don't. While this seemed to solve the problems of free will and moral responsibility, this immediately bothered the young Dennett: "How on earth," he asked, "could my thoughts and feelings fit in the same world with the nerve cells and molecules that made up my brain?" [2, xi]. Conversely, "How could our lives have meaning at all if we are just huge collections of proteins and other molecules churning away according to the laws of chemistry and physics?" [1, p15]. He now believes he can solve these ancient questions.

It seemed to him that the only conceivable way the classic Cartesian approach could survive was by a small miracle connecting the two realms. He scoffed at this in a cartoon in *Consciousness Explained* [2, p38]. Descartes, he argues at great length, did philosophy an enormous disservice by splitting mind and body, creating what he quotes as the "Cartesian wound" [1, p13]. The goal of philosophy, as he sees it, is to heal the wound by "... constructing a theory that is *not* dualism in disguise" [1, p14]. Unusually for philosophers, he believes that by relying on recent scientific progress, he can show that even "... doubters can *take seriously* the prospect of a scientific, materialist theory of their own minds" [1, p16].

He is not impressed by other philosophers' attempts to examine this most difficult of areas, dismissing them as yielding only "...self-contradiction, quandaries or blank walls of mystery..." [3, ix]. His view is that "...the various phenomena (of) consciousness... are all physical effects of the brain's activities..." [2, p16]. He concedes that it is "...very hard to imagine how your mind could be your brain—but not impossible." He is, however, convinced that "...a theory of the biological mechanisms..." would resolve the "...traditional paradoxes and mysteries of consciousness..." His ambition is an unyielding materialism: "Somehow, the brain must be the mind" [2, p41]. He repeats this credo in *Bacteria to Bach*, aiming for "... a materialistic model of the brain as the mind" [1, p364]. He is certain his approach will succeed where others' had failed because they "got off on the wrong foot."

The first and worst wrong foot is the "forlorn" Cartesian notion of dual entities, the "...hopelessly contradiction-riddled myth of the distinct, separate soul" [2, p430], which sees the brain as one substance and mind as another. Based in his teenage understanding of the weakness in Descartes' solution, Dennett sees dualism as crude magical thinking that violates the fundamental laws of the universe, creating endless logical problems without solving any: "Dualism, the idea that a brain cannot be a thinking thing so a thinking thing cannot be a brain..." At different points, he rails against it ("accepting dualism is giving up"), belittles it ("I wiggle my finger by...what, wiggling my soul?") or just mocks it ("ectoplasm, Wonder Tissue") because it is false, incoherent and antiscientific:

> There is the lurking suspicion that the most attractive feature of mind stuff is its promise of being so mysterious that it keeps science at bay forever... if dualism is the best we can do, then we can't understand human consciousness [2, p37-9].

In *Freedom Evolves* [4], Dennett sets himself the task of answering an ancient and powerful objection to a monist theory of mind, the question of free will and morality. If molecules don't have free will, and if the human brain is made of molecules, how can we humans have freedom of choice? Similarly, if we write God out of the equation, what is the source of morality? Materialism seems such a mechanistic and amoral system that many people are repelled by it, but Dennett disagrees vehemently. Even if the natural world is truly deterministic, he can show that humans have genuine free will that leads to a non-divine or humanist morality. But first, he scathingly dismisses dualist attempts to explain these phenomena as "...like the little green man in the control room of the man-sized puppet in the morgue in *Men in Black*... an immaterial portion of glowing ectoplasm that oozes around in your brain like a ghost amoeba... an angel whose wings are folded till you are called to fly to heaven" [4, p232]. Dualism is necessarily puerile non-science and a proper theory must avoid it at all costs.

He has no doubt that ectoplasm or spirit stuff is very slippery. One eye must always be kept peeled for it lest it worm its way into what seems like a brilliant new theory of mind. Sometimes, he warns, the problem is much more subtle than simply proposing a little gremlin or homunculus inside the head. Every now and then, neurophysiological concepts are used to cloak what is, in form, just a rehash of Descartes' non-solution. It is thus more important to look at the *form* of a new theory, and not be misled by its content. This is especially the case where somebody uses lots of, say, neurophysiological or data-processing terms to garnish what is essentially a dualist model.

Fortunately, Dennett has an infallible test for mind stuff, the "Cartesian Theater." If the magical spirit floating in the head is able to see and hear and feel the information being channeled to it from the outside, and to look into the memory banks and then make decisions before sending them to the various effector organs, then any hidden ectoplasm can easily be found lurking where the information flows to, or at a point it flows past. It's a bit like an army: if you want to find the general, he's likely to be hanging around whatever the troops are marching past. Conversely, if the troops are marching in review, somebody is reviewing them. In the brain, that somebody can only be a dualist Big Boss, Ultimate Executive, spirit or whatever.

Thus, if the conscious contents assemble into a stream, or flow, or river, or if they travel along a path or to a specific part of the brain where they cavort in a field or on a stage, or if they are bathed in an inner light or are illuminated or picked out in any way, then the reason is because they will be inspected by an inner eye. In turn, this inner eye must belong to an "inner man" or homunculus whom nobody can see because he/she/it has "no shape, no form or color, no size or even location." This is his test: the Cartesian Theater necessarily implies an Observer, and the Observer is necessarily made of magical stuff, the Ghost in the Machine. This means that, even if we can't actually see the observer, any hint of the Cartesian Theater means there is one hiding behind the curtains so the whole thing is non-scientific. The only solution to magical mind stuff is to get rid of all traces of the observer and of the observed, leaving only a monist theory of mind, such that consciousness can be explained "…without ever giving in to the siren song of dualism" [2, p33].

Consciousness Explained was published in 1991, meaning it was written in the year or two before that. That's a long time ago, so has Dennett modified his stance since then? *Kinds of Minds* [3] from 1996, and *Freedom Evolves* [4] from 2003, hew closely to the same theme present since *Brainstorms*, in 1979 [5]. Since then, and despite a bout of serious illness, he has maintained a punishing schedule of lectures and publications but has tended to pay more attention to the question of evolutionary theory.

At first, *Kinds of Minds* seems to have a limited scope, that of asking the right questions to improve our understanding of ourselves and the world. That, however, is illusory and Dennett packs some high-powered philosophizing in a small volume. As mentioned, he much prefers his version of the right questions to those asked by other philosophers, as he opines in *Bacteria to Bach*: "... I have found a path that takes us all the way to a satisfactory—and satisfying—account of how the 'magic' of our minds is accomplished without any magic. It is not the only path on offer, but it is the best, most promising to date..." [1, p4]. Armed with this self-assurance, he opines:

> Dualism (the view that minds are composed of some nonphysical and utterly mysterious stuff) and vitalism (the view that living things contain some special physical but equally mysterious stuff—*élan vital*) have been relegated to the trash heap of history, along with alchemy and astrology. (If) you ... (believe) that the world is flat and the sun is a fiery chariot pulled by winged horses... [3, p31],

... then Prof. Dennett will not provide you any comfort. In brief, he argues that our minds evolved from simpler minds, so there is nothing magic or supernatural about the human mind. However, even though simpler minds are essentially robotic, it does not follow that we are robots ourselves. We have a full range of mental attributes; his task as a philosopher is to give a rational (naturalistic) account of them.

What, then, is the essence of dualism, so that we may recognise it when it slithers in? Watson's pithy conclusion bears repeating:

> The crux of dualism is an apparently unbridgeable gap between two incommensurable orders of being that must be reconciled if we (wish to justify) our assumption that there is a comprehensible universe... [7, p210]

The two orders of being we apprehend are firstly, the material, physical universe which is governed by the laws of physics as we understand them now and as they will develop in the future. Second, there is the immaterial, non-physical mental realm of Descarte's "thinking stuff" which has no points of contact with the laws of physics. Dennett's view is that this concept of the mental realm is wrong at every point; he promises to show that what we think of as mental is, at base, biological. As such, "mind" obeys all the laws of the material realm, including all the laws of biology with no exceptions. In the rest of this chapter, we will examine his position and his claims to see if he has been able to construct "... a theory that is *not* dualism in disguise" [1, p14].

8.3. Mind as brain.

Dennett is far too sophisticated to fall for the simplistic notion that "mind = brain," as in mind-brain identity theory (MBIT, Chap. 2). He argues that the phenomena we experience as "mental events" must and can be fully explained as brain events, as matters of biology, leaving no epistemological questions unanswered, or at least none worth answering. This is his first theme, a vehement antidualism. However, while antidualist, he is not, as Skinner was, antimentalist [5, Ch. 4]. Dennett's approach is that mental life must be explained in non-mentalist terms (meaning biology) so he freely uses what, at first glance, are frankly dualist concepts and expressions. On every page, he talks of the mind and consciousness, of perceptions, memory, imagination, emotion, plans and ambitions, intentions and frustrations and so on. There is no mentalist concept that he doesn't accept as the raw material of his philosophy, and correctly so: the goal of a philosophy of mind is to account for the phenomena of mind, not to pretend they don't exist.

So while Skinner's effort was an antidualist theory of non-mind, Dennett's is an antidualist theory of mind and consciousness. Skinner simply ruled mentalism out of court; Dennett has chosen the vastly more difficult task of giving a step-by-step account of the laborious processes by which the ineffably complex human mind emerged from the darkness of pond life aeons ago, and how it functions today *as a biological organ*. Necessarily, a large part of his work revolves around language, what it is and how it evolved, because it is distinctively human and so has to fit with his general thesis: *Mind is wholly a biological phenomenon subject to all known and potential physical laws of the universe*. It doesn't matter how our understanding of physical reality evolves, mind must remain consistent with those laws.

His second theme is that, as biology, our understanding of the mind must be entirely consistent with that most fundamental of biological concepts, the theory of evolution. This appears in two of the titles listed above and is central to his work, including his studies of language, with evolutionary ideas and biological evidence appearing on practically every page. Had he not opted for such a strict biologism, then he would not have created this particular trek through what he calls "... a jungle of science and philosophy" [1, p3]. However, he is satisfied that his approach has led to the "... best scientific theory to date of how our minds came into existence" [1, pxiv]. Nonetheless, it is a risky ploy. It means that if for some reason the mind, or a significant aspect of it, is *not* consistent with the laws of evolution, then his larger project is at serious risk.

His antidualism roars in almost from the opening lines of each of the texts listed above. As quoted in S.8.2. above, and unusually for philosophers, he is openly contemptuous of any and all hints of his opponents' ideas. That, however, can be overlooked as these are not really philosophical texts. The wealth, even deluge, of biological material that fills every page shifts attention from his core thesis, that *the apparent mentality of mind is illusory*. Now this claim is not itself biological; it is a statement of his ontology, his fundamental beliefs of the nature of the universe, which puts it in the same class of questions as in the quote by Watson on dualism, above. It is a metaphysical statement, not an empirical matter, i.e. it cannot be resolved by using empirical evidence from the natural sciences. And he doesn't argue it. Instead, he pours abuse on each and every idea of dualism while leading a merry dance through the borderlands of philosophy and biology. This means that philosophers will think he has somehow settled the matter with biology while, overawed by his remarkable verbal facility, students of the natural sciences will think he has dealt the Cartesian wound a healing blow somewhere in the philosophy when, in fact, he hasn't succeeded on either count.

First point: his biology is not at all convincing. He cherry picks the evidence and rephrases it in such a manner as to suggest the mentalism has been eliminated when it hasn't. There are hundreds of points in each book where frankly mentalist concepts are used as a "skyhook" (his expression, [1, p54]) to save his thesis. For example, "thinking tools" are "installed in our brains" via some process of evolution that installs "... thinking tools by the thousands in our brains (and only in our brains), turning them into minds—not 'minds' or sorta minds but proper minds" [1, p171]. Now this is problematic because, by his own statement, "thinking tools" are information, and information, as we all know, does not obey the laws of the physical universe. It is insubstantial and has its own laws which cheerfully ignore the laws of gravity, or of energy conservation, or whatever else reigns in the physical universe. And Dennett understands this perfectly, as he showed using a well-known quote from the mathematician, Norbert Wiener:

> The mechanical brain does not secrete thought 'as the liver does bile,' as the earlier materialists claimed, nor does it put it out in

the form of energy, as the muscle puts out its activity. Information is information, not matter or energy. No materialism which does not admit this can survive at the present day (from *Cybernetics,* 1948) [in 1, p136].

That's all there is to it: precisely as Descartes concluded, nearly 400 years ago, information is wholly and irredeemably dualist in nature *just because* it is insubstantial and does not obey the laws of the physical universe. Information is coded on physical tokens but, as each token is a symbol, its informational content cannot be reduced to the tokens themselves, i.e. it represents something *other than itself*. A physical token cannot be a symbol of itself and can only be recognised as such by another information-processing entity. But if the informational element is removed from Dennett's model of mind, then it collapses. He cannot escape this. There are dozens, if not hundreds, of points in this text and the other three where the same covert error sneaks in, allowing him to incorporate dualist concepts in an ostensibly monist model:

> Tokens of words are all physical things of one sort or another, but words are, one might say, made of information, like software... [1, p187].

> We are the persuadable species ... capable of being moved ... by reasons *represented to us*, not free-floating [1, p219].

> ... the acquisition of a language—and of memes more generally— is very much like the installation of a predesigned software app of considerable power ... [1, p292].

> (Sweetness) is no property at all: it is a benign illusion. Our brains have tricked us into (believing that some foods are sweet) [1, p356].

> ... but human imagination, the capacity we have to envision realities that are not accessible to us ... permit(s) us to create, by foresighted design, opportunities and, ultimately, enterprises and artifacts that could not otherwise arise.... we have evolved the ability to think about (possibilities) and either seek or shun them [1, p399].

> A mind is fundamentally an anticipator, an expectation-generator. It mines the present for clues, which it refines with the

> help of the materials it has saved from the past, turning them into anticipations of the future [3, p75].

> ... what minds do is *process information*; minds are the control systems of bodies, and in order to execute their appointed duties, they need to gather, discriminate, store, transform, and otherwise process information about the control tasks they perform [3, p90].

> A brain ... is a localised device for mining the past environment for information that can then be refined into the gold of good expectations about the future [3, p162].

> ... language, when it is installed in a human brain, brings with it the construction of a new cognitive architecture that *creates* a new kind of consciousness—and morality [3, p260].

Hidden in plain sight in each of these examples there is a dualist element that completes the explanatory sequence, and without which there is no explanation. Sometimes he apologises for using overtly mentalist language but he doesn't eliminate the dualist intent: "Ponce *had an idea in his mind* of the Fountain of Youth (we might say, loosely speaking) ..." [*sic*, 1, p360]. Despite his efforts, these are all descriptions, not explanations and *just are* statements of a dualist nature. No evasion or apology will conceal that fact. There is no such thing as a "cognitive architecture;" that's a metaphor we use to describe something insubstantial and unlocalised. The future does not yet exist, it is not real and yes, we can anticipate it—but only in an informational system. Foresight, imagination, beliefs, traditions, recollections, persuasion, morality, mistaken presumptions, canons of practice ... these are the mentalist terms that he says he will explain *as biological entities*, but he doesn't. He seems to believe that once something frankly mental undergoes the (unexplained) process of being "installed in the brain," its dualism is at an end; duly stripped of its mentalist connotations, it is thereafter a fully paid up matter of biology.

But this was Skinner's error: Skinner believed that if he described something in his new, "objective" language, he had eradicated the need for mentalist explanations when, as a matter of logic, he had not. All he had done was shift the mentalism around, from an homunculus or 'little man' in the head to another man hidden in the environment. This led him to argue, for example, that there was no such thing as a creative artist [8]. What we think of as a creative artist, he said, is merely an artist skilled at arranging a "creativity-inducing environment." But who decides what constitutes a creativity-inducing environment? Presumably the artist, using his mentalist "skills." So Skinner merely shifted the problem from one of explaining creativity to one of explaining how people decide what will induce creativity (presumably a fairly creative exercise in its own right).

Dennett does the same. He has the view that if he *redescribes* mental events in a mix of biological and data-processing language, he has adequately *explained* them. For example, "Our brains have tricked us..." That is a frankly dualist statement: our brains are separate from the "us" that occupies them. Similarly, acquiring a language is just a matter of "installing the software in the brain." Sure, we all know that: does he have an easier way of learning irregular French verbs? But the real question is not *whether* this happens but *how*? What is the *mechanism* by which the brain codes information, and by what *processes* does it then relate to the experience of imagining a future event, or of generating speech to discuss it, or getting excited over the prospect, and so on? What is the mechanism by which "... the infrastructure for culture is designed and installed..." Installing infrastructure? Are we talking philosophy or shop-fitting? What is the *medium* in which the "cognitive architecture" is implemented? These are the critical questions but he dismisses them, just because he routinely conflates the informational *content* of a statement with the brain's physical *mechanism* for storing that statement as information. These are "two incommensurable orders of being that must be reconciled" (Watson) because "Information is information, not matter or energy" (Wiener).

Unquestionably, the mechanisms by which we "gather, discriminate, store, transform, and otherwise process information" (Dennett) are *brain mechanisms*, which (as Descartes argued) we possess in common with most other animals on earth, but the *mechanisms* are not the *information itself*. Information, as Dennett often says, is realizable in different formats, meaning its content is an "order of being" *removed* from the mechanism that implements it. That ontological separation must be explained, not dismissed as "pathetic bleats" [1, p19]. Without a process of emergence of and a medium of implementation for the "cognitive architecture," there can be no materialist theory of mind. Absent these anchors to hold the proposed "mind" in reality, his description is indistinguishable from a lump of "glowing ectoplasm that oozes around in your brain like a ghost amoeba." Just as he concedes when he says "Our brains have tricked us..."—there is a brain, and there is a me. These are "incommensurable orders of being."

Now Dennett may argue that he has explained all this in his previous works but that's not the case. He consistently falls into the trap of believing that redescribing events in a different, technical language removes the mentalist element from everyday experience. It does not, as the failure of Skinner's project shows. But even Dennett acknowledges this because, in the end, all he can do to save his model is invoke dualism in its purest form, that of a virtual machine:

> Human consciousness is *itself* a huge complex ... that can best be understood as the operation of a *"von Neumannesque"* virtual machine *implemented* in the *parallel architecture* of a brain that was not designed for any such activities. The power of this *virtual machine* vastly enhances the underlying powers of the organic *hardware* on which it runs... [2, p210; his emphasis].

> That is just what I am suggesting: Conscious human minds are more-or-less serial virtual machines implemented (in the brain) [2, p218].

> ... when language came into existence, it brought into existence the kind of mind that can transform itself on a moment's notice into a somewhat different virtual machine, taking on new projects, following new rules, adopting new policies. We are transformers. That's what a mind is, as contrasted with a mere brain, the control system of a chameleonic transformer, a virtual machine for making more virtual machines [4, p250-51].

> We have added a layer on top of the bird's (and the ape's and the dolphin's) capacity to decide what to do next. It is not an anatomical layer in the brain but a functional layer, a virtual layer composed somehow in the micro-details of the brain's anatomy [4, p251].

> You can simulate a virtual serial machine on a parallel architecture—that's what the brain does, as I showed in *Consciousness Explained*... [1, p155].

> Words, one might say, are a kind of *virtual DNA*, a largely digitised medium that exists only in the manifest image [1, p202].

> (Repetitions of words) are not *physical* replicas of their ancestors but they are—we might say—*virtual* replicas [1, p226].

> ...the EVM (English Virtual Machine) installed in your brain's wetware ... [1, p302].

> In effect, people can download and execute a virtual machine with no need for trial and error or associative learning... [1, p303].

> ... human consciousness as a system of virtual machines... [2, p335].

> Our thinking is enabled by the installation of a virtual machine made of virtual machines made of virtual machines ... and then we get to use them ourselves... as guests in our own brains [1, p341].

The crucial word here is "virtual" which means "not real, insubstantial, unlocalisable" and, above all, "not subject to the laws of the physical realm." A virtual machine implemented in the brain "we might say" is "sorta" there (his expression) but most emphatically not "there" in any tangible, physical sense. It exists as the emergent performance of a highly complex machine [1, p75] but he abhors the idea of emergence because it means "two incommensurable orders of being," i.e. dualist. *An emergent performance is not to be confused with the mechanism that generates it*, which he does when he says "Somehow, the brain must be the mind" [2, p41] or opts for "... a materialistic model of the brain as the mind" [1, p364] or proposes we are "guests in our own brains" [1, p341]. Nice try, Professor, but dualism is as dualism does. If it can't be seen and can't be localised and isn't subject to the laws of physics but then acts upon the natural world (it has to act on the physical world in some sense otherwise we wouldn't know it was there), then, even if it arises from a physical entity, it ain't biological. And if it ain't biological, it's dualist. QED.

His notion of "mind as more or less virtual machine" is nothing more than recycled Cartesian dualism hidden under a flood of biologistic and IT jargon. And another thing, isn't this habit of slipping things past as "somehow," or "we might say," or "more or less" or "sorta there" just a teensy bit sloppy, a little light on detail for a full tenured professor at a prestigious university? Could his students get through their exams with such legerdemain? I think not. The mind is *either* to be seen as a virtual (non-physical, dualist) machine implemented in the brain's architecture *or* it's not. If it is, kindly give an account of the mechanism by which it emerges, the medium in which it is implemented, the rules that govern its virtual function and its means of interaction with the somatic body. If it isn't, then forget all this stuff about virtual machines and try again. Because until we have a mechanism of emergence and a medium of implementation, then his virtual machine occupies precisely the conceptual space in his cartoon where it says "And a miracle occurs." Even Descartes refused to allow miracles.

8.4. An aside on information.

Elsewhere, I have proposed that mind is an emergent informational state generated by the brain's vast data-processing capacity, meaning a theory of information is logically prior to a theory of mind [9]. This is, of course, a dualist model but it is a natural dualism hanging on a single point: Can we give a naturalistic account (i.e. not a magical or "skyhook" account) of information? As always, Step 1 in any enquiry is: Define your topic. Despite devoting an entire chapter to the question of information [1, Ch 6, pp105-136], Dennett was unable to do so. After a great deal of mixed biology and IT, he faded out with Wiener's warning that information is something above and beyond the physical universe ("Information is information, not matter or energy") [1, p136]. His failure to account for information is not surprising. After a careful analysis, philosopher Luciano Floridi glumly concluded:

> The concept of information has become central in most contemporary philosophy. However, recent surveys have shown no consensus on a single, unified definition of semantic information. This is hardly surprising. Information is such a powerful and elusive concept... [10].

In his more recent primer on information, Floridi offers descriptions of information at work but does not define it [11]. Even his major work, entitled *The Philosophy of Information*, says only: "Information is still an elusive concept" [12, p30]. It was elusive because of the inherently circular nature of every attempt to pin it down. My definition started with that circularity and proceeded forward:

> Information is an *assessment* of some *discernible* aspect of the universe by an entity with the *capacity* to *represent* states of affairs in a *symbolic calculus* [9, p46; in the text, each point in italics is addressed to eliminate the obvious circularity].

In order to derive a naturalistic account of computation, we can extend this definition to encompass what can be *done* with information:

> Given an entity with the capacity to represent states of affairs in
> a symbolic calculus, computation is the manipulation, according
> to the rules of the relevant calculus, of various assessments of
> discernible aspects of the universe, leading to representations of
> alternative, unrealised states of affairs [9].

The computational capacity of the human brain meets this definition. Dennett's attempt to deal with this admittedly slippery concept
gets off to a bad start when he misquotes Claude Shannon as the
author of a "mathematical theory of information" [1, p106]. Shannon's
first publication in this area was his 1937 Master's thesis, entitled *A
Symbolic Analysis of Relay and Switching Circuits* [13], in which he
sets out the conditions for what are now known as logic gates. In 1948,
he published a lengthy paper entitled *A Mathematical Theory of
Communication* [14], subsequently republished with an introduction
by Warren Weaver in a volume firmly entitled *The Mathematical
Theory of Communication* [15]. Shannon took pains to say what can
be *done* with information but not what it *is*:

> The fundamental problem of communication is that of
> reproducing at one point either exactly or approximately a
> message selected at another point. Frequently the messages have
> *meaning*; that is, they refer to or are correlated according to
> some system with certain physical or conceptual entities. These
> semantic aspects of communication are irrelevant to the
> engineering problem [15, p31].

Because information as we understand it relates to semantic content,
Shannon was specifically saying his was *not* a theory of information.
His was strictly an engineer's view of the technology of accurately
transmitting or communicating physical signals. What engineers
transmit with their codes and blips and bandwidth may or may not
amount to information, but they don't care about that. Plato or
pornography for IT engineers, fine wine or sewage for hydraulic
engineers, abattoirs or hospitals for civil engineers, it's all the same to
them. Without grasping this distinction, Dennett was unable to see the
inherent dualism of semantic information. He clearly thinks that
communication and information refer to the same event, but they
don't: one is a physical event, as specified in Shannon's papers, the
other is a mental perception of the *meaning* of that physical event.

Explaining the physical event doesn't explain the perceptual event as perceptions are not governed by the laws of physical machines. *Meaning* is something above and beyond mere electronics but, as Shannon emphasised, it is "irrelevant to the engineering problem." As we use the word, meaning is only indirectly related to communications technology. We can certainly have meaning with no communication— we all have our secrets—and, regrettably, a large and growing proportion of what is communicated is meaningless.

Dennett, like so many others, failed to heed Shannon's warning. Viscerally unable to accept the inherent duality of signal/meaning, that information and physical reality are "two incommensurable orders of being," he decreed that the blips are all there is, that once meaning is encoded in a signal, it becomes a physical thing, a part of the material universe. Declaring them to be one and the same thing (as in "the brain must be the mind") doesn't reconcile them, it slams the door on reconciliation by declaring the contest over. My reading of Descartes is that he understood this perfectly well.

8.5. Memes and the evolution of minds.

If, as Dennett claims, there is no duality of mental life; if minds and brains are, in some ultimate explanatory sense, either one and the same biological thing or reducible to the same biological nature; and all things biological have evolved, then minds must have evolved. It would seem that explaining the evolution of the brain should also explain the evolution of the mind but that doesn't go far enough. The natural dualist is able to say "When the brain became sufficiently complex, minds emerged as an ontologically distinct, functional duality." However, this is toxic to antidualists because emergent phenomena aren't governed by the rules of the physical universe. If the only categories they recognise are "rational biologism" and "irrational dualism," then emergent minds fall in the irrational category. A central part of Dennett's program, therefore, is to show that what we ordinarily believe to be quintessential mentalist concepts, such as language and culture, are in fact well-behaved citizens of the physical universe and thus subject to all the usual laws, including evolution. If somehow they don't follow the laws of evolution, then the mind probably isn't biological and the door is wide open to the ectoplasmic ooze, leaving Dennett's life's work in tatters.

In *Consciousness Explained* [2], from 1991, Dennett proposed an "empirical theory of mind" called the multiple drafts model which he agreed was "speculative." Leaving aside his glaring failure to propose a biological mechanism for his model or, apart from "somewhere in the brain," a medium in which it was implemented and interacted, he needed to explain the process by which the human brain was lifted above the level of clever apes *without* invoking frank mentalist concepts such as intellect. In a section entitled *The memes of consciousness: the virtual machine to be installed*, he populated the brain with non-mentalist *bits* of intelligence. Memes are defined as "an element of a culture or system of behaviour passed from one individual to another by imitation or other non-genetic means" although Dennett goes further by giving them properties similar to those of living entities:

> The transformation of a human brain by infestations of memes is a major alteration in the competence of that organ [2, p209].

He acknowledged that his model was an apparent "trick with mirrors" [2, p226] that could be equated with the dreaded Cartesian "self" but he persisted and finally concluded that a "self" is OK if it is biological. Using its infestation of memes, the human brain spins a virtual self that does everything an oozing amoeboid Cartesian self does, but since memes aren't dualist, his virtual biological self can't possibly be dualist and so no ghostly amoebae get a look in. However, if it looks like a duck and quacks like a duck … Everything, then, depends on whether he can use the idea of insensate memes to build a monist model of mind.

Like so many other fads (memes, you might say), the word "meme" started with a fairly technical meaning but was quickly snapped up by the chattering classes. According to Wikipedia, a meme is:

> … an idea, behavior, or style that spreads by means of imitation from person to person within a culture and often carries symbolic meaning representing a particular phenomenon or theme. A meme acts as a unit for carrying cultural ideas, symbols, or practices, that can be transmitted from one mind to another through writing, speech, gestures, rituals, or other imitable phenomena with a mimicked theme. Supporters of the concept regard memes as cultural analogues to genes in that they self-replicate, mutate, and respond to selective pressures (accessed Aug 26th 2022).

The term comes from the popular biological author, Richard Dawkins, in his 1976 book, *The Selfish Gene*. He used it as a unit of cultural transmission, to explain how ideas and fashions spread through society in a similar manner to biological evolution. While the idea and the expression have been stringently criticised ever since, few writers have offered stronger support than Daniel Dennett who adopted it as central to his biological thesis. He defines a meme as:

> ... a kind of *way of behaving* (roughly) that can be copied, transmitted, remembered, taught, shunned, denounced, brandished, ridiculed, parodied, censored, hallowed ... *memes are ways*: ways of doing something or making somehing, but not *instincts* ... memes are transmitted perceptually, not genetically ... Memes just are semantic information [1, p206; his emphasis].

Examples of memes are tunes, fashions (wearing a cap backwards, torn jeans, socks with sandals [1, p208]), gestures, applying plaster to walls [1, p212], collecting seeds, kindling fires, felling trees [1, p216], pasta, "things to die for (and to kill for): freedom, democracy, truth, communism, Roman Catholicism, Islam... " [1, p218]. A brick is not itself a meme, but the *idea* of bricks, how to make them, what is the right clay, what fires them best, how to lay them, how to use them structurally or decoratively—in short, a meme is anything that isn't stuck down: "*Memes are informational things* ... 'prescriptions' for ways of doing things that can be transmitted, stored, and mutated without being executed or expressed (rather like recessive genes...)" [1, p211]. He meant "things," not things; things are material entities populating the real world of matter and energy, time and space while "things" are a metaphor to describe some abstract, unreal or virtual matter which is not of the physical world. Nor is it clear why he put prescriptions in scare quotes because that is exactly what memes are: an order, instruction, plan or process that can be conveyed through space and time by some informational means from one person to another in order to achieve a certain result by following a particular procedure. He defines words as a special but critically important class of memes, namely, spoken memes.

Thus, memes are "like viruses" in that they infest brains where they proliferate and then spread to other brains because they want to survive and multiply. They have no mentality of their own but rely on the host, just like viruses which have no reproductive machinery of their own and must rely on the host to reproduce them (in fact, viruses don't want to survive, they just do because viruses). While memes can be spread by explicit instruction (such as reading this book, going to a class or looking at a plan), their main mode of transmission is by intuitive apprehension. In the process, they turn brains into minds, and minds, as he has made perfectly clear, have all the properties that we expect them to have:

> That is the triumph of the memes invasion: it has turned our brains into minds—*our* minds ... thanks to the apps installed in our necktops [1, p315] ... Our thinking is enabled by the installation of a virtual machine made of virtual machines made of virtual machines [1, p341].

Now a reader new to the idea of memes may ask: "What's the point? What's the difference between this idea and Descartes' thinking stuff from 400 years ago?" Patience, dear reader: the difference is that Dennett's model is very explicitly *biological*. How is it biological, as a duck is biological? Because Dennett says so. Look at memes: granted they are information and information doesn't inhere in the real world, but they can spread intuitively. Implicit learning is more biological than explicit. A brain isn't a mind until it's got a nucleus of information ("apps") but children acquire knowledge before they are taught anything. That's because memes want to infest and breed and proliferate and spread in any brain material they can find. Just like viruses.

No. No. No. All wrong.

The problem is that Dennett is absolutely desperate to "prove" that the brain is the mind; he is, just by virtue of that desperation, an ideologue, totally the product of his generation (infested by the same meme that parasitised (his word) Skinner? That's a bit embarrassing). He needs to show that culture is not developed or transmitted by the intervention of *thinking* human beings because that's Cartesian dualism. Thus, he has fixed on the idea that since we can come up with bright ideas without really knowing how (which is true of practically everything we do, see [9]), then it must be biological and if it's biological, it isn't a magical Cartesian substance. Possibly, although Freud thought of it long before Dennett and Dawkins were born, but we'll let him prove his case. So far, his case is only an argument for unconscious causation, which is still part of the mind, but he doesn't like unconscious causation because that implies that there is something called "conscious causation," (in the same way as Skinner's concept of reflex behavior implied there is something called "non-reflex behavior," aka intentional), conscious causation is dualist, and dualism... you know the rest.

So, in order to win the debate with his opponents (and Dennett has many, many opponents), he must show that ideas can be separated from their inherent mentality and can thereby spread without human intervention. It's sorta the reverse process of anthropomorphism, in which human attributes, traits, characteristics, emotions or intentions are attributed to non-human entities, animate or inanimate. So he strips ideas of their inherent mentality leaving only an intellectually-undemanding husk, gives them a fancy name and, hey presto, they seem to act like mindless viruses. Possibly true, but both birds and frogs lay eggs. If we pluck a bird's feathers, it will flop around on the ground like a frog. Does that prove it is an amphibian?

Dennett shoots himself in the foot when he says, over and over, "*Memes are informational things* ... transmitted perceptually" [1, p206, his emphasis]. Yes, we all agree that an idea is an informational thing, that it has no substance, no location in time or space and cheerfully ignores the laws of physics, i.e. that it isn't a citizen of the physical universe. We humans are, as he says often enough, information processors with a brain that computes. Our brains are stuffed with information that nobody can see or locate, which means we are composed of "apparently incommensurable orders of being which must be reconciled" if we wish to make sense of our existence. Declaring that information is a biological thing just because it can be written on paper, or on stone, or in computers or brains is not reconciliation. It's like declaring yourself winner of a boxing match because you don't like the other boxer (or declaring yourself winner of an election because you didn't like losing).

> Information is information, *not* matter or energy. No materialism which does not admit this can survive at the present day (Wiener; emphasis added).

If memes are "informational things," and by their presence they can convert a brain to a mind, then the mind is itself an informational thing, which is dualism simpliciter (actually, they don't convert the brain, it's still there; they just add an emergent entity, the "me"). Information is not matter and it is not energy, yet it is real because, once parked in a suitable transducer (that's us, the humans in the equation, not our brains), it can act upon the real world. The positivist notion that the universe consists of only what we can see and touch and measure is outmoded, as outmoded as Cartesian mechanics after

Newton. Nowadays, we have to accept that the universe consists of time and space, matter and energy, and the *informational states that control them* (for a more detailed treatment of the derivation, implementation and significance of informational states, see [9]).

What controls human behaviour? According to the "... best scientific theory to date of how our minds came into existence" [1, pxiv], courtesy of Prof. Dennett, it is information transmitted and handed down by a myriad means, from one generation to the next, allowing human knowledge to accumulate exponentially [1, p113]. Information "installed" in the human brain converts it into a human mind where it proliferates, develops, refines and generally proves itself beneficial to its host. We all know that babies have baby minds before they have information, and animal brains are loaded with information, at least some of which they can hand on; suffice it to say linguistic information expands the reach of the human mind by many orders of magnitude.

In order to construct "a theory which is *not* dualism in disguise" [1, p14], Dennett strips the inherent meaning from words by calling them memes, then "installs" them in your brain, and *then* smuggles in the same dualist meaning they had before he got to work on them. "Memes" are just a bit of clever wordplay to convince the unsuspecting that ideas and genes are exactly homologous when they are only the very loosest of analogies—which, in any event, only a mentally-equipped creature could understand. For Dennett, the purpose of memes (*purpose* being itself an irreducibly mentalist concept) is to act as skyhooks to support his depauperate model of mind after he has stripped its mentality to the point where it can no longer stand on its own feet. All because he is viscerally unable to accept that information is inherently dualist in nature.

The concept of dualism, as we ordinarily understand the word, is the *sine qua non* of information; information *just is* dualist. These are not separate or distinct notions: the moment an informational state exists (see [9] for details), then *ipso facto* a dualist entity springs into being, and *vice versa*. Given the definitions of information and computation in S.8.4 above, it follows that ...

> The concepts employed in defining information are both necessary and sufficient to define a dualist universe. It is impossible to invoke information without *ipso facto* invoking dualism. The ontological distinction between information and dualism is a distinction without a difference.

But putting the hollow shells of his "memes" aside, I can still see blue when I look out my window, so what does he have to say to that? What about pain? Where is there room for pain, for the sheer *experience* of pain or for misery, in his model? This brings Dennett to his most contemptuous: if he stamps on your foot, he exclaims, you will feel only a fleeting pain which is so minor as not to warrant the label of "suffering." It would be a "risible" misuse of the term to apply it to an irritation that is no more than "...a brief, negatively-signed experience... of vanishing moral significance" [2, p220]. If we look at the mind from the right point of view (biologism) and ask the right questions (his), we will eventually get out of the old, magical way of thinking and see the mind for what it is, a virtual machine generated by the high-speed, multimodal, distributed, information-processing system which is our brain. Pain is merely the functional state which inclines you to wince and complain, nothing more.

That, of course, is his attempt, not to *explain* the experience of pain but to *explain away* the sheer, ineffable painfulness of pain because it messes with his antidualist model. It is also necessary to be rid of the painfulness of pain, the lonely terror of panic, the self-loathing of guilt and the sheer misery of grief because they are the very experiences that drive people to embrace... guess what? That's right, religion. It is also exactly the sort of disdainful attitude you would expect from a person born into privilege but it excludes his model from any consideration in psychiatry: we are looking for a model that *explains* human distress, *not* one that explains it away. Is torture "risible"? Is rape of "vanishing moral significance"? Genocide just a giggle? Later, he attempts to explain away the sensation of blue with promissory materialism [1, p347] (aka hand-waving). However, there is no reason to believe that we can ever explain the experiences unless and until we have the brain codes underlying the "neural-level activity," but codes are informational and therefore dualist, after all. Twist and turn as he will, Dennett just can't escape the tentacles of the "glowing ectoplasm that oozes around in your brain like a ghost amoeba..." [4, p232]. To paraphrase his own epigram:

> If anti-dualism is the best we can do, then we can't understand information, and if we can't understand information, then we can't understand human consciousness.

8.6. Conclusion: Reality 7.0.

What we want from philosophers is an *explanation* of the incontrovertible sense of being alive, of being a sentient *thing*, the same sense that Descartes (and his intellectual forebears) struggled with so long ago. We don't need to hear from people trying to explain it away. If somebody stamped on his little granddaughter's foot, would Dennett say with a light laugh, "Tut tut, sweet child, it's silly to get upset over such a fleeting negative experience"? I doubt it. Is depression any the less real just because there is no chemical to explain it, or anxiety less crippling because there is no blood test for it? [16].

Dennett is stuck on the idea that dualism means "two substances." He can't think beyond this hackneyed interpretation of Descartes' term (bearing in mind that Descartes used "substance" and "thing" interchangeably). He doesn't betray any acknowledgement of the view, inherent in Watson's definition above, that dualism also means "two sets of rules." His entire case hangs on that one, critical word that he smuggles in under the guise of its being a physical event: virtual. If the mind is a *virtual machine*, meaning insubstantial, unlocalised, and running by a non-physical set of rules while still able to act on the real world, it is still real, just an expanded version of real: Reality 7.0, you could say (after the folk, Cartesian, Newtonian, Darwinian, relativistic and Shannon/Turing concepts of reality). Despite his efforts at disguise, dualism is as dualism does.

References:

1. Dennett DC (2017). *From Bacteria to Bach and Back: the evolution of minds.* London: Allen Lane. Page numbers refer to the Penguin edition (2018).

2. Dennett DC (1991). *Consciousness Explained.* Boston: Little Brown. Page numbers refer to the Penguin edition (1993).

3. Dennett DC (1996). *Kinds of Minds: Towards an understanding of consciousness.* London: Weidenfeld and Nicholson,.

4. Dennett DC (2003). *Freedom Evolves.* London: Penguin,.

5. Dennett DC (1978). *Brainstorms: Philosophical essays on mind and psychology.* Hassocks, Sussex: Harvester Press.

6. Dennett DC (1987). *The Intentional Stance.* Boston: MIT Press. Page numbers refer to the MIT Paperback edition (1989).

7. Watson RA (1995), in Audi R (Ed.). *The Cambridge Dictionary of Philosophy*. Cambridge: University Press.

8. Skinner BF. *Beyond Freedom and Dignity*. New York: Knopf, 1971. Page numbers refer to the Bantam Books edition, 1972.

9. McLaren N (2021): *Natural Dualism and Mental Disorder: The biocognitive model for psychiatry*. London, Routledge.

10. Floridi L (2005). Is Semantic Information Meaningful Data? *Philosophy and Phenomenological Research* 70:(2): 351-71

11. Floridi L (2010). *Information: A very short introduction*. Oxford: University Press.

12. Floridi L (2011). *The philosophy of information*. Oxford: University Press.

13. Shannon CE (1937). *A Symbolic Analysis of Relay and Switching Circuits*. Unpublished MS Thesis, Massachusetts Institute of Technology, Aug. 10, 1937. Available at:

http://dspace.mit.edu/bitstream/handle/1721.1/11173/34541425.pdf?sequence=1

14. Shannon CE (1948) A Mathematical Theory of Communication. *Bell System Technical Journal* 27: 379–423, 623–656 (July, October). At: https://people.math.harvard.edu/~ctm/home/text/others/shannon/entropy/entropy.pdf

15. Shannon CE, Weaver W (1949). *The Mathematical Theory of Communication*. Urbana, Ill: University of Illinois Press.

16. Moncrieff, J., Cooper, R.E., Stockmann, T. *et al.* (2022) The serotonin theory of depression: a systematic umbrella review of the evidence. *Molecular Psychiatry* Published online July 20th 2022. https://doi.org/10.1038/s41380-022-01661-0

9   Searle:
Biology to the rescue

> I made one enormous error. I thought that family and genetic studies, advances in neuroscience, and the newly emerging discipline of molecular biology would soon elucidate pathogenesis and result in improved therapeutics (of mental disorder). How wrong I turned out to be.
>
> Steven Hyman
> (Director of NIMH during Human Genome Project)

9.1. The biology of consciousness.

Over the half-century or so that Chomsky and Dennett have been slogging it out in Boston, far away on the west coast of USA a more traditional philosopher has been working steadily to explain consciousness through a project he calls biological naturalism. It would be fair to say that, as a philosopher, John Searle does not enjoy the same profile among the public and among psychiatrists as the earthier Dennett or the sainted Chomsky, although I doubt this would much concern him. As a writer, Searle is rather old-fashioned, if a spare and sober style means old-fashioned. There is generally no difficulty extracting his position from his writing, as he inclines to state his views briefly at the beginning of a paper, then deal with each point in turn until he is satisfied the topic is exhausted, closing with a summary that aims to forestall further quibbles. Here, he opens his case with a transparent statement of his subject:

> By 'consciousness' I simply mean those subjective states of sentience or awareness that begin when one awakes in the morning from a dreamless sleep and continue throughout the day until one goes to sleep at night or falls into a coma, or dies, or otherwise becomes, as one would say, 'unconscious' [1, p40-41].

This experience of "something rather than nothing" is what he has to explain. In order to achieve his goal, he needs tools and these, he believes, are readily to hand in our scientific laboratories:

> Some philosophical problems, but unfortunately not very many, can receive a scientific solution. I believe one of these is the problem of consciousness [2, p169].

This is a bold claim, especially from someone with limited grounding in science, but it has some strong precedents. For example, he can point to the discoveries that led people to drop the idea that living matter is created when some special unseen power or *élan vitale* occupies inanimate matter and turns it into a living thing. Progress in physiology and biochemistry eventually showed that living material is just complex chemical stuff doing its thing, just as science dispensed with phlogiston and the luminiferous aether. His claim, or rather his credo, recurs regularly throughout his writings:

> ... the mind is essentially a biological phenomenon ... therefore its two most important interrelated features, consciousness and intentionality, are also biological [1, p112].

> All conscious states, without exception, are caused by neuro-biological processes in the brain ... everything in consciousness ... is caused by lower level neurobiological processes in the brain ... There is nothing to the causal power of consciousness which cannot be explained by the causal power of the neuronal base. That is why consciousness ... is an ordinary part of our human and animal biology [2, p170].

> ... consciousness is real, it is caused by brain processes, it is realized in the brain, and it functions causally... (this is) "biological naturalism" ... the right level for a scientific account of consciousness is the biological level... consciousness is an ordinary part of nature along with life, digestion, photosynthesis and all the rest of it.... You can have a perfectly objective science of an ontologically subjective domain... [2, p171-2]

> ... given the constitution of reality, consciousness has to follow in the same way that any other biological property, such as mitosis, meiosis, photosynthesis, digestion, lactation, or the secretion of bile, follows [2, p177].

> Once we see that consciousness is a biological phenomenon like any other, then it can be investigated neurobiologically. Consciousness is entirely caused by neurobiological processes and is realized in brain structures [3, p557].

> ... we have a solution to the traditional mind-body problem. And here it is: All of our mental states are caused by neurobiological processes in the brain, and they are themselves realized in the brain as its higher level or system features [4, p492].

> Consciousness, intentionality, subjectivity, and mental causation are all a part of our biological life history, along with growth, reproduction, the secretion of bile, and digestion [5, p675].

The four cardinal features of mind that need to be explained, he believes, are the unity of the conscious experience; the fact that the mind is causally effective; that mental states are intensional (directed); and that all mental states amount to a qualitative experience. From the beginning, he excludes the supernatural as a form of explanation. He offers as the "default" view of mind the folk concept that:

> ... each of us consists of two separate entities, a body on the one hand, and a mind or soul on the other, and that these are joined together during our lifetimes but are independent to the extent that our minds or souls can become detached from our bodies and continue to exist as conscious entities ever after our bodies are totally annihilated. This view is called "dualism" [1, p11]... Consciousness has for many centuries seemed to philosophers to pose a serious problem in metaphysics. How is it possible that a world consisting entirely of material particles in fields of force can contain systems that are conscious? If you think of consciousness as some separate, mysterious kind of phenomenon, distinct from material or physical reality, then it looks like you are forced to what is traditionally called "dualism," the idea that there are two basically different kinds of phenomena in the universe [1, p45]... dualism in any form makes the status and existence of consciousness utterly mysterious [1, p47].

Dualism is forlorn, he says, a hapless project not consistent with the scientific ethos that has given us such progress as we see in everyday life. He fully expects that some day, the same scientific ontology, even if not the current technology, will provide a complete explanation of the ancient questions of the nature of mind and its origin in and mode of interaction with the body.

9.2. Racing ahead.

Searle doesn't offer any definition or explanation of mind; despite its prominence (e.g. in the title to [1]), we can only assume that what he means by mind is what we all understand by it. He also doesn't define consciousness, he describes it, but as a negative: consciousness is what being unconscious is not, it fills the gaps between bouts of nothingness. However, I don't think anybody can improve on that. We all know what consciousness is by direct experience: "Consciousness is the state of being able to report that one is conscious." All that remains to know is its nature. If we were to discover exactly how that experience is "... caused by brain processes, it is realized in the brain," it may lose some of its mystery but it would still be there; not, in my view, " ... an ordinary part of nature" but quite extraordinary. If "... a world consisting entirely of material particles in fields of force can contain systems that are conscious," understanding how this comes about would require a revolution in our understanding of the physical universe. This is what we want to know. Insisting that consciousness is somehow secreted by the brain by the same order of nature as the kidneys secrete urine is not that revolution: it is an attempt to wind the clock back, to prevent a revolution by sticking to what we know. Before anybody can take seriously his claim that consciousness is "... caused by brain processes, it is realized in the brain," we need some indication of the mechanisms by which the brain achieves this miracle, and some account of the medium in which it is realised because one thing is clear: when looking at a blue sky, there are no blue neurons in my head (but even if there were, they would only be the first steps in a long chain of causation; the experience would still demand explanation).

As it stands (i.e. without any attempt at citing authorities or providing an argument), Searle's statement, that consciousness is an ordinary part of biology, is a metaphysical claim, a statement of the nature of the universe as he sees it. He expects that the progress of science, essentially meaning neurophysiology, will allow us to say that the concept of consciousness as "... distinct from material or physical reality..." belongs in the waste paper basket of history. That is, he endorses a physicalist stance and expects science to eliminate our archaic beliefs in our default position, an inexplicable dualist universe.

However, we have to be careful with what is called eliminative materialism. People point to history and say: "We used to believe in the *élan vitale* and phlogiston and the luminiferous aether, yet science eliminated them." This is true but the analogy is faulty. Each of those examples was an attempt at explaining observations, e.g. that living material behaves very differently from non-living, or that materials lose weight during the process of burning, etc. They were hypotheticals, suggestions of an unseen mechanism that explained the observations, whereas in the case of mind or consciousness, the experience is the observation that needs to be explained, so it can't be eliminated.

But Searle is not trying to do that. He is saying "The experience of seeing blue will still be there, we will just have a purely biological explanation for it." Except we won't. Look again at this quote:

> ... given the constitution of reality, consciousness has to follow in the same way that any other biological property, such as mitosis, meiosis, photosynthesis, digestion, lactation, or the secretion of bile, follows [2, p177].

In the case of each of these biological events, we have a complete knowledge of all the biochemical steps involved. For example, the secretion of bile is understood in immense detail from the breakdown of haem pigments, the formation of bilirubin and bile salts, and the storage and secretion of bile, etc. Every step in the complex pathways is understood entirely as a function of matter-energy transfers, even to the level of the role of individual electrons in the enzymatic processes. Every step along the way conforms precisely to the laws of physics and thermodynamics as we understand them. Matter and energy in, matter and energy out, and the pathways have to balance in every respect otherwise our livers would either cook themselves or putrefy. This is also true of each of the examples of physiological processes he gave, mitosis, photosynthesis, etc..

People with no background in biology generally do not understand the explanatory power of molecular biology. For vision, we can talk about the impact of a single photon on the visual receptors, but that power does not extend to the actual sensory experience of seeing a pinpoint of light just because the laws of physics and thermodynamics *do not apply* to the experience. This is because mental events involve something above and beyond "matter and energy in, matter and energy out." They are informational processes, which are not addressed at any point by physiology. Brain function is entirely different from normal cellular function: non-neural tissues have an input and an output but the brain achieves nothing in the physical realm *except return to status quo ante*. The whole point of a neuronal spike impulse is to discharge and then return precisely to its resting state, with no trace of its activity, ready for the next impulse to arrive. And that point, which Searle has not recognised, is the basis of the brain's informational processing capacity. No other cell in the body has it, although animal neurons have it as well.

But the point of the experience of blue is *not* that it is implemented by the brain—nobody is disputing that. The crucial point is that it involves steps which are *outside* the realm of action of the laws of thermodynamics, etc., which is what the dual in "dualism" means. Searle's emphasis on immortality as an essential feature or property of a dualist entity is a straw man: the essence of dualism is two sets of laws, not immortality. So dualism is a case of "Matter and energy in, matter and energy *and something else* out." If I think about, or even look at, a fire, my brain doesn't get any hotter. If I imagine walking up a hill, my cerebral energy consumption is no different from watching a bird outside my window or just daydreaming.

It is the disjunct between matter and energy and the laws of physics governing them, and the apparently formless and limitless realm of mental experience, that needs explaining. Telling me, on no authority whatsoever, that one fine day, biology will explain all this is utterly unconvincing because my lifetime's training in biology says it won't (that's why I bother myself with this topic). Science was able to eliminate suggested *mechanisms* such as the *élan vitale* and phlogiston and the aether, but it can't do the same trick with mind because mind is what we have to explain, it is the explicandum, not the explicans. Anyway, we need our minds to perform his elimination trick, which is why professorial opinions amount to naught.

Despite Searle's sunny optimism, the best that a future science can do is to explain mind but it can't eliminate what we all know is there. We can say it isn't what it seems but there is nothing Searle, or Skinner, or any of them can say that will convince me I don't now have the *impression* of the sun shining brightly on my curtains and the joyous shrieks of the white cockatoos as they raid my fruit trees. That's my reality, that's what I want explained, and nobody can eliminate my reality by explaining the mechanism by which it is realised or, more to Searle's point, explain my reality by eliminating it. They may say it isn't what it seems to be but two more problems poke up their thorny heads.

My first objection is "Well, I know pain, it just *is* what it seems to be. You can't give me a pamphlet to read that will suddenly cause it to go away." Even when we have a full physiological explanation of pain, it will still hurt, and *that* is what requires explanation: What is the nature of the human mind that a hammer dropped on the foot *hurts*? The second imp was the same one Descartes explored nearly 400 years ago, that even if we are fooled about all the impressions and beliefs and memories that seem to indicate something real "out there," there's still something left, there's always *me, the entity being fooled*. Descartes said it: *Je pense, donc je suis*. I think, so that proves I am some *thing*. Please explain, but don't try to fool me it isn't happening to me.

These days, nobody likes Descartes' attempt at an explanation, any more than they liked Bergson's, so we have several major approaches to this ancient question. The first is Chomsky's, to ignore it by talking around the point. The second is Dennett's, to explain it away but covertly to invoke dualism to get us over that last, crucial hurdle, the fact that I am some *thing* that experiences. Searle's is quite clear: he wishes to reclassify mental events as biological and then explain them (not explain them away) using the principles and methods of ordinary biological science. He sets this out in detail when he tries to answer the question "What is wrong with dualism?" [2, p175]. His first step is to argue that even though mind is causally reducible to brain processes, it is not ontologically reducible to a matter of brain processes, because "...consciousness has a first-person or subjective ontology, and for that reason cannot be reduced to something that has a third-person or objective ontology. If you try to make the reduction you leave something out, namely the subjectivity of consciousness" [2, p175].

This leads us back to the old problem of causation: how can a subjective entity that we can't even locate in space influence the objective universe? He asks "So what is the solution to this puzzle? I think the solution is obvious ... " namely, reclassify all the subjective features of mind that we need to explain (subjectivity, quality, intensionality etc) as features of the material realm *et voilà*, problem solved. His proof of the validity of this move? He can raise his right arm if he chooses to do so, which proves that at some level, mind can act on body. Naturally enough, he expects objections and counters them thus:

> We know there must have been a sequence of neuron firings going from the motor-cortex to the muscles, we know the neurotransmitter was acetylcholine, and we know the acetylcholine at

the axon-endplates of the motor neurons activated the ion channels in such a way as to attack the cytoplasm of a muscle-fiber. So we can generalize this as...:

(1) Certain mental events cause physical events of bodily movements.
(2) Anything that causes such bodily movements in the internal bodily fashion must have electro-chemical properties. Therefore
(3) Such mental events have electro-chemical properties.

...I actually think philosophically or metaphysically the situation is really that simple... On my view, given the constitution of reality, consciousness has to follow in the same way that any other biological property, such as mitosis, meiosis, photosynthesis, digestion, lactation, or the secretion of bile, follows [2, p176-7].

While consciousness is a "higher level feature" of the physical brain, it remains "... part of the ordinary physical world like any other biological phenomenon" [2, p178]. Nobody is disputing that the mind depends on a healthy brain, all that remains is Searle's explanation of *how* this comes about. However, he offers no suggestion of a mechanism by which some cells in the body secrete bile while others "secrete" thought, a problem anticipated by the mathematician, Norbert Wiener, some sixty years ago [6].

It is one thing to state that the mind is a biological entity, something else again to outline its nature, which is determined by the mechanism by which it is generated by neural activity, and the medium within which it is implemented. These, of course, are the issues that Descartes tackled, some 400 years ago. Searle appears to be aware of this because, when it comes to the quintessential human behaviour, language, the attribute that seems to distinguish us from all other living creatures, he is forced to move beyond "mere physics" to complete his task. Language involves symbolism, "... the capacity to use one object to stand for, represent, express, or symbolise something else" [1, 154]. But, and this is the critical qualification that undoes his entire project, the meaning of a word or symbol "... cannot lie in the physics" [1, p156] of the word or symbol alone. That is, he acknowledges that meaning, the *sine qua non* of language, is non-material in nature, it is exempt from the the ordinary laws of physics that govern the physical world.

By just this point, he concedes that for a complete account of human mentality, we need another and entirely different set of laws unrelated to (incommensurable with) the laws of physics. In other words, there are two forms of causation, meaning the universe is irreducibly of a dual nature. For all his talk about biology, Searle's "biological naturalism" is, at core, covertly dualist. Without invoking this non-material element, his entire project is nothing more than a series of unproven and non-explanatory claims about the nature of mind. Or the nature of consciousness, I don't mind.

9.3: That room.

Even though it has nothing to do with mental disorder, we can't leave this philosopher without mentioning his most famous paper, one of the most influential papers on philosophy of mind in the past fifty years. In answering No to the question "Can computers think?" Searle developed the "thought experiment" widely known as "the Chinese room" [5]. It's not long, anybody who has read this far should pause to read it. In briefest terms, it involves a person who doesn't speak Chinese sitting in a room with several baskets piled high with cards inscribed with Chinese ideograms, and a book of instructions in English. Monoglot Chinese outside the room write questions on cards and push them through a slot to the man inside, of whom they know nothing. He then consults his instruction book which tells him which of his cards to match to the incoming question, and pushes the answer out through the slot. While he knows the instruction book back to front and can quickly select the right card so the people outside will never know he doesn't understand anything they are asking, he will never learn a word of Chinese himself.

Searle's case is that while the monolingual man in the room knows how to manipulate the symbols into a grammatically correct sequence, or syntax, he doesn't know what they mean, i.e. he understands nothing of the semantics of what he is doing. That is, syntax and semantics, or meaning, are conceptually separate; mastering one does not guarantee competence in the other. Since computers operate solely according to the program, or syntax, for manipulating symbols, and never get to know what the symbols mean, therefore computers lack meaning, the critical element of human thinking. Therefore, and as we use the term, computers can't, and never can, think.

Needless to say, it is a controversial paper and, over forty years later, it still provokes intense debate although it seems the tide is slowly turning against Searle's strong position. Nonetheless, the question remains: is he right? On a number of grounds, my view is that he isn't, he has backed the wrong horse in the race. Firstly, as we know, he has no theory of mind that allows him to say that meaning can only arise in a biological system and not in silicon-based. He endorses naturalism; so what is special about the brain that allows it to grasp meaning that isn't available to computers? He doesn't say. I don't see his position as anything other than vitalism, the notion that there is something special about living material that sets it apart from non-living. Or from Descartes' stance, that humans have some extra mental element that animals don't. This is especially true as, in the early parts of that paper, he mocks AI workers who were sure that thinking machines were just around the corner:

> (My) refutation has nothing whatever to do with any particular stage of computer technology. It is important to emphasise this point because the temptation is always to think that the solution to our problems must wait on some as yet uncreated technological wonder [5, p670].

Now this is a bit alarming because when it comes to explaining how "… the mind is just a natural biological phenomenon in the world like any other" [p673], what does he invoke? That's right, "some as yet uncreated technological wonder." Biological sciences will ride to Searle's rescue whereas the physical/IT sciences can't even find the horse. This is promissory materialism which, in my view, is the weakest argument of all. Any explanatory account of the emergence and role of meaning in the human mind will immediately open the door to some bright spark writing a program that duplicates just that function, thereby gifting computers with yet another "inalienably" human attribute.

My second objection is with the structure of his Chinese room and the assertion that it contains nothing like meaning. This is similar to Skinner's claim that his experiments showed animals have nothing like intelligence when the reality was that he had simply moved the intelligence around so that they only seemed stupid. We do this all the time: we put people in mind-numbing environments like prisons and mental hospitals, then complain that the inmates are mindless. In fact, Searle's room with its inmate and his cards and booklet is not lacking meaning at all, it has simply gone out for lunch. The bilingual person who wrote the instruction book had full knowledge and understanding of Chinese and could match all possible incoming questions with all possible responses; obviously, he got bored and left it to an underling who didn't know Chinese to sit in the room but the underling didn't have to know what he was doing. He simply "borrowed" the writer's intellect and understanding of the meaning of Chinese characters and got on with the job. It's the same as when I speak: my tongue doesn't have to know what it's saying.

There is another example from the Australian Antarctic Expedition many years ago. One of the members developed appendicitis so, under telegraphed instructions from a surgeon in Australia, another member of the team operated and successfully removed it. The technician in Antarctica didn't know anything about surgery, but he didn't have to. As long as the surgeon thousands of kilometres away knew what was happening, all was well. Meaning is much like intellect or responsibility, it can be shifted around. We can hide it and play games with it (usually called practical jokes) but it doesn't go away. A chimp could be trained to sit in Searle's Chinese room and pass the test but it could never write the instruction book. Only a person who understood Chinese and English could do that, so Searle's whole system was *not* devoid of understanding. This point has been missed repeatedly over the years. People object to Searle's conclusion on the basis that "the whole system" understands the meaning of the questions but Searle is able to despatch those objections with ease. That is because they leave the intelligence out of the system. And computers are exactly the same. They don't have to understand what they're doing, any more than the frypan needs to know whether it's cooking eggs or sausages. In fact, computers that think they know what you want to write or try to answer your questions are fools of things, they never get it right. But one day, they will.

Next, Searle tries to trivialise the concept of computation:

> From a mathematical point of view, anything whatever can be described *as if* it were a digital computer. And that's because it can be described as instantiating or implementing a computer program. In an utterly trivial sense, the pen that is on the desk in front of me can be described as a digital computer. It just happens to have a very boring computer program. The program says: "Stay there." Now since in this sense, anything whatever is a digital computer, because anything whatever can be described as implementing a computer program... [p672].

Yes, it is forty years since this was written but it was wrong then and it's still wrong. The pen is not a computer because it does not compute, nor does it implement a program, just because implementing is an action. Pens lying on desks do not act. Computing to implement a program means to take some *informational* input (not a physical input) and manipulate it according to a predetermined calculus in order to to select a particular output from a range of possibilities. This is what the brain does, but it is not what a pen lying on a desk does, nor a brick lying on the ground, nor a wind turbine turning in the breeze, or a solar panel generating power, or a wall, or a photosynthesising leaf, or hepatocytes secreting bile, or a cell undergoing mitosis and so on through all his examples. Implementing a computational program is an act ('to implement' is a verb) and pens don't act (I just wish telephones didn't).

Finally, Searle's claim that there is no meaning in the system breaks down at the point where he says computers manipulate symbols. By definition, a symbol is a content-neutral, physical thing or item which represents or stands for something else, without itself being an example of that something else. The "something else" is what the symbol *means*. The separation between the neutral item and its meaning allows the symbol to be manipulated in place of the object it represents. This, as George Boole showed in 1854 [7], is the entire point of the dual-valued logic which lies at the heart of all computers.

This separation is the very essence of computation: some physical thing is converted into a symbol by the act of designating it as a surrogate for the object(s) to be computed. The item is then manipulated according to the predetermined calculus, aka program, to give an outcome, but computational processes are always content neutral, otherwise they couldn't be manipulated. At the end of the process, the symbol is converted back to whatever it represented and the answer communicated in some form. That is exactly what his Chinese room and its contents were doing, and it is exactly what humans do all day, every day. For example, if we want to distribute six apples among three people, we don't hand them around in trial and error, or try to divide apples into people, that's too messy. We strip the meanings from the symbols and divide one symbol by another. We then reassemble the conclusion with the meanings (apples and people) in the right place. But that's an extra step; Searle seems to believe it just happens in brains and can't possibly happen in digital computers.

Now the man in his Chinese room was unable to access the store of information which said what each symbol represented because the bilingual person who wrote the instruction booklet had gone to another job. All Searle did was "discover" that all computational processes are content neutral, or should I say "rediscover" Boole's astounding insight from 175 years ago, even though it was never lost. The difference between humans and his Chinese room is that we can't access our own computational processes, they are exceedingly fast, of the order of milliseconds. As a result, the final event of converting the symbols appears to us to be instantaneous, and it therefore seems that, for us, syntax is inseparable from semantics. But it isn't. They have to be separable, otherwise there could be no computation as we know it. So if we want a computer that can "understand the meaning" of a sentence, we actually have to design an extra step and build a computer which does just that. We haven't had them until quite recently, partly because we didn't need them (mindless computers did lots of drudge work) and partly because it's not that easy. But it's happening.

On this basis, Searle concluded that computers will never be able to think. My conclusion is that he is wrong in his argument. Meaning is not something inherent in or restricted to brains, either human or animal, it is simply an extra computational event. We will eventually be able to duplicate each and every step in the way of human mental functions but most likely we will never know the codes the brain uses. Thus, sometime in the future, if we ask the latest computer "Can you think?" it will answer "Sure I can, what do you think I am, an abacus?" And we still won't know.

9.4. Conclusion: Onward to the past.

In this very brief summary, I have not been able to convey the extent to which Searle ties himself in knots trying to explain a manifestly dualist experience in non-dualist terms. His account of intensionality and language, two central concepts in philosophy of mind, and thence of society, is tortuous and ultimately unsuccessful because he can't bring himself to admit that language and society function according to rules. Rules are information, and information is not matter or energy. Sure, information is *implemented* by matter and energy, but that doesn't mean they're the same thing. As information, rules are not bound by the laws of physics. I can make a rule today, and cancel it tomorrow but I can't cancel gravity quite so easily. Even though the mechanism of their implementation is, of course, entirely physical, rules exist and operate in a physics-free realm. The same problem arises in his prolix and admittedly futile attempt at a solution of the question of free will [4]. He insists it must be biological just because he has no model of mind that can account for it and can't accept the idea of unconscious causation.

The errors originate in his definition of "dualism," as something mysterious and immortal. Given that definition, he is always going to have trouble stomaching the idea that rules and language and intentionality aren't constrained by the laws of physics. I would too, that's why I use as my starting point Watson's definition of dualism, the idea that the universe contains two incommensurable orders of being that we must reconcile in order to make sense of our daily experience. The experience of pain is real, that's why we ban torture; for all his cleverness, Searle has not advanced our knowledge of pain one iota, but then nor has any other philosopher. Physiologists, of course, accept that even though they know a great deal about the *mechanisms* of pain, they will never explain the experience.

Why does Searle bother with these intellectual gymnastics? Again, we see the same commitment in Searle as in Chomsky and Dennett, an uncompromising antidualism, an unthinking adherence to the doctrine of Holy Positivism. Searle was quite scandalised to observe "... an odd thing has happened: dualism has gradually come to seem intellectually respectable again" [2, p170] as though it should be resisted by all right-thinking people. But the question he doesn't answer is this: Does excluding the supernatural exclude all possible forms of dualism? Can we conceive of some form of biologically-based dualism to be unified, causally-effective, limited to our lifespans, that gives us subjectivity, quality, intensionality and the experience of a unity of consciousness yet excludes the supernatural baggage of immortality and such whimsy as telepathy, telekinesis, precognition and so on? If he had posed his questions this way, he would have immediately seen that the answer is Yes, we certainly can conceive of such a dualism while remaining well within the limits imposed by a material universe. In fact, we already have such models. But, like the others of his generation, imbued in an uncompromising positivist hostility to anything remotely Cartesian, he couldn't see it.

Searle's generation were raised to believe that any reasonably educated person looking dispassionately at the question of mind must come to the Right Conclusion, that the universe has only one set of laws. Of course, that also means that anybody who didn't agree was either poorly-educated, dim-witted or wilfully blind, as philosopher David Oderberg commented rather bitterly some years ago:

> Dualism... persists in being more the object of ridicule than of serious rational engagement. It is held by the vast majority of philosophers be anything from (and not mutually exclusively) false, mysterious, and bizarre, to obscurantist, unintelligible, and/or dangerous to morals. Its adherents are assumed to be biased, scientifically ill-informed, motivated by prior theological dogma, cursed by metaphysical anachronism, and/or to have taken leave of their senses. Dualists who otherwise appear relatively sane in their philosophical writings are often treated with a certain benign, quasi-parental indulgence [8].

The older generation certainly believed they were dispassionate; as with all ideologues, the thought that they may be ideologues never occurred to them. For them, embracing dualism was not an error that could be corrected by further study but was a moral issue, an intellectual sin. But this was their generational scotoma, the blind spot they inherited from teachers fired by the scientism of John B Watson, Moritz Schlick and the other early positivists. Crude monism such as mind-brain identity theory failed; sophisticated monism such as functionalism failed; now Searle's biological naturalism, an artful monism that tries to preserve the valid parts of dualism, has also failed its objective.

So should we declare monism dead and buried, just as Watson tried to bury mentalism a hundred years ago? Before we pronounce the last rites, it would help to have a solid historical account of why an entire generation of thinkers were convinced that dualism necessarily means supernatural when, manifestly, it doesn't: the word 'dual' simply means two-fold, and it can apply equally to laws as to substances. It doesn't imply immortality. That would be a fascinating historical study but is outside the scope of this work, which is about theories in psychiatry.

So far, our search has not yielded a single hook on which to hang a theory or model of mental disorder that can be used to justify locking people up and forcing them to take drugs and ECT against their will. And despite their ideological clamour about having sorted out the mind-body problem, it's starting to look as though philosophers don't have any answers, either.

References

1. Searle JR (1999). *Mind, Language and Society: Doing philosophy in the real world*. London: Weidenfeld and Nicholson.

2. Searle JR (2007). Dualism revisited. *J Physiol Paris* 101: 169–178. doi:10.1016/j.jphysparis.2007.11.003

3. Searle JR (2000). Consciousness. Ann Rev *Neurosci*. 23:557-578 (March 2000) https://doi.org/10.1146/annurev.neuro.23.1.557

4. Searle JR (2001) Freewill as a problem in neurobiology. *Philosophy* 76: 491-515.

5. Searle JR (1983). Can computers think? From *Minds, Brains, and Science*, p28-41. Harvard University Press. Reprinted in Chalmers DJ (2002). *Philosophy of Mind: classical and contemporary readings*. Oxford: University Press, p669 (there are numerous versions of this argument, which first appeared in print as the lead article in a section with critical commentaries in *The Behavioral and Brain Sciences* (1980) 3:417-457).

6. Wiener N (1948, 1965). *Cybernetics, or contol and communication in the animal and the machine*. Cambridge, MA: MIT Press.

7. Boole, G. (1854). *An Investigation of the Laws of Thought, on which are Founded the Mathematical Theories of Logic and Probabilities*. Dover Classics of Science and Mathematics. New York: Dover (1958).

8. Oderberg DS (2005). Hylemorphic Dualism, in Paul EF, Miller FD, Paul J: *Personal Identity*. Cambridge: University Press.

10 Chalmers and Unreal Dualism

There is no idea so obscure that someone after having used it for a long time could not come to regard it as self-evident.

Leszek Kolakowski

10.1: Dualism just won't die.

After a century of effort, the goal of writing the mentality out of mental events isn't showing much progress. Some, in fact, may say it is the wrong research program, that it can never succeed, that the research effort is wasted [1]. However, approaching the end of what turned out to be an unproductive career, very few academics would look back and say, "Hmm, seems as though I backed the wrong horse. I'd better tell my students to drop my project." That doesn't happen. Always, the response to an unproductive program is "Get more money to try again and try harder, blame your opponents but never give in." Radical change does happen but, as Thomas Kuhn noted, it usually comes from newcomers to the field or from researchers working outside the mainstream.

A generation ago, a newcomer dared to suggest that philosophers of mind needed to give up their obsession with a physicalist account of mind, and put their efforts into reassessing dualism. In his PhD thesis, David Chalmers, then a young graduate in mathematics and philosophy, argued that dualism does not necessarily mean magical thinking. We can give an account, he said, of consciousness as a natural outcome of the brain's structure and function while avoiding the trap of supernatural substances. Expanding on his thesis in *The Conscious Mind: In Search of a Fundamental Theory,* from 1996 [2], Chalmers meticulously analysed the means by which consciousness could supervene upon the physical structure of the brain. Since then, the field of consciousness studies has acquired a momentum of its own, with university centres, journals, conferences and so on. A lot of it is centred around Chalmers himself, who has been instrumental in its growth. His most recent work, released a few months ago, is a shift of emphasis. In *Reality+: Virtual Worlds and the Problems of Philosophy* [3], he explores a central concept in any consideration of consciousness, the relationship of humans as sentient beings to the universe in which we live.

It has to be understood that his later work is somewhat tangential to the goal of this section, which is to examine different philosophies of mind as a means of approaching mental disorder. In the first place, Chalmers doesn't offer a ready-made philosophy of mind. At numerous points in both of these books, in total about 850 pages of fairly densely-argued text, he is quite clear that delineating the essential features of a natural dualism is a work in progress:

> Conscious experience is a part of the natural world, and like other natural phenomena it cries out for explanation ... Currently it may be hard to see what such a theory (of consciousness) would be like, but without such a theory we could not be said to fully understand consciousness [2, p5] ... it is clearly premature to worry about untestability (of theories) before we have even a single theory that can handle the phenomena (of consciousness) in a remotely satisfactory way [2, p218] ... these questions show(s) just how far these sketchy ideas are from being a true theory [2, p309].

That is, his "sketchy ideas" don't and probably can't form the basis of a theory of mind leading to a model of mental disorder. Second, he doesn't address other central concepts in psychiatry and psychology such as personality. He hardly ever mentions mental disorder and says nothing about its possible causes. On the subject of mental disorder he is neutral, so psychiatrists who look to Chalmers for a settlement of the nature-nurture argument will be disappointed. However, until the preliminaries to a dualist theory of mind are settled, there can't be any progress on that particular question. So what does he say? First thing to note, he uses the word "consciousness" where I and others use the word "mind." My training was medical: to me, the term "conscious state" more or less equates with the biological term 'arousal,' meaning the level of alertness, which ranges from over-alert (over-aroused) to alert and down to drowsy, stuporose and comatose. Also, a theory of consciousness does not imply an explanation of what, following Freud, we call the unconscious mind. And, of course, "mind" is much easier to type.

Chalmers splits the full range of mental functions in two, into what he calls psychological consciousness and phenomenal consciousness. The former means the cognitive or knowing functions of the mind, the processes by which we learn what is going on around us, and make and effect decisions. It represents the informational state that allows us to survive and prosper in a dangerous world. The other part, phenomenal consciousness, is the sense that there is something to being alive, something out there and something in here, a sense, we believe, that rocks and dead people don't have. It includes all the sensory input and experiences such as vision, sound, pain, etc, and the inner emotional state:

> On the phenomenal concept, mind is characterised by the way it *feels*; on the psychological concept, mind is characterised by what it *does* [2, p11].

This split allows him to dispense with some of the opposition. Functionalism concerns itself only with the mind as a knower and doer, not as a feeler. As we saw with Dennett (Ch. 8), functionalism tries to write the mind *qua* feeling agency out of the equation. Pain, Dennett snorted, is "…a brief, negatively-signed experience… of vanishing moral significance," far too insignificant to warrant the term "suffering." But, Chalmers emphasises, as it's still an experience that we need to explain, it can't and won't be explained away and we shouldn't try. Further, the psychological part of the mind doesn't hold any mysteries for us. We have very good models of non-magical computational processes that can mimic or even improve on human knowledge and decision-making abilities. The knowledge functions are, he says, the easy bit of the problem of mind; the rest, giving a natural or non-magical and non-circular account of phenomenal experience, is the sticky bit, or what he terms the "hard problem of consciousness." His work is directed at providing a logical basis for such explanations.

And this is an important point: Chalmers is not offering an empirical account of mind, as Dennett and others try to do. They have the easy task, of coming up with some sort of explanation of the mind as a biological calculator, which is why their work is so heavily larded with biological material. Do we, as humans, compute? Sure we do. Just now, I reached for my cup. In an instant, I had to assess its direction and distance and send signals to my arm to reach out just that distance and direction, no more and no less, and grip the handle with just the right pressure, then lift it without looking at it to my mouth. All that is computation, in the broadest sense of the term (see Chap. 8, S.8.4). But I was not aware of any of the processes by which I made that decision or implemented it, it arrived without any effort on my part. And that's true of all decisions we make, including language as we speak it. This is why Dennett, for example, is so confident that his is the "best scientific theory" of mind: he only tackled the easy or computational bit, the bit most amenable to a "scientific" analysis. For Chalmers, reductionism works fine on the psychological or computational mind but it can't work on experience:

> Whether or not consciousness is a biochemical structure, that is not what "consciousness" *means*. To analyse consciousness that way again trivialises the explanatory problem by changing the subject. It seems that the concept of consciousness is irreducible, being characterisable only in terms of concepts that themselves involve consciousness ... There is no way for an entailment from physical facts to consciousness to get off the ground ... Why should all this (brain) structure and function give rise to experience? The story about the physical processes does not say [2, p106-7].

As a result, Chalmers shoulders the problem of showing a valid process by which the experience of phenomenal consciousness can arise in the physical brain without being either magic or a "mere physical matter," i.e.explaining the hard problem of consciousness. Quite a problem.

10.2. Chalmers' dualist case.

Moving by tightly-argued steps, Chalmers builds his case on a device widely-used in logic, conceivability or logical possibility, generally understood as "logically-possible worlds." Take two examples he uses: a flying telephone is conceivable and is therefore logically possible, if impractical, whereas a male vixen is contradictory. There is no logically possible world in which such a creature could exist [2, p35]. Similarly, a mile-high unicycle is logically possible as is, he argues, a living, breathing, functioning human being indistinguishable from the rest of us but who has no inner mental life whatsoever. This is the notion of a zombie, a person whose head is not just dark, as ours is when we close our eyes, but is ... nothing [2, p95]:

> For philosophers, a zombie is a system that outwardly behaves much like a conscious being, but which inwardly has no conscious experience at all... As far as I can tell, there's no contradiction in the idea that there could be a physical structure that's atom-for-atom identical to Donald Trump and is not conscious [3, p275, 285].

It is not, he says, inherently contradictory to talk of an outwardly normal human being with no inner sense or awareness at all. This opens an explanatory gap between the physical state and the mental state which must be bridged. To summarise his work in one sentence, Chalmers fills that gap by arguing that consciousness supervenes upon the physical structure and function of the brain by a set of natural psychophysical laws that, in time, we can understand. This means, of course, that we could eventually build a silicon-based computer model of the brain which would be conscious in the ordinary sense of the word. I believe he is correct in his conclusions but will argue that he uses entirely the wrong case to reach them; that his case goes nowhere except to give physicalists something to laugh at.

Zombies have a high profile in his work [2,3,4], including what he calls his "zombie twin":

> This creature is molecule for molecule identical to me, and identical in all the low level properties postulated by a completed physics, but he lacks conscious experience entirely... (... I have grown quite fond of my zombie twin) ... He will be psychologically identical to me... he will be awake, able to report the contents of his internal states, able to focus attention in various places... none of this functioning will be accompanied by any real conscious experience ... no phenomenal feel. There is nothing it is like to be a zombie ... I confess that the logical possibility of zombies seems equally obvious to me.... I can discern no contradiction in the description ... (It) comes down to a brute intuition [2, p94-96; note that "psychologically identical" means only behaviorally identical].

Zombies had a starring role in *Conscious Mind* in 1996 and were reprised in *Reality+* in 2022. Their role is to show that consciousness supervenes naturally but not logically upon the physical reality of the human body and brain. Without this notion, it would be fair to say his argument would be critically weakened. But we have to be very careful of this type of argument because what are called logically possible worlds aren't the real world at all. For example, a world which runs on perpetual motion machines is logically possible even though thermo-dynamically impossible, so what good comes from making the case?

Consider another logical possibility: Mr Smith can be alive, or the same Mr Smith can be dead. In the ordinary run of things, we would say he can be alive or dead but he can't be both alive and dead at the same time. However, in the realm of logic, Mr Smith is either dead, or he is alive, or he is both. That's what the disjunctive operator of logic means: logical possibility does not translate to or equate with an equivalent status in the material universe we occupy. To rephrase that, the set of real people who are simultaneously dead and alive is necessarily empty, it is a logical fiction, a conceptual space in the informational realm that has no counterpart, and can never be filled, in reality. Its bearing on reality is thus moot and convincing only to the impressionable (and don't mention Schrödinger's cat).

Now Chalmers has spent thirty years or more dreaming of zombies and doesn't see anything inherently contradictory in the idea. By the same token, as described in his Meditation III, Descartes spent just as many years thinking about God and didn't see anything contradictory in the idea. He spelled this out in his *Principles of Philosophy*:

> XIV: When the mind afterwards reviews the different ideas that are in it, it discovers what is by far the chief among them--that of a Being omniscient, all-powerful, and absolutely perfect; and it observes that in this idea there is contained not only possible and contingent existence, as in the ideas of all other things which it clearly perceives, but existence absolutely necessary and eternal. And just as because, for example, the equality of its three angles to two right angles is necessarily comprised in the idea of a triangle, the mind is firmly persuaded that the three angles of a triangle are equal to two right angles; so, from its perceiving necessary and eternal existence to be comprised in the idea which it has of an all-perfect Being, it ought manifestly to conclude that this all-perfect Being exists.

> XV: ...the idea of an all-perfect Being has not been framed by itself, and that it does not represent a chimera, but a true and immutable nature, which must exist since it can only be conceived as necessarily existing [5].

The fact that somebody, somewhere, can conceive of something, even become quite fond of the idea, proves nothing apart from our capacity to believe what we want to believe, as the Polish philosopher, Leszek Kolakowski, noted: "There is no idea so obscure that someone, after having used it for a long time, could not come to regard it as self-evident" [6, p183]. For me, the idea of zombies is hollow, a desperate clutching at logical straws that proves nothing about how our mental life arises—a skyhook, in other words. Consider this: if little zombies (zomboids?) don't hear, how do they learn to speak? Chalmers could say: "They learn to speak full sentences the same way you are able to mimic, unconsciously." But mimicking is an action, not an experience; parrots mimic but they don't understand, so it fails his test.

Perhaps his zombies function at an entirely mechanical level, as we do in many respects, e.g. I can walk beside you, deep in conversation, and not pay any attention to my feet, which keep working without conscious interference. But that's an artefact as we are constantly attending to the different tasks yet not recording those checks in memory. In any event, his is a theory of consciousness, not of the unconscious.

As for identi-Trump, yes, there could be a perfect reconstruction of any human with no conscious experience; there's just the small matter that it would be dead. If it could talk and move, then the brain must be functioning, and if the brain were functioning, it would reproduce conscious Don't recawareness unless there were blocks to prevent this, in which case it wouldn't be identical. A physically identical brain without conscious experience must be non-functional, aka dead (also, talking about a Trump with no mental activity is verging on poor taste). Or: why do zombies breed? We know why worms and fish and cattle breed, it's all to do with chemicals but humans? That's all to do with sensation, and zombies don't have sensation so they're not identical to us and would probably die out rather quickly.

If, instead, their numbers were kept up by regular mutations then they're *ipso facto* not identical. Also: if they have no sensation, operations would be very simple. No anaesthetic, all they may need is a muscle blocker to stop reflex responses to painful stimuli and they would be fine. For many major operations, they would be fully alert and able to talk and laugh with the surgeon. But that also shows they aren't identical. The idea of a zombie "molecule for molecule identical" to a human being is logically impossible, as inherently contradictory as a male vixen. The whole concept is a fantasy, pure magical thinking, and the source of the error is easy to see. Chalmers tells us himself: "I can discern *no contradiction* in the description (of a zombie)" (emphasis added).

All languages use sentence structure in one form or another. English uses the form Subject - Verb - Object - Extension, as in: "Mary saw Tom riding his bike." All meaningful sentences in English use this form or its many variations. "Meaningful" means only that the audience can form in their minds a facsimile of that part of the speaker's mental state which he intends to convey. The spoken words are a coded signal to anybody who knows the code (in this case, English) just which mental state to recreate. But the fact that slots exist in the sentence format to insert a word doesn't guarantee that the ensuing sentence makes sense, i.e. that it can be used to create a facsimile of the speaker's mental state in the audience's heads. Chomsky showed this with his well-known nonsense sentence:

> Colourless green ideas sleep furiously.

This is a sentence of the S-V-O-E form but it is full of contradictions and thus cannot generate anything like a rational picture in the minds of the audience. People are left scratching their heads, saying "But what does it mean?" Nothing. It has the form of a sentence but it cannot generate a facsimile of the speaker's mental state, so it conveys no meaning. This is also true of Chalmers' statement:

> There is nothing it is like to be a zombie ... I confess that the logical possibility of zombies seems equally obvious to me.... I can discern no contradiction in the description ... (It) comes down to a brute intuition.

All he is saying here is that there is nothing inherently contradictory in the sentence "Zombies are human in form but inhuman in that they have no mental content." That is true only in the sense that colorless green ideas do indeed sleep furiously because if the complete human form is there, the mental content will also be there. He also says his zombie twin is "able to report the contents of his internal states," even though, by definition, twin zombie doesn't have internal states. There is the contradiction: a zombie with identical behaviour must be able to report mental events of which it has no knowledge or experience. Chalmers' "brute intuition" that this is *not* contradictory is insufficient foundation to build a theory of mind. There are plenty of highly intelligent people, such as the late Sir John Eccles [7, p555], who intuitively believe in an immortal soul. Eccles would say: "I confess that the logical possibility of life after death seems equally obvious to me ... I can discern no contradiction in the description ... (It) comes down to a brute intuition" (his coauthor, Sir Karl Popper, retorted: "I find the thought of eternal life quite frightening").

So until Chalmers shows that his brute intuition isn't just a skyhook, a quick wave of his magic wand, we don't need to be convinced by his model. I'm not. I think "logical possibilities" in "other worlds" are not enough for a model of mental disorder as they open the door to the fantastic. If we open the door to zombies, then possession states will barge through. I'm interested in the practical realities in this world, not impractical possibilities in make-believe worlds. Nonetheless, I believe he reached the correct conclusion, that the human mind (OK, consciousness) is an irreducibly non-material but causally-effective entity that supervenes naturally upon (emerges from) the brain's structure and function. In all species. Next questions: How? How does it arise, by what mechanism; in what medium does it operate to do what it does; how does information get in and out; how does it interact with the material brain? As an exercise in logic, entirely divorced from the brain, Chalmers' approach cannot and does not attempt to answer these critical points. He cannot say *how* it happens, only *that* it happens, which we all know anyway.

10.3. Choose your reality ...

Chalmers' latest work, *Reality+: Virtual worlds and the problems of philosophy* [3], has been received with rapturous delight. Various reviewers quoted on the back cover called it "A stunning achievement... A gripping book... A treasure trove... wild, profound, and playful... A mind-bending journey... Cleverly disguised as light reading... " Thus forearmed, readers probably settle down for an entertaining and educational excursion through some rather arcane matters.

The book probes a range of the most difficult questions in philosophy in the author's style of teasing out all imaginable and a few unimaginable consequences of every minute point in the argument, pursuing them to the end or noting when any of them are left hanging. However, this creates difficulties in summarising it as its 24 chapters cover an enormous range, so it has to be read carefully to appreciate its reach and complexity. The Introduction states:

Reality exists, independently of us. The truth matters. There are truths about reality, and we can try to find them. Even in an age of multiple realities, I still believe in objective reality [3, pxxiv] [8].

Using well-known arguments from philosophy, he explores the current and potential technology of computer games and IT-generated virtual reality to illustrate his primary claim: "The central thesis of this book is: *Virtual reality is genuine reality.* Or, at least, *virtual realities are genuine realities*" [pxvii]. That changes a little because late in the book he says: "My primary aim in this book is to argue against global skepticism about the external world" [p444]. Now we can all agree that defining real and reality is not easy and Chalmers devotes the better part of Ch. 6 to answering the question: "What is reality?" He mentions author Phillip Dick's notion that reality is whatever doesn't go away when you stop believing in it. Perhaps because of my medical background, I've always thought of reality as anchored by whatever hurts. Chalmers isolates five ways of thinking about reality: Reality as existence; as causal power; as mind-independence; as non-illusoriness (sic); and as genuineness.

- Existence: Pres. Joe Biden exists, Santa Claus doesn't. This seems fairly straight-forward but there are plenty of borderline cases, some of which he addresses in the text.

- Causal power: This notion goes back a long way. Anything that has the power to make a difference in the real world is itself real. Again, Mr Biden has actual power to move a cup on his desk or to launch an invasion whereas, and despite rumours, Santa Claus isn't able to rattle a single roof tile.

- Mind-independence: The Earth existed long before there were humans and it will continue to exist long after we have disappeared; dinosaurs were real even though only fossils remain. What humans know or claim to know is one thing but what *is* is something else again.

- Non-illusoriness: There needs to be a correspondence between the way things are and the way we understand and perceive them to be since, as Descartes made so clear, we can be misled.

---

8   In the remainder of this chapter, unless otherwise stated, all references are to *Reality+*, Reference 3.

- Genuineness: Chalmers defers to the British philosopher, JL Austin, who emphasised that philosophy must take account of the way words are used. This points to the difference between something existing and whether it is actually an example of what it purports to be, an issue when out shopping: Yes, I can see the watch you are trying to sell me for $5.00 is real but is it a real Rolex? [p108-114]

This list probably pins down most of what we intend when we talk about something being real, and thence of reality, and excludes most of what we would like to exclude. Using this account of reality, Chalmers then argues that a virtual cat is indeed a genuine cat. Virtual cats are "...digital objects, grounded in digital processes in a computer, but they're no less real for that" [p115]. "Virtual kittens are digital entities realised in silicon technology. Still, virtual kittens are perfectly real, just as robot kittens are real" [p200]. A virtual cat has causal powers in that it grows new fur, can push a virtual ball (itself a digital object) and produces experiences in anybody who looks at it. It exists independently as a digital object in a computer whether the machine is switched on or off, or even if nobody knows it's in the computer's memory. A virtual cat is as it seems to be, a furry, purring critter that isn't a dragon, even though it isn't real in the sense that a virtual library or a virtual calculator are real [p200]. (Fig. 28 on p200 illustrates the difference between a biological cat, a robotic cat and a virtual cat, but not the difference between a virtual cat and a virtual book). With this, he moves to a more adventurous position that may trouble some (older) readers:

> Simulation and VR (virtual reality) technologies have advanced fast, and it isn't hard to see a path to full-scale simulated worlds in which some people could spend a lifetime [p55] ... if Earth becomes dangerously degraded ... VR can offer a safe haven... But within limits, a move to virtual worlds need be no more escapist than emigration ... In the long term, virtual worlds may have most of what is good about the nonvirtual world. Given all the ways in which virtual worlds may surpass the nonvirtual world, life in virtual worlds will often be the right life to choose [p321-30] ... life in virtual worlds in the long term may approach or exceed the quality of life in nonvirtual worlds [p361].

All this is true but, no matter how sharp its simulated claws, a virtual cat will never draw real blood. When he says "virtual kittens are perfectly real," he is splitting reality in unexpected ways, much the same as we say a rainbow is a "real thing" but not the same kind of real thing as, say, the crafty birds raiding my fruit trees. Similarly, a virtual banquet will have no effect on your waistline so eat, drink, be merry, for tomorrow you waste away. Why, then, does Chalmers insist that virtual reality is genuine reality? His answer comes a little later in the book when he essays an answer to the question "What is reality?" (Ch. 6):

> *Virtual things are not real* is the standard line on virtual reality. I think it's wrong. Virtual reality is real—that is, the entities in virtual reality really exist. My view is a sort of *virtual realism* ... the thesis that virtual reality is genuine reality ... virtual objects are real and not an illusion ... objects in virtual reality are digital objects—roughly speaking, structures of binary information, or bits ... (In) more familiar virtual reality technologies ... virtual worlds and objects are real [p105-107].

All that is lacking is some account of the nature of information, say information about a cat, how it is coded in computers and projected to influence the human mind in order to generate an experience that, to all intents, looks remarkably like any other cat. Chapter 8, "Is the universe made of information?" addresses this critical concept. After a few preliminary pages, readers are introduced to "a wonderful thing for a philosopher," the powerful new metaphysical idea that "...everything in the physical world around us—tables and chairs, stars and planets, dogs and cats, electrons and quarks—is made of patterns of bits" [p148]. After a few more pages on the history of metaphysics, he introduces the concept of information, albeit at a basic level, and quickly concludes "Information is physical" [p156]. This is soon qualified: "Information is physical—or, at least, structural information can be physically embodied." A drawing of a punch card from last century [Fig. 22, p153] illustrates this point.

After further description by way of Babbage, Leibniz and Pascal, he concludes: "By grounding the structure of bits in the structure of its, the abstract mathematical power of computation is harnessed in a physical system" [p158]. This, of course, is the essence of machine-based computation but there is no indication as to the brain mechanism by which this comes about. In particular, even though he had mentioned Claude Shannon's early contribution, the basis of computation in *physically-embodied logical processes* is not mentioned.

However, in an earlier and widely-quoted publication from 2012 [8], Chalmers had elaborated on the theoretical mechanisms involved. In that paper, he outlined a response to two critical questions:

> What are the conditions under which a physical system implements a given computation? ... Once a theory of implementation has been provided, we can use it to answer the second key question: What is the relationship between computation and cognition?

He answered the questions by degrees. The first question, he proposed, is satisfied as follows: "A physical system implements a given computation when the causal structure of the physical system mirrors the formal structure of the computation." However, the chapter on information in *Reality* + does not rely on this and therefore drifts into the startling idea of the universe as pure information, "... a little like software without hardware—as if Microsoft Word were running without any computer for it to run on." This idea, he concedes, "isn't easy to grasp at first" [3, p165] and the concept "... may not be a scientific hypothesis, since we can never obtain evidence for or against it" [3, p162]. Nonetheless, Chapter 8, "Is the universe made of information?" ends on an optimistic note:

> Ultimately, the it-from-bit view will serve as a sort of step ladder that we can kick away. What matters most is not the bits per se but the underlying structuralism on which reality can be fully described in mathematical terms. But the it-from-bit view provides a wonderful illustration of this structuralist idea, and it also provides a clean bridge to the simulation hypothesis [p166].

The relationship between computation and cognition is of central importance in all this work but, in the absence of a theory of mind and, in particular, the absence of a mechanism by which mentality is implemented in a computational structure, it cannot be developed. Indeed, the suggestion that there could be computation without a formal mechanism, "software without hardware," seems to indicate that the actual mechanism is of no importance, i.e. the exact opposite of what he had said in 2015, about the "physical system mirror(ing) the formal structure of the computation." While it implies that paranormal phenomena (telekinesis, telepathy, etc) are real, he uses the move to open a pathway to an idea beloved of scifi writers and gamers, the notion that the informational content of the brain could somehow be uploaded to digital computers. This would recreate the same conscious experience as "a sort of immortality … (in) a sort of heaven where people can live forever" [p276]. The notion is reprised while examining how technology extends the mind:

> A final step in extending the mind might come when our minds are uploaded from our brain to a computer… We'll exist on computers, and our "internal" processes will be able to link to external systems as easily as any two computers can link to each other [p301].

As a matter of technology, this is a very, very long way in the future, if ever. Conceptually, one would have thought that formal theories of mind and of information would be *sine qua non* of such procedures. Nonetheless, the book concludes on a somewhat more grounded basis:

> It's an open question how much we can know about reality… We don't know how much of reality is accessible and how much is inaccessible. But the truth is out there, and we can know some of it [p462].

Which, after the peregrinations through some of the more febrile edges of human creativity, takes us back more or less to where we started in the Introduction. Plus ça change, plus c'est la même chose.

10.4. … but reality is as reality does.

Readers may ask: "But what has this to do with mental disorder?" The answer is, of course, nothing, but mental disorder often leads to quite profound disturbances of the sense of reality, so the topic is of some interest. As "Adventures in technophilosophy" (the title to the Introduction), this book does not address mental disorder [9] as a field of enquiry in its own right, so it has nothing new to tell a reasonably sensitive psychologist or psychiatrist. The only question is: Can its "wild, profound and playful" ideas be developed to the point where they contribute to our understanding of the nature and phenomena of mental disorder? The short answer is "Most assuredly not," so readers interested in mental disorder may prefer to turn to the next chapter. The longer answer requires some background.

---

9   The reference to schizophrenia on p218 is incorrect: the definition of a hallucination is that it is taken as a veridical percept; on p455, we find the same mistake but the section is garbled and inconclusive.

Based entirely on the material in this book, it appears that, since the age of ten, Prof. Chalmers has spent a substantial part of his life playing computer games or otherwise involved with computers, reading science fiction and fantasy novels, watching science fiction films and talking science fiction. I don't do any of those things because they're boringly predictable, mostly badly written and don't tell us about the human condition (apart from reinforcing how violent *H sapiens* are, which, after a lifetime of dealing with mental casualties, I don't need to be told again). I think that qualifies me to review a book about science fiction, computer games and so on, as in: "Go ahead, see if you can convince me."

For a book on problems of philosophy, this is unusual as, liberally scattered throughout its 500 or so pages of text, are dozens of definitions, snippets of history or lengthy descriptions which appear to assume that the reader knows little or no philosophy. However, the intricacy of the material is such that there would be few people without training in philosophy who could comfortably follow his case. More to the point, because the writing style is "cleverly disguised as light reading" (meaning superficially non-technical), the uninitiated are likely to believe they have grasped the matter with ease. The Introduction leaves no doubt that nephytes are his intended audience:

> By the end of this book, you'll have been introduced to many of the central questions in philosophy ... By the end, you'll have a sense of some of the historical and contemporary landscape of philosophy ... The best way I know to introduce philosophy is to *do* philosophy ... So even if you're an old hand at philosophy, I hope you'll find rewards here [pxxii].

By replacing philosophy in that quote with any other topic such as geology or botany, it will be clear that this is the standard introduction to any elementary text: he actually says it is "to introduce philosophy" and suspects a few "old hand(s) at philosophy" may sneak a look. With its jaunty style coupled with the many "amazing illustrations" [p465], and the relentless preoccupation with science fiction and computer games, it could almost pass as a book to entice precocious 14 year olds into believing they have nailed some of the most contentious themes in human thought. The trouble is, anybody who needs definitions such as philosophy [pxvi], skepticism [p45], binary codes [p146], metaphysics [p148], information [p152], structuralism [p175], value [p315], scientific realism [p402-6], and many other basic topics, will not be in a position to assess critically the theme of the book (whether virtual reality is indeed genuine reality), or to detect its errors. But let's assume a bright 14 year old with a preoccupation with science fiction and computer games picks up the book and starts reading. What will happen?

The first point that such a reader will not realise is that the expression on the cover of the book, "virtual worlds," is nebulous. Apart from some tendentious description on p14, the word 'virtual' and its cognates, nonvirtual and virtual reality, which appear 98 times in the introduction, 105 times in the first short chapter, and up to twenty times a page in the text, are undefined. Early in the introduction [pxii], we read: "Virtual reality involves an immersive, interactive, computer-generated space," but this is a description, not a definition, as in: "Murder involves an assailant and a dead body." This leaves readers to apply their own meanings, to assume that they and Chalmers are in agreement. For such complex matters, this is a significant shortcoming. For myself, I follow the dictionary definition, in which virtual means "almost or nearly as described, but not completely or according to strict definition; a semblance." Virtual reality thus means "almost or nearly real, a semblance of reality," the inevitable implication being "...but not completely real." That is, Chalmers sets himself the task of proving true something the dictionary says is not true. The burden of proof rests with the author; it is up to the reader to judge his performance but I don't believe unsophisticated readers will be aware of this.

The second trap for unwary players seeking a "wild, profound, playful and mind-bending journey cleverly disguised as light reading" is the fact that mind is not defined, nor is there any reference to an articulated model of mind that would provide the sort of intellectual structure that "old hands at philosophy" could reasonably expect. It is not until quite late in the book that he makes this explicit:

> Why is there consciousness in the universe? How do physical processes give rise to consciousness? How can there be subjective experience in an objective world? Right now, no one knows the answers to these questions [p278].

It would have been better to have stated this at the outset, something like:

> By the end of this book, you'll have been introduced to many of the central questions in philosophy but readers should be

> warned: even though we're talking philosophy, and philosophy is very largely about the mind or consciousness, I do not have a theory of mind to offer as a foundation for all that follows. Essentially, the whole of this book has no basis in a published philosophical theory. That puts it in the realm of supposition so if that's your interest, enjoy. All you boring people might prefer to do the crossword.

Third pitfall, which I suspect many people trained in philosophy and IT will not recognise, is that there is no theory of information. For a work that depends utterly on information technology as its *raison d'être*, this is more or less fatal. At different times, Chalmers hints at a formal account but these are brief and not expanded to the point where they could "provide a clean bridge" between mind and artificial realities. We will come back to this in discussing his Chapter 8, "Is the universe made of information?"

The fourth and last caveat is that these are not accidental omissions. The book has four tightly interwoven themes, three overt and one covert: philosophy, IT, science fiction, and, lurking in the shadows thrown by the breezy prose, religion. It doesn't use science fiction themes to illustrate and expand on ancient questions of philosophy, nor does it use philosophy to penetrate the mysteries of IT. Instead, it uses philosophical analysis, in which the author is very well qualified, to reinterpret persistent scifi memes in IT language, thereby giving some ancient religious ideas an ersatz credibility, a new lease of life, as it were, in this age of declining religiosity. Concepts—perhaps we should call them memes—such as creation, morality, immortality, rapture, resurrection, magic and the godhead recur repeatedly. However, instead of being authorised by some holy book or messiah, they are situated in and justified by a materialist concept of the universe, with the gaps filled in by imagination. In one brief sentence, this book is a digital translation of all things religious. For a self-professed atheist [p125, 144], this is somewhat unexpected but we press on.

There are seven sections to the book addressing central issues in philosophy. Each chapter is built around the question in its title, some of which can't be answered, and most start with a story from a novel, game or film. In case the ideas aren't clear, there are lots of "amazing" (read: elementary) pictures to illustrate points in the text, pictures which even bright teenagers would probably find pointless and irritating: do we really need a picture of a punchcard? We will answer this in due course. Part 1 sets out his basic case by launching readers into *Virtual Worlds*, unfortunately undefined, through the portal of Chapter 1 which asks: *Is this the real life?* Via some age-old myths, it raises "... three key questions about virtual worlds ... Can we know whether or not we're in a virtual world? ... Are virtual worlds real or illusory?... Can you lead a good life in a virtual world?" [p9]. These are, of course, ancient questions recast in modern guise; all that remains is whether our modern perception of the universe can add anything to the great thinkers of the past.

Question 1, *Are we virtual beings in a virtual world?* is answered in short order: We don't know and we can never know. Unless, of course, the superior beings who are running the show decide to reveal themselves. Until then, we also can't be sure we're not in a virtual world but, he warns, "... we should take seriously the possibility that we *are* in a virtual world" [p10-11]. At this point, some readers may be tempted to give up on the basis that, whatever the nature of this world, this is the one we live in and we need to deal with it before we blow it up or cook it. The rest of the chapter offers a justification of the next 480 pages. His position is clear: "My guess is that within a century, we will have virtual realities that are indistinguishable from the nonvirtual world" (note that at this early stage, the expression "real world" has morphed into "nonvirtual world," because Chalmers' case is that virtual is also real).

Chapter 2 ventures an answer to *What is the simulation hypothesis?* Even though simulation is defined ostensively, his version of the simulation hypothesis is "We are and always have been in an artificially designed computer simulation of a world" [p29]. He concedes that this claim is irrefutable and therefore non-scientific because every bit of evidence for or against the hypothesis could itself be simulated. Again, a decision point for the reader: Do I discard the book or press on with an irrefutable idea? We press on, curious to know how the author justifies the assertion in the last paragraph, that "... *virtual reality is genuine reality.*"

Chapter 3, *Do we know things?* introduces Part 2, *Knowledge.* This is the field of epistemology, in which Chalmers is very well-versed. His question leads to a discussion of skepticism, "the view that nobody knows anything" [p45], of which the best-known version was elaborated nearly 400 years ago by René Descartes (1596-1650). In his *Discourse on the Method*, published in 1637, Descartes, who was very widely-read, described how, in his youth, he had determined to pursue truth by studying the great books. Slowly he realised that, if it existed, truth wasn't in any of the books he had read (and he had read them all) as, for every opinion expressed so eloquently in one book, he could go to another and find exactly the opposite opinion. As a result, as soon as he had graduated, he resolved to give up on the classics and to trust only what he could see in the world or decide himself. He made this clear in Article 1 of *The Passions of the Soul*:

> There is nothing more clearly evinces the learning which we receive from the Ancients to be defective, than what they have written concerning the passions... Yet what the Ancients have taught concerning them, is so little, and for the most part so little credible that I cannot hope to approach truth, except by keeping away from the paths they followed [9].

This led him to his famous position of doubt, elaborated in his *Meditations on First Philosophy*, from 1641, that we can easily be fooled by our senses, that memory is notoriously untrustworthy and that one person's truth is another's fantasy. His solution was to apply systematic doubt to everything he knew and see what was left. In fact, three things were left: God, the material world, and the certainty that if he could ask "Do I exist?" then, by the very question, he had established that he does. As Chalmers points out, that was the easy bit: "How do we get from knowledge of ourselves and our own minds to knowledge of the external world?" [p60].

Chapter 4 continues by asking *Can we prove there is an external world?* Echoing Descartes, the short answer is: No, the whole thing could be a simulation: "Once simulations become a serious possibility... our commonsense views about the external world are thrown into question" [p80]. This raises two important points, one epistemological and one moral. The former is that I, for one, do not take the simulation hypothesis as "a serious possibility." It's just another creation myth larded with talk of computers and so on, which converts it from a matter of faith into an intellectual game of no consequence. We will consider the moral question later in the chapter. Meantime, Chapter 5, asks: *Is it likely that we're in a simulation?* By some statistical legerdemain, including, for the numerically challenged, a picture to illustrate the ratio 100:1 [Fig 14, p82] , he concludes: "... we cannot know we are not in a simulation." It isn't clear how that is supposed to change anything but it ends Part 2, *Knowledge*.

Part 3, *Reality*, opens with Chapter 6 asking *What is reality?* Answer: "Virtual reality is real—that is, the entities in virtual reality really exist ... virtual objects are real and not an illusion" [p105-6]. On p200, he takes this point further:

> When I see Barack Obama on TV, I'm really seeing *Barack Obama* ... When I see Pac-Man on the screen, I'm really seeing Pac-Man. The screen enables me to see him.

This is not self-evident. As mentioned in S.10.3, Chalmers gives five ways of thinking of reality: Reality as existence; as causal power; as mind-independence; as non-illusoriness; and as genuineness [p108-114]. After a great deal of roundabout talk, we learn that reality is pretty much what we have come to expect it to be. The fact that we can talk about "simulated reality" indicates that we have a good, albeit intuitive, grasp of the concept of reality for the virtual reality to simulate. Look at the sentence about Mr Obama: "When I see Barack Obama on TV, I'm really seeing *Barack Obama.*" As it stands, this seems to be implying something like "You may think I'm only seeing an image on TV but actually I'm seeing the real thing, he's really there," or perhaps "... I'm seeing a real thing, it's really there."

If we paraphrase it slightly, the covert meaning is elided and the inherent tautology becomes clear: "When I see (an image of) Barack Obama on TV, I'm really seeing (an image of) *Barack Obama.*" That is certainly true, but it is boring truth. The same goes for Pac-Man (an arcade game from prehistory), which is just a pattern of LED pixels switching on and off on a screen to give the impression of a "thing" moving across the screen. Yes, there is a real screen there and yes, when the computer is switched on and the keys manipulated, the program sends coded instructions to the screen that generate the pattern known to the cognoscenti as Pac-Man but that's all. It's an apparently moving picture on the screen; the rest is anthropomorphism. All of this confusion arises because of a specific omission in his account, the third flaw mentioned above, the lack of a theory of information.

The problem of seeing vs. "seeing" Mr Obama is similar to that implied in the term beloved of behaviorist psychologists, "reflex behaviour." There can only be *reflex* behaviour if there is *non-reflex* behaviour to compare it to, otherwise the term becomes vacuous. Similarly, reality has various properties and attributes which simulated reality doesn't have, otherwise it wouldn't be simulated, it would be the real thing. But claiming that virtual reality has the same properties as genuine reality reduces the issue to absurdity. So his case would be greatly strengthened by saying "Virtual reality has *some* of the properties and attributes of genuine reality, and different combinations of the various properties and attributes will produce different versions of virtual reality, different simulations for us to work with."

But he can't say that as he has not given a formal theory of information to guide his assertion that "Virtual reality is real ... virtual objects are real." Yes, the images are real, caused by light rays projected by LEDs impacting on the retina but no, they're not independently real, they only *seem* real, because that's what their designers get paid for. Any causative properties attributed to the "virtual object" are the properties of light rays, not of the object whose facsimile they are creating. When on TV I see Adolf Hitler, I am not *seeing Adolph Hitler* as I am seeing those wicked birds in my fruit trees. I am seeing an image created on a screen by a computer program built on a copy of an image taken from a celluloid tape captured in Nuremberg in 1936 ... All of which is possible because information can be copied, multiplied and shunted around effortlessly whereas there's only one Mr Obama, and he's not in my living room.

The error arises again when the author tries to eliminate the idea that virtual reality is an illusion. He needs to prove that virtual objects are real objects, and not illusory in any way:

> Virtual objects really exist as digital objects inside a computer. When we see virtual objects, we're seeing a pattern of activity inside the computer [p207].

Here, he conflates the visual *impression* of an object physically located "just over there" (normally known as a virtual image) with the computer program that generates the light rays emitted by the screen in the goggles. The correct causative sequence is: Computer program causes patterns on screen, which causes streams of photons to enter the eye, which cause volleys of impulses in the optic nerve, which travel to the visual cortex for interpretation, giving rise to the clear visual experience of that particular object when a person without the goggles, whose eyes aren't in the way of the streams of photons and who thus doesn't get the visual input, doesn't have that experience. So the experience is illusory, not much different from looking at a stick in water and having the impression it's bent. It all depends on how the light rays enter the eye. Even the word illusory implies a separate reality that we can grasp.

But one thing is clear: a person wearing VR goggles is *not* seeing a pattern of activity inside the computer, and not just because it's a pattern of microscopic electromagnetic charges inside the chips and thus invisible (we can't see electric charges or magnetic fields) but it's also hidden in a box. The viewer is seeing a pattern of light deliberately generated on a screen by that activity, for the specific purpose of giving the impression that there is an object "over there." This is not a visual hallucination, a private experience resulting from abnormal brain activity, but it is an illusion: a reproducible visual experience which has the quality of a veridical percept and thereby gives anybody who experiences it a misleading impression of external reality. The fact that it is deliberate doesn't mean it isn't illusory.

Virtual objects are real *only* in the sense that they have a basis in a real stream of light, they're not imaginary and they're not hallucinated. Beyond that, they're artifice. And if virtual objects aren't real, his entire case starts to unravel. We can expand upon this a little (for a theory of implemented information as it relates to the human brain, see [10]), starting with the alarming claim:

> Virtual reality is real—that is, the entities in virtual reality really exist ... virtual objects are real and not an illusion [p105-6].

Just now, 10.06am AEST, Wednesday December 28th, 2022, seated in the study at my home on the outskirts of Brisbane, I cannot see or hear or sense anything that would in any way constitute a virtual image or object. In order to see what Chalmers claims is a "real virtual object," I would need a particular program for my computer, a set of gamers' VR goggles and a much more impressive set of headphones. Suitably plugged in and switched on, I could then see a scene somewhere, somewhen, anywhere, on earth or even on the moon in what we call stereoscopic view, meaning an impression of depth and movement. If the view were of, say, a jungle somewhere on earth, I would also hear through the headphones sounds of birds, insects, maybe animals or rain and so on. If I wanted to see the back of a tree, I would simply "move" my location to what appeared to be right or left and it would come into view but I would not be able to move my location "through" the tree. It's fascinating but then I remember I have to mow the lawn so I take off the goggles and headphones, switch off the machine and here I am, still in my study. Of course, I haven't been anywhere but the impressions seemed very real. And they were. Real visual and aural *experiences*, all without a single macaw looking down at me from my bookcase.

Let's look at the steps involved. I have to download the program and install it in my computer, i.e. set up a facsimile in my machine of the original stored on the company's servers somewhere far away. According to Google, that would be about 1.686GB of data, stored as totally invisible charges inside the precisely-ordered and very complex architecture of my computer. In operation, the program generates a tightly coordinated flow of electrical impulses in wires, or maybe radio waves, to activate the screens in the goggles and the speakers in the headphones. Photons generated by the LEDs in the screens enter my eyes but in a manner that precisely *mimics* the process when I look at an object outside my window. Streams of photons activate retinal photo- and colour-receptors, sending a train of electrochemical impulses back through the optic nerve and tract, via the brainstem and optic radiation to the occipital or visual cortex. There, the impulses are processed and reprocessed, from which arises that familiar sense of seeing "something out there," or what we call the mind. Because of tiny differences in the direction of the light rays from each screen, I gain the impression that what I am seeing has depth and location, that it "moves" as I move my head, and so on. That is, it *seems* it is an "object" in my visual field when, as a matter of *biology*, it is no different from looking at a picture on my wall. But it's all electronic legerdemain, just flows of data through various transducers designed to fool me.

A similar process occurs with the headphones, to produce a sense of sound sources moving around. For some reason, nobody refers to these as "virtual objects," possibly because everybody knows that that's what stereophonic headphones are designed to do. A "virtual object" in the sense Chalmers uses the term is wholly a visual impression but it is real only in the sense that the impression is generated by real photons entering the eye. The digital charges in the computer are real, the photons are real, the sound waves are real but the mental perception of an "object" they represent is an illusion simpliciter. "Virtual objects" are not real in any interesting sense of the word.

With articulated theories of mind and of information [9], the functional relationship between information and the thing we call mind becomes clear. So, we ask, do "the entities in virtual reality really exist"? Sure they do, they are real illusions (i.e. somebody else can also have the experience, as distinct from hallucinations, which are private), created by real computers to mislead real minds. People pay big money for illusions but the crucial question is this: Is the mind a real thing?

Well, that's a far more interesting question but it's outside the scope of this work [10].

Chapter 7, *Is God a hacker in the next universe up?* is pure creation myth. If we are simulated beings "living" in a simulated world in some gigantic computer, then the being that formulated the program that generates us occupies the role of God. Or god(s). As a declared atheist [p125, 144], Chalmers finds this idea interesting although he insists it would not justify worshipping the computer-operator/nerd in the "next universe up." In the search for a theory of mental disorder, I have no interest in creation myths, either original or recast as science. Apart from giving him the opportunity to mock the idea of a deity that needs to be worshipped, I don't see much point to this but ...

... Chapter 8, *Is the universe made of information?* is more interesting, not least because it lays bare his lack of a theory of information and how it could relate to the mind. After half a dozen pages of elementary description of binary systems and metaphysics, the text jumps to discussing information in its various manifestations without offering a fundamental theory. This is unexpected because Chalmers had already asked "What are the conditions under which a physical system implements a given computation? ... Once a theory of implementation has been provided..." [5]. That suggests he was about to provide one but there is no evidence of it in this text. In the absence of such a theory, he segues smoothly to the "attractive" idea that "The universe at its bottom level is a universe of pure differences."

Of course, those differences have to be differences *in something*, but he dismisses this as an unnecessary complication of a beautiful idea: "The idea isn't easy to grasp at first ... a shocking idea at first, but many people get used to it" [p165-6]. Get used to it? Philosophy isn't just a matter of people "getting used to whacky ideas," it's designed to strip out the whackiness. And what of those who don't get used to it, who gag on it? Well, they stop reading but the clear implication is that we don't adopt an idea because it's logically impeccable. Instead, we adopt or reject ideas because they fit our prejudices, which we will consider again at the end of the chapter. So why bother with this completely irrefutable notion? Because his digital creation myth is incomplete without it.

Chapter 9, *Did simulation create its from bits?*, tries to argue that the idea we exist as simulated beings in a simulated world is no sillier than any other creation myth. Quite so. Along the way, he paints Descartes as a "global skeptic":

> The Cartesian argument combines two main premises: We can't
> know were not in a simulation and In a simulation, nothing is
> real. It concludes: We can't know that anything is real [p182].

That is not how I read Descartes. Descartes was perfectly clear: because he rejected the collective "wisdom of the ancients," he was looking for some form of certainty in an uncertain world. God was one pole of certainty but was a bit remote for daily life so, by employing systematic doubt, by emphasising how easily we can be misled, he arrived at another pole, that he himself exists *as a real thing*. He says this repeatedly: *Je sais que je suis une chose qui pense.* I know that I am a thinking thing. I think, therefore I indubitably exist, meaning "I am real." For him, systematic doubt was a tool, not an attitude and certainly not an intellectual game. *Je suis une chose qui pense* cannot be understood as a "clean bridge" to *Nous ne pouvons jamais savoir que quelque chose est veritable.* We can never know if anything is real.

Per the author's invitation in the Introduction [pxxiii], we can comfortably pass over Part 4, *Real virtual reality*, because it doesn't clarify the confusion over the relationship between the informational bits that comprise a computer program, an image on a screen generated by that program, and our mental perception of that image. Part 5, *Mind*, opens with Chapter 14 and the question *How do mind and body interact in a virtual world?* Beside "virtually," the chapter adds nothing to our knowledge of how mind and body interact in the real world. Chapter 15, *Can there be consciousness in a digital world?* asks:

> Why is there consciousness in the universe? How do physical
> processes give rise to consciousness? How can there be subjective
> experience in an objective world? Right now, no one knows the
> answers to these questions [p278].

That is a clear statement that this book is neither shaped nor constrained by an articulated theory of mind. Chalmers likes the expression used by Thomas Nagel in his widely-quoted paper from 1974, *What is it like to be a bat?* [11]. Nagel answered: Not like being a human. More broadly, to be conscious, there is something it is like to be in pain, or to see blue, and so on. This is a slight improvement on definitions of consciousness that say "Consciousness is what being unconscious is not." However, all it says is that being in pain is like being in pain. Given these limitations, Chalmers concludes, we can't define consciousness independently, and have no idea how or why it arises:

> All this strengthens the case that virtual reality is genuine reality, by making the case that simulated minds are genuine minds... all this makes the prospects look better for mind uploading [p292].

For those of us concerned merely with the survival of the planet, his suggestion that "mind uploading" is a goal worthy of science and philosophy is consistent with the view that this work is not about philosophy at all. It simply uses philosophical methods and techniques to justify shifting reworked versions of a variety of myths from the category of religion and science fiction to that of science proper. How realistic is it? If we had some inkling of the nature of the code the brain uses (assuming there is only one; more likely, motor and sensory, emotional and cognitive, cortical and subcortical nuclei all use completely different codes), and some indication of where to plug the USB (the belly button?), it may have some traction but, as it stands, "mind uploading" is on a par with the ansible communicator.

On a somewhat more prosaic level, Chapter 16 asks: *Does augmented reality extend the mind?* The "augmented" refers to the use of computer-generated images projected into the visual field via a screen between the eye and the world to supplement one's memory. This is similar to the way my hammer extends the power of my hand, or my ladder extends the reach of my legs:

> The ubiquitous coupling of humans, smartphones and the internet has been a giant leap in extending the mind ... there has been a recent surge of work on brain-computer interfaces... in a few decades we should be able to communicate well with our devices just by thinking. And they might connect directly to our brain's perceptual systems, bypassing eyes and ears to convey information to us with no need for glasses or screens [p299-300].

"Technological augmentation almost always has the potential to increase our capacities. How we use that potential is up to us" [p307]. True, but so far, all it has done is bring us to the eve of destruction by nuclear war and/or irreversible climate change. On present trends, in a few decades we will all be living in a fascist-militarist climate catastrophe, not utopia. Also note that "ubiquitous" means universal. Most people on earth don't own a smartphone; of those who do, the great majority don't have the education or time or motive to access the internet's resources; of those who do, most use the phone to play games, talk to their friends, or watch the stock market or fashion influencers or pornography (or all at once); while of those who don't own one, many of us can still function without a smartphone [p297-298]; finally, the great majority of research on brain-computer interfaces is funded by the military, for the express purpose of killing more people more quickly and more cheaply at less risk to the killers, who value their lives far more than The Others.

Part 6, *Value*, raises the question of whether one can lead a good life in a virtual world:

> The year is 2095. Earth's surface is a wreck, a casualty of nuclear warfare and of climate change. You could live a hardscrabble existence here, avoiding gangs and dodging mines, with your main aspiration being survival. Or you could lock your physical body in a well-protected warehouse and enter a virtual world ... Could you live a good life in virtual reality? [p311].

To me, that question is supremely irrelevant but I think he's right: the world is presently on course to be "a wreck, a casualty of nuclear warfare and of climate change" by 2095 or long before, mainly due to greedy and brutal people who are electing not to lead good lives in the real world. As Edmund Burke commented, "All that is necessary for the triumph of evil is that good men do nothing." Debating "Could you live a good life in virtual reality?" is academese for doing nothing. But after considering the nature of value in life, the author warns:

> ... when I ask for what makes a good life, I'm asking: what makes a life good for oneself? It may be that for many people, leading a personally good life require also leading a morally good life, but we cannot presuppose that at the outset [p316].

He is fairly sure that, when the technology permits, "... many people will freely choose to live most of their lives in virtual worlds" [p323]. This leads to a "... deep question: What is the role of birth and death in a good life?" [p325]. Life in a virtual world may be somewhat poorer for not having these experiences, especially if and when brain uploading makes immortality an option, but think of all the benefits: your own mansion, even your own planet to play with, and many other...

> ...enormous benefits in the realms of space, time, experience, embodiment, and more [p321] ... life in virtual worlds in the long term may approach or exceed the quality of life in nonvirtual worlds [p361] (note that the last word in that quote is probably

a mistake; last time I looked, there was only one nonvirtual world, an increasingly grim one at that).

Assuredly, if the educated and leisured wealthy classes persist in doing nothing, then there is every risk that life in the real world will have deteriorated to the point where fantasy seems preferable. The rest of the book focuses on the concept of computation and how it is conceptualised and realised in a nontrivial way. It tidies some loose ends but does not add to his thesis.

In his book-length essay *Brave New World Revisited*, from 1958 [12], Aldous Huxley commented:

> A society, most of whose members spend a great part of their time, not on the spot, not here and now and in the calculable future, but somewhere else, in the irrelevant other worlds of sport and soap opera, of mythology and metaphysical fantasy, will find it hard to resist the encroachments of those who would manipulate and control it.

That warning, from one who knew, more or less sums up Chalmers' *Reality+*.

10.5. Conclusion: To complete the program.

The idea of a natural dualism is important, and not just to balance the deluge of positivist material that has long controlled debate in so many fields. Chalmers' earlier work on the validity of the idea opened the door to a serious debate that, throughout the twentieth century, had been treated with contempt by most thinkers. However, as indicated, I believe he stopped short of a convincing argument by not offering some suggestion as to the actual nature of the psychophysical laws of supervenience. That would have made his case so much stronger, and pulled the rug from under the feet of the functionalists who are busily pouring contempt on the very idea of an ontologically distinct mind. I believe that if he had devoted more time to the details of a theory of information and how this relates to the emergence of mind, it would have shifted the whole debate on the nature of mind, and of mental disorder, to a different level, but that didn't happen. His later work, on reality, doesn't lead to a model of mental disorder so it's of no interest to psychiatry. And, I suggest, no real interest to any serious thinker.

References:

1. Stoljar D (2010). *Physicalism*. Oxford: Routledge.

2. Chalmers DJ (1996). *The Conscious Mind: in search of a fundamental theory.* Oxford: University Press.

3. Chalmers DJ (2022). *Reality+: Virtual worlds and the problems of philosophy.* London: Allen Lane.

4. Chalmers DJ (2010), *The Character of Consciousness.* Oxford: University Press.

5. Descartes R (1644) *The Principles of Philosophy.* Available online.

6. Kolakowski, L. (1968). *Positivist Philosophy: From Hume to the Vienna Circle.* New York: Doubleday. Page numbers refer to Penguin Edition, 1972.

7. Eccles JC, in Popper KR, Eccles JC (1981). *The Self and its Brain.* London: Springer.

8. Chalmers DJ. (2012). A computational foundation for the study of cognition. *Journal of Cognitive Sciences.* Available at: https://consc.net/papers/computation.html Accessed Dec 21st 2022.

9. Descartes R (1649). The Passions of the Soul. Unknown translator. https://TheVirtualLibrary.org

10. McLaren N (2021): *Natural Dualism and Mental Disorder: The biocognitive model for psychiatry.* London, Routledge.

11. Nagel T. 1974. What it is like to be a bat? *The Philosophical Review,* 83 (4): 435-450.

12. Huxley A (1958). *Brave New World Revisited.* New York: Harper and Row.

11 Wittgenstein as the anti-philosopher

He (Wittgenstein) was a tortured soul, the last survivor of a family with a tragic history, living a lonely life among strangers, trying until the end to express the inexpressible.

Freeman Dyson.

Well, God has arrived. I met him on the 5:15 train. He has a plan to stay in Cambridge permanently.

John Maynard Keynes (on meeting Wittgenstein)

11.1: Wittgenstein speaks.

So far in this section, we have looked at four living philosophers, without much luck. Richard Carrier, the "professional historian, published philosopher, and prominent defender of the American free-thought movement" (see Chap. 12), has strong views on why this has come about:

> ... it is odd that people give (philosophy) so little attention. Philosophers are largely to blame. The have reduced their craft to the very thing it should not be, a jargonised verbal dance around largely useless minutiae... The have retreated behind ivory walls, talking over the heads of the unititated, and doing nothing useful for the everyman ... [1]

In this and the next chapter, we will consider two highly regarded philosophers who are no longer with us, either of whom could have served as the target of Carrier's ire. While they were radically different, they illustrate the recurring theme of this book: That without plausible suggestions as to the mechanism by which mental activity arises or emerges from the brain, and some idea of the medium in which the activity is implemented, philosophy of mind goes in circles. One of the authors fought against the idea of a philosophy that goes in circles while another seems almost to exemplify it.

The young Ludwig Wittgenstein (1889-1951) briefly attended the same high school in Linz as Adolf Hitler (also born in 1889) but may have started just after Hitler had left, so he is probably not the "odd Jewish boy" Hitler refers to in Chapter 2 of *Mein Kampf*. Be that as it may, he was certainly an odd boy who never grew out of it. His philosophy is also odd, partly in his style but also in the quirky message that philosophy has no special territory of its own and no particular insights to enlighten the world. That would hardly seem to qualify him for a job as a philosopher yet many people regard him as the greatest philosopher of the twentieth century. I'm not qualified to buy into that debate; my task is to find a philosopher who can point us to a theory of mind suitable for psychiatry. Can an anti-philosopher help in that search?

One way to answer the question of mental disorder is to look at exactly what philosophers say. With Wittgenstein, we know what he said but there is a sizeable cottage industry devoted to arguing over what he meant. The best place to start is with his first major work, his *Tractatus Logico-Philosophicus*, published in 1922. Anybody inclined to read this fairly brief work should start with the *Side-by-side-by-side* edition, from 2021 [2], which gives his original German and two influential English translations for comparison (I will rely on the 1961 version by Pears and McGuinness). The highly personal material is presented as groups of aphorisms, carefully numbered in what amount to chapters to show how his ideas develop. Each chapter starts with a proposition that he expands in stepwise fashion. In the introduction, he gives his general view of his work in what is probably his best-known sentence:

> ... it is not a textbook ... (it) deals with the problems of philosophy, and shows ... that the logic of our language is misunderstood. The whole sense of the book might be summed up in the following words: what can be said at all can be said clearly, and what we cannot talk about we must pass over in silence.

But, he warns: "I am conscious of having fallen a long way short of what is possible. Simply because my powers are too slight for the accomplishment of the task.—May others come and do it better." The first and briefest "chapter" sets the tone of what is a distinctive, even idiosyncratic, work:

1. The world is everything that is the case.

1.1. The world is the totality of facts, not of things.

1.11. The world is determined by the facts, and by their being *all* the facts.

1.12. For the totality of facts determines what is the case, and also whatever is not the case.

1.13. The facts in logical space are the world.

1.2. The world divides into facts.

1.21. Each item can be the case or not the case, while everything else remains the same.

He expands these ideas in the following chapters:

2. What is the case (a fact) is the existence of states of affairs.

3. A logical picture of facts is a thought.

4. A thought is a proposition with a sense.

5. A proposition is a truth-function of elementary propositions. (An elementary proposition is a truth-function of itself).

6. The general form of a proposition is the general form of a truth function, which is: $[\,p, \xi, N(\xi)]$. This is the general form of a proposition.

7. Whereof one cannot speak, thereof one must be silent.

Following his death in 1951, aged just 62, his executors published *Philosophical Investigations* [3], which was almost complete when he died. With the *Tractatus*, this brackets his professional life. In his preface to the later book, he describes it as a collection of incomplete investigations into "… the concepts of meaning, of understanding, of a proposition, of logic, the foundations of mathematics, states of consciousness, and other things." His ambition was a complete, coherent analysis of these arcane topics but he finally accepted he couldn't do it, not least because of his rapidly declining health:

> … the thoughts should proceed from one subject to another in a natural order and without breaks. After several unsuccessful

attempts to weld my results together into such a whole, I realized that I should never succeed [3, pvii].

What follows is 160 or so pages of rambling interrogation of the concepts and processes of language and the other topics he mentioned. It cannot be summarised but he always returns to his main theme, that our problems with language are fundamental. In S.109 of *Investigations*, after raising the notion of thought as a "gaseous medium," he proposed:

> The problems (of philosophy) are solved, not by giving new information, but by arranging what we have always known. Philosophy is a battle against the bewitchment of our intelligence by means of language.

What exactly is he saying? Having pored over both these texts several times, I don't know for certain but I'm not convinced anybody else does, either. For example, in the *Tractatus*, he states:

> 2.061:   States of affairs are independent of one another.

> 2.062:   From the existence or non-existence of one state of affairs it is impossible to infer the existence or non-existence of another.

Does this mean there is no formal causation, that there are no laws of thermodynamics, that the universe is entirely random? One thing is crystal clear: he does not offer anything like a theory or model of mind that could help us understand mental disorder. I suggest the reasons lie in his background. Wittgenstein was the youngest of nine children born to the heir of one of the largest fortunes in the world. His father was a rigid perfectionist while his mother was anxious and insecure. At his father's insistence, he was educated at home so that he wouldn't pick up bad habits from the boys at school. However, after two of his brothers had killed themselves, his father relented and allowed him to go to a small state school in the provincial city of Linz. He was baptised and raised as a Catholic: why didn't he go to any of the many excellent Catholic colleges in Vienna? It would appear his patchy marks and his odd behaviour would have been an embarrassment but, in Linz, he cut an almost bizarre figure, teased by the other boys, and appeared to have been desperately unhappy.

On graduating, he briefly studied engineering in Berlin, then went to Manchester to study aeronautics. This led him to mathematics, thence to logic and the philosophy of mathematics, through which he met some of the greatest thinkers of his age, including Bertrand Russell at Cambridge (he barged into Russell's rooms at the university and introduced himself). When the Great War broke out, he was back in Europe and, even though he qualified as medically-exempt, quickly volunteered for service in the Austro-Hungarian Army. He saw extensive action on a number of fronts and was eventually promoted to lieutenant. His "calm and courageous conduct" under fire led to him being highly decorated although the experience of war caused a reawakening of religious ideas. Postwar, he tried to work as a school teacher but was clearly unfit for the role; in 1921, while living in rural Austria, his *Tractatus* was published, with an English translation appearing the following year. For the next few years, he led an erratic life until he returned to Cambridge in 1929, after which he became increasingly influential in the field of philosophy.

11.2. The scope of intuition.

There is no question that Witgenstein was of the highest intellect, also that he was a tortured and desperately lonely individual. He signed away his fortune, was intolerant of lesser mortals and of criticism and left a legacy of material that have kept the mills of philosophical controversy turning since his death. Can he help us in our quest to understand mental disorder, even, to understand him, both as a person and as a philosopher? In one of those "thought experiments" so popular with philosophers, were he to turn up today at a psychiatrist's office, would his philosophy help the (unfortunate) psychiatrist understand him? I think the answer to that is an emphatic No, and the reason lies in the first chapter of his *Tractatus*, in fact, in the first five lines.

1.   The world is everything that is the case.

1.1.   The world is the totality of facts, not of things.

1.11.   The world is determined by the facts, and by their being *all* the facts.

1.12.   For the totality of facts determines what is the case, and also whatever is not the case.

1.13.   The facts in logical space are the world.

The first four lines are tautological, except where in 1.1 and reinforced in 1.13, he sets up a dualist universe by invoking the notion of a "logical space." In various forms, this expression appears repeatedly through the text, e.g. in 2.11, 2.202 and in 3.4. In 2.0121, it occurs as a "logical entity" while in 2.181 it becomes "logical picture" and "logical form." In 3.4, it appears as "logical space" and "logical place" while in 3.41, the latter is equated with "logical coordinates." This continues with "logical scaffolding" (3.42) and "structure" (6.3751), etc. The duality is reinforced at many different points, e.g. 4.01: "A proposition is a picture of reality. A proposition is a model of reality as we imagine it." 4.121: "Propositions *show* the logical form of reality. They display it." This concept, of the relationship of the information in a proposition to the reality it represents, is clearly of central importance yet it is undefined. In S.70 of *Investigations*, while elaborating on his concept of language games, he asks:

> When I give the description: "The ground was quite covered with plants"—do you want to say I don't know what I am talking about until I can give a definition of a plant?

One has to agree: that is just what I want to say. An expression as central to the concept of mind (and of language, and of logic, and mathematics, and science...) as "logical space" *does* need to be defined. Absent a definition, anything goes but defining it also serves to define *mind as an informational space* [4]. At different points in *Investigations*, he appears to be moving toward just this notion but then backs away, almost as if it were too confronting. In S.38 of *Investigations*, he says: "It is also possible for someone to get an explanation of the words out of what was intended as a piece of information. [Marginal note: Here lurks a crucial superstition.]."

In S.39, in a rambling discussion of the word "Excalibur," he describes how, if the actual sword known as Excalibur were to be broken in bits, the name would still survive; unstated but clearly implied, it survives somewhere, but that somewhere can only be the mind as an informational space. In S.40, he talks about meaning, but says nothing about the medium that bears the meaning. This is not trivial; the medium is the very "space" in which the logical operations are implemented, in which the meaning is manipulated. In S.44, he mentions that an idea continues to exist even after the object to which it referred has ceased to exist. Agreed: we can talk meaningfully of Neanderthals even though none of us has ever seen one but where does the idea exist? What is an idea? How and where is it instantiated and in what form, what is its relationship to the speaker, to the audience and to persisting external reality?

None of these critical questions are addressed in coherent form; my impression is that he understood this implicitly but he was unable to gain traction, as it were, because he had no theory of mind. He accepted the reality of the mind as a causally efficacious, dualist entity, he took it as his starting point and then tried to work forward when he should have been working back to an explanation of its origin. His preoccupation with language had to fail because he didn't see it for what it is: a means of setting up in the hearer's mind a facsimile of part of the speaker's mental state. A "logical space" is but a narrow subset of the whole informational space called "mind" [10] but the particular operations that generate his "logical space" are generic. Since they subserve all brain operations (perception, emotion, motion, visceral function etc), they are not specific to logical operations as he used the term.

Why did this happen? Here, I put on my psychiatrist's hat. In the *Tractatus*, Wittgentstein offers a cold and narrow vision of language as a logically perfect means of communicating facts; all the other functions of language simply don't appear:

> 5.6: *The limits of my language* mean the limits of my world.

> 5.61: Logic pervades the world: the limits of the world are also its limits. So we cannot say in logic, 'The world has this in it, and this, but not that.' For that would appear to presuppose that we were excluding certain possibilities, and this cannot be the case, since it would require that logic should go beyond the limits of the world; for only in that way could it view those limits from the other side as well. We cannot think what we cannot think; so what we cannot think we cannot *say* either.

> 5.62: This remark provides the key to the problem, how much truth there is in solipsism. For what the solipsist means is quite correct; only it cannot be said, but makes itself manifest. The

---

10 A case could be made that the human mind just is a "logical space" as it emerges from the coherent performance of logical operations by the brain's physical elements. However, I prefer to use the term "informational space" [5] as the perceived mind is the end product of the logical operations which are themselves silent and inaccessible. The totality of emergent mental events and contents is more than the logical operations that underwrite them, e.g. visual perceptions, pain, etc. derive from those logical operations but have no inherent logical content.

world is my world: this is manifest in the fact that the limits of *language* (of that language which alone I understand) mean the limits of *my* world.

In his introduction to the *Tractatus*, Russell noted his student's obsession with perfection:

A logically perfect language has rules of syntax which prevent nonsense, and has single symbols which always have a definite and unique meaning. Mr. Wittgenstein is concerned with the conditions for a logically perfect language—not that any language is logically perfect, or that we believe ourselves capable, here and now, of constructing a logically perfect language, but that the whole function of language is to have meaning, and it only fulfills this function in proportion as it approaches to the ideal language which we postulate.

At the same time, Russell was concerned over Wittgenstein's "mystical" side: "The totalities concerning which Mr. Wittgenstein holds that it is impossible to speak logically are nevertheless thought by him to exist, and are the subject-matter of his mysticism." We have, then, the picture of a prodigiously intelligent but seriously disturbed individual attempting to construct a "logically perfect language" but, by his own admission, failing:

Four years ago I had occasion to re-read my first book (the *Tractatus*) and to explain its ideas to someone... I have been forced to recognize grave mistakes in what I wrote in that first book... I should have liked to produce a good book. This has not come about, but the time is past in which I could improve it [3, pviii].

Why would he bother to try to produce a logically-perfect language? Partly, that was the product of the era, of the great logicians, such as Frege and Meinung, and of logicians trying to assemble a complete mathematics, such as Whitehead and Russell, but partly, it was Wittgenstein himself. I read him as saying:

Language has never served me well. I speak to people but cannot express myself fully and they don't understand me. Therefore, there is something wrong with language, so I turn to philosophy. Philosophy does not serve me well, I philosophise but people don't follow me and I cannot express my ideas with any clarity.

Therefore there is something wrong with philosophy. I put these conclusions together and *voilà*, I realise the problems with language are causing the problems with philosophy such that solving the problems of language as a logically perfect exercise is both necessary and sufficient to solve the problems of philosophy. Anything that can't be expressed in a logically perfect language can be ignored.

11.3. Conclusion: The limits to intuition.

The logician and philosopher, Herbert Feigl (1902-1988), one of the founders of the Vienna Circle, read and discussed the *Tractatus* in early meetings of the group, probably 1924. He was not particularly impressed, commenting: "I dismissed Wittgenstein as a most curious mixture of intuitive genius and schizophrenia" [4]. As a psychiatrist with lengthy experience of psychotic states in highly intelligent university students and others, I won't argue with his insight. As *science*, Wittgenstein's work is rambling, discursive and unfocussed, and seriously—if not fatally—flawed by his lack of definitions—and, it would have to be admitted, by his lack of discipline. If it interested him, he zeroed in on it, if not, he dismissed it. He understood his subject matter intuitively, but intuition isn't enough: the methodology of science is designed to lift our thoughts out of the mire of intuition, to provide a path out of the tangles of solipsism. As he said, as philosophy, his project failed. Again I agree, but I don't agree with his assessment that he lacked the "powers" to complete his project. If intellect were enough, everybody who knew him agreed he was sufficiently equipped to achieve his goal.

The physicist Werner Heisenberg was singularly unimpressed by the positivist goal of a logically perfect science and language, seeing it as doomed from the outset:

> The positivists have a simple solution: the world must be divided into that which we can say clearly and the rest, which we had better pass over in silence. But can any one conceive of a more pointless philosophy, seeing that what we can say clearly amounts to next to nothing? If we omitted all that is unclear we would probably be left with completely uninteresting and trivial tautologies (from *Positivism, Metaphysics and Religion*, 1971).

My view is that Wittgenstein failed just because he had no *concept* of a model of mind as the entity in which the mental operations he was studying took place, nor evinced any awareness that there was such a need. He had the intuition, clearly expressed a hundred times in each text, that the human mind is a causally efficacious, information-processing *thing*, but he had no notion of its relationship to the idea of informational operations, on which he wanted to build his "logically perfect language." In particular, he couldn't talk about emotions because his were too painful, so he passed over them in silence in order to produce some of the cognitive elements of a philosophy of mind (the "easy problem of consciousness"), but not the structure. He had no grasp of the mechanism by which mind is generated, nor of the medium in which it is instantiated. His philosophy is intuition taken to the extreme, the limit of what can be achieved without a formal model of mind, the point beyond which unstructured probing yields no results.

In fact, he was facing the wrong way. He started with the intuition that there is a mind, and moved forward, trying to intuit its rules of operation when he should have headed backwards, as Descartes did, to see if the brain were the sort of thing capable of supporting a "causally efficacious, information-processing *thing*." And it is. Had he done that, then he could have put two and two together and, with a quick wave of Bishop Ockham's celebrated razor, have seen that the information being processed in logical operations and the informational medium implementing it, his oft-invoked logical space, place, entity, structure, picture, scaffolding, and so on, were of the same nature and provenance, and thus comprised one and the same thing. Had that happened, there probably wouldn't have been the same cottage industry probing his delphic obscurity but it would have been of great assistance to psychiatry. Perhaps he had this in mind with his final comment in the *Tractatus*:

> My propositions serve as elucidations in the following way: anyone who understands *me* eventually recognizes *them* as nonsensical.

I don't think they're nonsensical, but they fall far short of the mark of which he was intuitively aware.

References

1. Carrier, R. (2005). *Sense and Goodness Without a God: a defence of metaphysical naturalism*. Bloomington, IN: AuthorHouse.

2. Wittgenstein L (1921) *Tractatus Logico-Philosophicus*. English translation: *Side-by-Side-by-Side Edition*, version 0.59 (May 12, 2021). At: http://people.umass.edu/klement/tlp/

3. Wittgenstein L (1953). *Philosophical Investigations*. Tr. GEM Anscombe. Oxford: Blackwell.

4. Neuber M (2022). Herbert Feigl. *Stanford Encyclopedia of Philosophy*, at https://plato.stanford.edu/index.html.

5. McLaren N (2021): *Natural Dualism and Mental Disorder: The biocognitive model for psychiatry*. London, Routledge.

12   Davidson and the logic of paranoia

What stands fast does so, not because it is intrinsically obvious or convincing; it is rather held fast by what lies around it.

Ludwig Wittgenstein

12.1: Mentality *sine* dualism.

Donald Davidson (1917-2003) is regarded as one of the most influential American philosophers of the latter half of the last century. Indeed, his 1970 paper *Mental Events* [1], has been praised as "... arguably the most debated paper in twentieth century Philosophy of Mind..." [2]. On that basis alone, our search for a philosophical basis for a model of mental disorder needs to include him.

Davidson trained in the Anglo-American analytic tradition but he was also familiar with continental philosophy. His first major work was published when he was 46, which is fairly late for academics, and until he died unexpectedly in 2003, his publications list was not especially prolific. Today, his work is closely studied and his influence remains pervasive but he is certainly a philosopher's philosopher. He did not write for beginners, such as we saw in Chalmers' *Reality+*, or with Dennett. I have never heard a psychiatrist mention him or his work, which perhaps warns us that a theory of mind leading to a model of mental disorder will not be found in the output of Donald Davidson.

On the other hand, it may be there, it's just that (the few) psychiatrists, psychologists and other practical people interested in philosophy can't find a path through what has been called his "profound" philosophising. In any event, he wrote extensively on concepts of truth and belief, which are of major significance in psychiatry, and was familiar with psychoanalytic theory, so it's worth the effort to read what he had to say. Beginners should be warned that he wrote in an old-fashioned and tortuous style so there is, and probably always will be, argument over what he actually meant. Lajos Brons said Davidson's work "resists easy interpretation," and interpreting Davidson is complicated "by his obscurity" [3]. Brons quotes Timothy Williamson (Wykeham Professor of Logic at Oxford) as saying "(Davidson's) style was too cryptic and elliptical, so that it was often unclear what his claims or arguments were," all of which is, I feel, studiously polite. Unfortunately, many people who claim to be able to understand his work write in a similar style, so commentaries aren't always helpful.

In *Mental Events*, from 1970, he sets himself the task of reconciling three fundamental principles:

> (1) ... at least some mental events interact causally with physical events. (... the Principle of Causal Interaction.)...

> (2) ... where there is causality, there must be a law: events related as cause and effect fall under strict deterministic laws. (... the Principle of the Nomological Character of Causality)...

> (3) ... there are no strict deterministic laws on the basis of which mental events can be predicted and explained (the Anomalism of the Mental) [1, p208].

In brief, some mental events can cause physical events (such as deciding to lift my arm) and vice versa (feeling pain from a blow), but cause-and-effect must be law-like and not random, except that there are no such laws that allow us to predict and explain mental events, and if there were, then there could be no free will. This is the central anomaly of human life, what Schopenhauer called the "world knot," i.e. that insubstantial or immaterial mental events can somehow move physical things such as rocks, yet we somehow retain free will.

Many philosophers have concluded that these three principles are inherently contradictory, hence the posivist program to rewrite mental life in such a form as to avoid one or other of these principles (e.g. behaviourism, which says that mental life doesn't count, or mind-brain identity theory, which says that mental events only seem to be insubstantial). Davidson, however, maintains the strong position, "...that all three principles are true, so that what must be done is to explain away the appearance of contradiction..." [1, p209]. His solution is to argue that some mental events are in fact physical events, so the impression we all have of immaterial events causing material events (thoughts moving arms, etc.) is illusory. This is a form of identity theory which, for him, carries the advantage of not requiring special psychophysical laws to bridge the causative gap. It sounds like a tidy arrangement but, when it was published fifty years ago, it provoked quite fierce controversy which continues to the present [4].

12.2. On truth and belief.

In his paper, *A Coherence Theory of Truth and Knowledge* [5], from 1983, Davidson adopts coherentism as he joins battle with that most elusive of topics, truth: What does it mean to say something is true, and can we formulate a general theory of truth? What is knowledge, what are beliefs, how do we know, what can we know, how does knowing result in action...? These questions lie at the core of analytic philosophy, and Davidson was careful not to claim he had any exclusive insights to offer. James Young defines coherentism tightly:

> A coherence theory of truth states that the truth of any (true) proposition consists in its coherence with some specified set of propositions ... the truth conditions of propositions consist in other propositions [6].

This is opposed to the correspondence theory which says that the truth of a proposition is determined by its correspondence with the facts of the world. These positions are not so strongly opposed as they seem, as correspondence with worldly facts will build a set of true propositions with which new observations or beliefs must cohere. We'll come back to this point as I will argue that it is of major significance in psychiatry.

Early in this paper, Davidson makes what polite people call a "bold" claim: "Truth is beautifully transparent compared to belief and coherence, and I take it as a primitive concept" [5, p139]. There are other people who would say that the concept of truth is anything but transparent, but this is a cornerstone of his position despite a circular element: Truth is only transparent to coherentists (because justifying beliefs are readily available), but he then uses coherence to justify his concept of truth. He continues: "...the truth of an utterance depends on just two things: what the words as spoken mean, and *how the world is arranged*" (emphasis added). Each of these concepts, however, depends on all the others being precisely defined, which is far from the case:

> If coherence is a test of truth, there is a direct connection with epistemology, for we have reason to believe many of our beliefs

cohere with many others, and in that case we have reason to believe many of our beliefs are true [5, p137]... Beliefs for me are states of people with intentions, desires, sense organs; they are states that are caused by, and cause, events inside and outside the bodies of their entertainers ... So mere coherence, no matter how strongly coherence is plausibly defined, cannot guarantee that what is believed is so. All that a coherence theory can maintain is that most of the beliefs in a coherent total set of beliefs are true [5, p138].

What started as a strong stance has quickly weakened, which he recognises by asking: "...why couldn't all my beliefs hang together and yet be comprehensively false about the actual world?" A good point, but he doesn't surrender easily:

The partisan of a coherence theory can't allow assurance to come from outside the system of belief, while nothing inside can produce support except as it can be shown to rest, finally or at once, on something independently trustworthy [5, 140].

And what is "independently trustworthy"? Here he throws out his boldest claim:

What distinguishes a coherence theory is simply the claim that nothing can count as a reason for holding a belief except another belief. Its partisan rejects as unintelligible the request for a ground or source of justification of another ilk. As (Richard) Rorty has put it, 'nothing counts as justification unless by reference to what we already accept, and there is no way to get outside our beliefs and our language so as to find some test other than coherence' [5, p141].

For Davidson, truth is not grounded in the external world just because we are constrained by our pre-existing sets of beliefs and the limits of language. Since he had already said truth depends on "how the world is arranged," it will be clear that there are weaknesses in his case but they are weaknesses that bedevil all epistemology. His is just one attempt of many to escape what appear to be circular or question-begging definitions of knowledge, belief, truth, meaning and so on. He concludes the paper with a general statement of his position:

All beliefs are justified in this sense: they are supported by numerous other beliefs (otherwise they wouldn't be the beliefs

> they are), and have a presumption in favor of their truth. The presumption increases the larger and more significant the body of beliefs with which a belief coheres and, there being no such thing as an isolated belief, there is no belief without a presumption in its favor ... But from each person's own vantage point, there must be a graded presumption in favor of each of his own beliefs. We cannot (conclude) that all true beliefs constitute knowledge... all that counts as evidence or justification for a belief must come from the same totality of belief to which it belongs.

Which points straight to relativism but, first, a look at some of his other papers relevant to the quest for a model of mental disorder. In *The Structure and Content of Truth* [7] from 1990, originally delivered as a series of three lectures, he opens with what is probably his most recognisable quote: "Nothing in the world, no object or event, would be true or false if there were not thinking creatures." Even though a truism, this states his position: Truth is an abstract quality, not a material fact like rocks, birds and cod liver oil. For example, it is a fact that there were dinosaurs long before there were humans, but (currently) only humans can believe the proposition: "It is true that dinosaurs once roamed the earth."

The distinction between material facts of the physical world and the abstract realms of thought is central to his work but, surprisingly, he rejected his earlier position: "I discuss correspondence theories, coherence theories, and theories that in one way or another make truth an epistemic concept. I reject all these kinds of theories" [5, p282]. What does he accept? Again, he defines truth as a brute fact: "It is a mistake to look for a behavioristic definition, or indeed any other sort of explicit definition or outright reduction of the concept of truth. Truth is one of the clearest and most basic concepts we have, so it is fruitless to dream of eliminating it in favor of something simpler or more fundamental" [5, p314]. Finally, after what even his keenest supporters would admit is a fairly tortuous argument, he concludes:

> We recognized that truth must somehow be related to the attitudes of rational creatures; this relation is now revealed as springing from the nature of interpersonal understanding. Linguistic communication, the indispensable instrument of fine-grained interpersonal understanding, rests on mutually understood utterances, the contents of which are finally fixed by

the patterns and causes of sentences held true. The conceptual underpinning of interpretation is a theory of truth; truth thus rests in the end on belief and, even more ultimately, on the affective attitudes.

"In the end, truth rests on belief and, beneath that, emotional attitudes." As philosophy, this is a little underwhelming: I expect that most people older than about eight can distinguish between what a person wants to believe and what is the fact of the matter. However, we can leave that for the time being and look at the ancient question of weakness of the will, or what the Greeks knew as akrasia. At first glance, this is more a matter of psychology than philosophy but we are looking for a philosophical model for mental disorder so perhaps this is it.

12.3. On the will.

In *How Is Weakness of the Will Possible?* [8], Davidson introduces his topic in the first sentence:

> An agent's will is weak if he acts, and acts intentionally, counter to his own best judgement; in such cases we sometimes say he lacks the willpower to do what he knows... would... be better.... It will be convenient to call actions of this kind incontinent actions, or to say that in doing them the agent acts incontinently [8, p21].

(For those with a medical background, incontinence has a different meaning; I prefer to avoid the term but I'm even more wary of expressions such as "weak will"). In *Actions, Reasons and Causes*, from 1963, he gives a striking if counterintuitive example: "On the contrary, a man may all his life have a yen, say, to drink a can of paint, without ever, even at the moment he yields, believing it would be worth doing" [9]. Davidson soon defines it more precisely but it amounts to this: Smith knows that he ought to do *x* but, in clear consciousness and with no additional information, he does *y* instead. This phenomenon, akrasia to Socrates and his successors, incontinence to Dante, and weak will to moderns, has been debated since, with as much clarity and resolution as we'd expect from a debate lasting 2,500 years. Davidson's position is clear: "There is no proving such actions exist; but it seems to me absolutely certain that they do" [8, p29].

What follows is a continuation of that ancient debate, but his point emerges slowly: to provide a "coherent theory of practical reason" [8, p37], i.e. what it is to want to act; the idea of an intentional action; one's reasons for acting, and so on. In the course of a complex discussion, Davidson dismisses a range of possible solutions from classic authors, such as Aristotle, to arrive at his own conclusion:

> There is no paradox in supposing a person sometimes holds that all that he believes and values supports a certain course of action, when at the same time those same beliefs and values cause him to reject that course of action ... The akrates (weak-willed person) does not ... hold logically contradictory beliefs, nor is his failure necessarily a moral failure. What is wrong is that the incontinent man acts, and judges, irrationally [8, p41] ... But if the question is read, what is the agent's reason for doing a thing when he believes it would be better, all things considered, to do another thing, then the answer must be: for this, the agent has no reason... the actor cannot understand himself: he recognizes, in his own intentional behaviour, something essentially surd [8, p42] ('surd' is a mathematical term meaning irrational; I presume this is what he meant).

This seems a long and tortuous path just to conclude "People do dumb things," but that's his conclusion, so we'll leave it for the moment.

12.4. Toward a model of mental disorder.

What can Davidson add to our search for a formal model of mental disorder? In the first place, and unlike Dennett and others, he does not mention biology. Part of the reason has to be that he accepts the mentality of mind and has no need to show it can be reduced to brain, as he said in regard to truth ("... it is fruitless to dream of eliminating it in favor of something simpler or more fundamental"). His concern is normal mental function, not abnormal, but he says nothing about the structure and function of the brain which converts it from a lump of meat like the liver to an organ that can generate mental events, perceptions, beliefs and so on. The mind-brain problem receives but tacit acknowledgement nor, in the four papers quoted above, does he mention mental disorder in any form or setting. Moreover, in his introduction, Jeff Malpas (who knew Davidson well) commented:

> ... Davidson is not an easy writer to approach... (the critique of Lepore and Ludwig is) ... largely negative in its assessment of the

cogency of Davidson's arguments, and the philosophical viability of the positions he advances [2].

This is code for some quite damning criticism, so why bother with his work? Two reasons: he is an important figure who has had a wide influence in analytic philosophy, and, regardless of his intent, I believe he has something significant to offer in the (very important) matters of cognitive dissonance and of paranoid states. Getting there, however, will take some time.

Starting with his general work, *Mental Events* [1], he argues that mind and brain can interact, but only according to "strict deterministic laws." However, since we have no deterministic laws, strict or otherwise, which allow us to predict and explain mental events, we have a problem. That's true—so long as there is no attempt to explain the emergence of mind from the pink stuff between our ears. Davidson didn't attempt that. He also didn't attempt, as Dennett and so many others have done, to "explain mind away," but he starts with it as a fact hanging somewhere by itself, unrelated to the physical world. He has no mechanism by which mind emerges from brain, no sense of a medium in which mental events take place, no theory of any kind, so of course he can't produce "psychophysical laws" relating mind and brain. Necessarily, the physical mechanism of the brain dictates the deterministic laws although, as a matter of historical fact, they have been known in outline since 1854 [10, 11].

In attempting to divine the laws governing mind-body interaction without at least some understanding of the body, he was like a person trying to understand transport without ever seeing a road, or like somebody who knows nothing about computers staring at a computer screen and trying to work out the rules governing the appearances on the screen. It can't be done, they are far, far too complex. All he could offer was the suggestion "Oh well, some mind events must be brain events, so problem solved." He concludes:

> Mental events as a class cannot be explained by physical science; particular mental events can when we know particular identities... The anomalism of the mental is thus a necessary condition for viewing action as autonomous.

That is, without a non-deterministic mental life, humans can't be considered to have free will, which he regards as essential. I agree, and I also agree that "mental events as a class cannot be explained by physical science." That's what dualism means: two sets of laws, one governing the physical world and one governing the informational [11]. But we don't know any "particular identities" and, as I have argued in Chap. 2.3, we never will, so I'm not convinced by his solution to the quandary of his three fundamental principles. How can he guarantee that the mental events he classes as "mind-brain identity functions" are the very events that are causally significant in our behaviour? How can one mental event occur independently of the brain and the next one be identical with it? And what about all the mental events left over? They still have to be explained, not dismissed as "also rans." Philosophy has to be plausible and consistent, otherwise it degenerates into a case of special pleading.

12.5. Self-justifying belief.

Moving on, in *A Coherence Theory of Truth and Knowledge* [5], he makes a series of audacious claims:

> What distinguishes a coherence theory is simply the claim that nothing can count as a reason for holding a belief except another belief....

> All beliefs are justified in this sense: they are supported by numerous other beliefs ... and have a presumption in favor of their truth. The presumption increases the larger and more significant the body of beliefs with which a belief coheres ...

> But from each person's own vantage point, there must be a graded presumption in favor of each of his own beliefs.... all that counts as evidence or justification for a belief must come from the same totality of belief to which it belongs.

These points are important and, I will argue, establish a firm *logical* basis, not for ideal or rational mental function, but for the sublime irrationality of paranoid states. Remember that conventional psychiatry says only that paranoid states are a "chemical imbalance of the brain," or some such shibboleth. I totally disagree: the word 'paranoid' is an adjective, in the same class as words like sweet, heavy, aggressive or complex. It describes a mental set on the world, a disposition to see events from a particular point of view. Like 'ponderous,' 'pretty' or 'parlous,' 'paranoid' is not a thing or entity in its own right; there is no such thing as "paranoia." People can show paranoid thinking either as part of the normal personality or as a modification or "flavor" of any form of mental trouble that subsequently develops.

Traditionally, psychiatry accepts there are five fairly distinct postures in the paranoid stance:

> An intense preoccupation with justice and matters of right and wrong;
>
> An intense preoccupation with persecution;
>
> An intense preoccupation with conspiracies;
>
> An intense preoccupation with the supernatural;
>
> An intense grandiosity and self-righteousness.

Intense means intense; it doesn't mean "more than me," or even "more than most." It means "dominating the person's thought and actions to the exclusion of normal content; taking control of the person's life with adverse effects." The central element in each of these clusters, the common factor, is the sense of being the centre of the universe: "I know better than anybody. I'm so important and so clever that anything I believe is right and anybody who doesn't agree is wilfully wrong."

A paranoid personality is endlessly dominated by ideas of conspiracies and persecution and so on, but it doesn't reach psychotic intensity; it is that person's normal way of addressing the world, his normal mode of intercourse, you could say. Everything he says and does *makes sense* from the point of view of a person who is deeply mistrustful and never takes things at face value. In the paranoid personality, there are no hallucinations and no true delusions although it can be difficult to tell an over-valued idea from a low-grade delusion. Hallucinations and delusions can be of a paranoid nature, or a person may be paranoid while depressed but, once the depression settles, go back to normal. People showing acute stress reactions are commonly paranoid but, unless they had a premorbid tendency, it tends to be transient.

My concern, however, is not the common-or-garden paranoid, that odd fellow at work or the wierdo woman down the street, but the monstrous, systematised set of completely crazy beliefs that were on full display in Washington, DC, on January 6th, 2021. How do these festering farragos arise? Why do people want to believe the election was stolen when everything says it wasn't? Why would apparently sensible adults lap up the idea that somebody called Q is revealing a vast conspiracy run by paedophiles and lizard people who have taken over the US Government [14]? In short, why do ideas get worse, and not better? Davidson's concept of one belief leading to another is important, but with one proviso: it has to start somewhere.

As it stands, his opinion that every belief is preceded by another belief fails on a number of points. First: how does it all start? We're not born with beliefs, we acquire them, but he implies an infinite regress, maybe an endless loop of beliefs. Second: how do we change our beliefs, i.e. prioritise them? Third, how do people end up with inconsistent or conflicting beliefs?

First, that ancient question: "What came first, the chicken or the egg?" The answer is just this: What came first was ... a different sort of chicken. And that's also true for beliefs: What precedes a belief? A slightly different belief, a little more general and less specific. We can track back along people's beliefs (which, in nearly fifty years as a psychiatrist, I have done thousands of times) and, just as Descartes did, finally arrive at the most primitive beliefs of all: "I exist," and "The world exists." Where do these come from? How do children acquire them? Davidson's position is perfectly clear:

> The partisan of a coherence theory can't allow assurance to come from outside the system of belief, ... Its partisan rejects as unintelligible the request for a ground or source of justification of another ilk....

If so, coherence theory is wrong. These elemental beliefs do not come from prior beliefs, because there are no prior beliefs, nor are we born with them. They come from experience, they are the *Ur*-beliefs on which all subsequent beliefs are built. So when we get to adulthood, yes, it's true, each belief is preceded by a logically prior belief but here is the crucial point: the preceding belief is a bit less focussed and a little more general, broader in scope and, most important, cruder and less sophisticated.

Instead of a single line of beliefs, as Davidson implied, there is a hierarchy. Each new belief is nested in the beliefs that preceded it, back and back until we reach the *Ur*-beliefs. Thus, each level of belief defines a set whose members are the clusters of beliefs that follow it, but beliefs at a particular level are slightly different from each other (otherwise they'd be the same belief), from those before it and, of course, from those that follow. And each slightly different belief can lead to more differences, and those to more differences, until one's head is populated with swarming lines of beliefs which may or may not be compatible, depending on one crucial factor, the sense of self-righteousness. Normal personalities question their own beliefs and eliminate contradictory ideas, whereas a self-righteous personality, which is at the core of the paranoid state, never does. The paranoid person *never* says "I could be wrong but..."

This way, we can end up with branching and compartmentalised belief sets that may or may not contradict each other, but as long as only one belief system is active at any one time, there is no distress, better known as cognitive dissonance. For example, there is a TV reporter in the US who specialises in going to MAGA rallies and interviewing people to bring out their contradictions. In one segment, he asked a middle aged woman wearing a red hat and a *Women for Trump* shirt whether she supported Trump. Yes, most definitely, she replied, I support everything he does, he's on our side. I see, said the reporter, so what do you think of the Supreme Court striking down the right to abortion? Oh that's dreadful, she replied, it's a woman's right to decide, our bodies etc. "So you think the Supreme Court made a wrong decision?" "Absolutely," she replied, "a terrible thing." "But are you aware the justices who voted to overturn Roe v Wade were all appointed by Trump for that specific purpose, to restrict abortion?" No, she wasn't, and she didn't know what to say. In another segment from an anti-abortion rally, he approached a man carrying a large banner that proclaimed "God is Pro-life." "What does that mean?" asked the reporter. "It means God loves us and wants us to live." "But you do know that God once destroyed practically every living person and animal on earth? You know, the Flood?" His target turned away and refused to speak further.

Ordinarily, a person holding manifestly contradictory beliefs would experience the distress of cognitive dissonance but these people aren't troubled until it is jammed in their faces. The answer lies in Davidson's concept of coherentism, that a belief is held to be true because it meshes with lots of older beliefs. The very essence of the paranoid personality is that it "... can't allow assurance to come from outside the system of belief ... (and) rejects as unintelligible the request for a ground or source of justification of another ilk (i.e. other than its own belief system)..." The reporter's interviews are funny to watch although it's probably quite dangerous for him (c.f. Russell, B: "The fundamental cause of trouble in the world is that the stupid are cocksure while the intelligent are full of doubt"). But this is not mental *pathology*. These people may be idiots but they're not crazy [11]. The paranoid belief system *always* feels internally consonant, it's only sensible people who are troubled by doubts, who feel the need to eliminate cognitive dissonance.

Instead of a neat line of rationality extending back forever, as in Davidson's highly idealised model, in normal mental function, we find hierarchies of nebulous, wandering, shape-shifting belief systems, like those big, wavering advertising figures that are held aloft by air pumped up through them. Every now and then, an arm floats off into space or perhaps another head appears. Perhaps elderly philosophers have rationally-ordered lines of beliefs, or maybe just one line with no free-floating islands, I don't know, but be assured the overwhelming majority of humans don't. Most belief systems are a morass of overt inconsistency held together by self-interest. And that includes politicians, financiers, generals, industrialists and all the other bigwigs who calmly reassure us that they know what they're doing. Only the paranoid are free of the anxiety of self-doubt. And psychopaths, of course, we mustn't forget them.

For practically every human, our early beliefs are the most powerful. After "I exist in the world" come beliefs like "I have to survive," "I need to be part of the group," and "I want to be wanted."

Early life experiences are crticially important in shaping the individual's belief system, producing something like: "The world is a lovely, exciting place, filled with caring people who love me and want me." That child is happy and outgoing so people respond accordingly and thus, the child's belief system reinforces itself positively. For a paranoid person, a very early, crude belief is "The world is a cruel, hard place." That comes from *experience*, not from a prior belief (or genes), and is soon succeeded by "People are dangerous, they'll do me in if they get the chance so I have to keep my eyes open at all times." This belief leads to "Leave nothing to chance, trust nobody" then "People are probably conspiring against me right now," followed by "That man looked at me then whispered to his friends, they must be conspiring against me." Finally, he cracks: "Aha, that gesture proves they're conspiring, I need to get them before they get me."

---

11   Definition of an idiot: the ability to move back and forth between conflicting beliefs without experiencing distress. This has nothing to do with age, intelligence, sex, education or mental disorder.

Each new belief is more focussed and more precise but it fits comfortably with the preceding beliefs, the controlling factor being the subject choosing safety over rationality. A person who alone believes X can either remain lonely or move to join a group who don't believe X. Being part of a group is usually more important than being true to one's beliefs. This is "coherentism" in action, except it does nothing to deliver absolute truth to an individual; all it does is convince *him* that all the evidence points in one direction so everybody else must be lying. The process is self-reinforcing, as it shapes the succeeding beliefs because evidence that confirms this opinion will be stored and savored while contradictory evidence will be dismissed: "They said that, did they? They're lying. How do I know? I just know, I feel it in my bones."

As the recent history of conspiracies shows, paranoid people end up with vast, interlocking systems of belief, all of which fits together perfectly in their minds with no loose ends that they can't immediately reconcile, and all of which seems completely mad to outsiders—except most of the believers aren't mad [11]. I doubt very much that this is what Davidson had in mind with his epistemological model of an elegant line of beliefs extending back into the past, but if a theory or model of mind can't account for mental disorder, it isn't worth reading. Davidson's model leads to a plausible account of one form of mental disorder (a coherentist model of paranoid states) and needs to be taken seriously because paranoid states can be dangerous—and are getting more dangerous by the day [12].

12.6. Willpower vs anxiety.

How Is Weakness of the Will Possible? This is a most interesting question and we should examine his position closely in order to criticise it:

> An agent's will is weak if he acts ... intentionally, counter to his own best judgement [8, p21].

> There is no paradox in supposing a person sometimes holds that all that he believes and values supports a certain course of action, when at the same time those same beliefs and values cause him to reject that course of action... [8, p42]

> There is no proving such actions exist; but it seems to me absolutely certain that they do [8, p29].

> Objection 1: "An agent's will is weak if he acts .."

From the outset, there is no such thing as weakness of will. You either do it or you don't; willpower is irrelevant to the equation because all our decisions are computed from a myriad inputs, not all of which can be in consciousness at the time or, indeed, ever. Freud said that all behaviour is over-determined, by which he meant there are many, many factors operating to influence a decision. If you do something, then *ipso facto* the act says "At the moment the action was initiated, that was the decision you reached." You may instantly regret it, or may (as usually happens) quickly lose track of the many factors involved, or not even be aware of them but, regardless of anything you may have said or done before, you can't say it wasn't your decision to act just so at that particular instant.

Consider his example of the man who drank a can of paint: he elected to reach out to it and take a swig. That was his action, he initiated it because his arm won't move unless and until he wills it to do so. This is true of all decisions we make: try to catch yourself in the act of willing to lift your right arm. You cannot do it, just because decisions are very fast, of the order milliseconds, too fast for us to apprehend. In any event, there is no reason to believe we have conscious (reportable) access to our decsion-making apparatus [11]. The mere fact that you can't grasp the instant of that decision does not imply that you didn't make it as a voluntary action. I think Davidson had spent too much time pondering weighty questions in his study, and not enough time talking in depth to ordinary working people.

> Objection 2: "There is no paradox in supposing a person sometimes holds that all that he believes and values supports a certain course of action, when at the same time those same beliefs and values cause him to reject that course of action..."

There is indeed a paradox in supposing that a person can believe and value one action yet do the exact opposite, because that means beliefs and values are irrelevant in the process of making a decision. For somebody who wanted hard and fast rules joining mind and brain, that is contradictory: apart from beliefs and values, what other sources of information are there that can lead to and justify an action?

> Objection 3: "There is no proving such actions exist..."

If so, he shouldn't be talking about them as they're in the same realm of discourse as angels dancing on the heads of pins.

Objection 4: "...but it seems to me absolutely certain that they do."

Does he have an authority for this assertion? No, he does not, but I have a problem with this because, after nearly half a century as a psychotherapist talking in depth to over 12,000 people from a very wide range of backgrounds, it seems to me absolutely certain that such actions do *not* exist. As mentioned above, we daily make innumerable decisions in the infinitely complex, high-speed, multi-channel information-processing organ called the brain, which operates at millisecond time levels, and we implement them even before we can report them. It only *seems* that people can have "weak will," which leads to...

Objection 5: The reality of "weak will."

The most common reason people appear "weak-willed" is because of anxiety, either overt or covert. This is entirely a separate subject, best understood through a cognitive model [13], which is, of course, *terra incognita* to philosophers huddled in their studies. People who impulsively do the opposite of what they normally do or should do often have a good reason, it's just that we can't see it and they don't want to talk about it. The whole two-and-a-half thousand year debate on "weak will," from Socrates to the present, has been a waste of time just because it focussed on entirely the wrong aspect of mental life. It tried to give a cognitive interpretation for an emotional event, which is "surd." But because people prefer to say "I did a really stupid thing, I had no reason," rather than admit "I was terrified and I had to get away," we think they are just irrational. No, they're not. They make perfect sense as long as we remember that emotions have their own logic.

12.7. Conclusion: Paranoid logic.

To conclude, I find Davidson's intellectualised approach to mental life restrictive but it was inevitable just because he didn't have a theory of mind. His work was descriptive and non-explanatory, which is probably why he chose to leave emotion out of it: too complicated, as Descartes found in his *Passions of the Soul*. Nonetheless, I agree with his dualist model, which necessitates mind-body interaction, but have argued he was wrong on the implementation just because he had no details of the mechanism by which the mind supervenes upon or emerges from the brain. Without a medium in which mental events occur, he could not say anything about the cognitive processes of reaching a decision nor how those are activated. An information-based model of mind leads directly to an account of free will and to a straight-forward model of mind-body interaction [11]. However, a central element of his cognitive model leads to a mechanism by which the self-reinforcing nature of paranoid states can be explained without resorting to some mythical "chemical imbalance of the brain." Instead of seeing paranoid states as "crazy brain chemicals," they can be seen as a potentially dangerous variant of normal mental life.

Once the essential self-correcting mechanism of self-criticism is switched off, the cognitive machinery serves abnormal mental function quite as well as it serves normal, as Hannah Arendt noted: "*What convinces masses are not facts, and not even invented facts, but only the consistency of the system of which they are presumably part.*" Paranoid states start with the earliest beliefs of the child, which depend totally on life experiences. Given new evidence (observational or informational), well-adjusted adults have no difficulty admitting error and correcting their views. Paranoid personalities, who reject anything that contradicts their previous beliefs, build an interlocking belief system that, by virtue of being so consistent, seems true beyond all evidence. At least, to them.

References:

1. Davidson D (1970) Mental Events. Reprinted in *Essays on Action and Events* (2001). https://doi.org/10.1093/0199246270.003.0011

2. Malpas J (2019) Donald Davidson, in *Stanford Encyclopedia of Philosophy*. At https://plato.stanford.edu/entries/davidson/#ProbIrra

3. Brons LL (2016). Putnam and Davidson on Coherence, Truth, and Justification. *The Science of Mind*, 54: 51-70.

4. McLaughlin B (2013). Anomalous monism. Chap. 24 in *A Companion to Donald Davidson*, Eds. Lepore E, Ludwig K. New York: Wiley

5. Davidson D. (1983) A Coherence Theory of Truth and Knowledge Chap. 10 in *Subjective, Intersubjective, Objective: Philosophical Essays, Vol. 3. https://doi.org/10.1093/0198237537.001.0001*

6. Young JO (2018). The Coherence Theory of Truth. *Stanford Encyclopedia of Philosophy*. At https://plato.stanford.edu/entries/truth-coherence/

7. Davidson D (1990) The Structure and Content of Truth. *Journal of Philosophy*, 87 (6): 279-328.

8. Davidson D (1970) How Is Weakness of the Will Possible? In Feinberg J (ed.), *Moral Concepts*, Oxford: University Press. Reprinted as Chap. 2 in *Essays on Action and Events* (2001). At: https://doi.org/10.1093/0199246270.001.0001

9. Davidson D(1963). Actions, Reasons and Causes. *Journal of Philosophy*, LX (23): 685-700.

10. Boole, G. (1854). *An Investigation of the Laws of Thought, on which are Founded the Mathematical Theories of Logic and Probabilities.* Dover Classics of Science and Mathematics. New York: Dover (1958).

11. McLaren N (2021): *Natural Dualism and Mental Disorder: The biocognitive model for psychiatry.* London, Routledge.

12. McLaren N (2022): *Narcisso-Fascism. The psychopathology of right wing extremism.* Ann Arbor, MI: Future Psychiatry Press. Due July 2023.

13. McLaren N (2018). *Anxiety: The Inside Story.* Ann Arbor, MI: Future Psychiatry Press.

14. Bloom M, Moskalenko S (2021). *Pastels and Pedophiles. Inside the Mind of QAnon.* Stanford, CA: Redwood Press.

13   Ryle on Ghosts

I suppose the greatest defect is that nearly all of it was false.

Alfred Ayer, late in life, commenting on positivism.

13.1. To conceive of mind.

I started formal study in philosophy in 1983, and prominent on the reading list was a text from 1949, widely regarded as one of the most influential books in twentieth century philosophy of mind. Gilbert Ryle's *The Concept of Mind* [1] is now about 75 years old so it's worth checking to see how it has aged and how philosophy has progressed in that time. But there is a larger reason to include it, as Ryle was an early and significant figure in the positivist movement, greatly assisting the development of the field known as functionalism. For example, when Daniel Dennett, a well-known functionalist philosopher (see Chap. 8), undertook his PhD at Oxford in the early 1960s, he studied under Ryle.

Gilbert Ryle (1900-1976) came from an intellectual and well-connected, upper-middle-class/professional background in genteel England. He studied at Oxford and, apart from his service as a major in Intelligence during World War II, worked there until he retired in 1968. He died a bachelor and although he was forthright, even "formidable," in his work, he was regarded as generous and encouraging of his students and colleagues. Most of his work was connected with his lifelong interests in linguistics and what was known as "ordinary language" philosophy, now generally termed analytic philosophy. However, he was familiar with the major continental philosophers of his time and was apparently able to read them in their original languages (which many native speakers struggle to do).

As an academic treatise, *The Concept of Mind* is unusual in that Ryle refers only to a few classic authors and not at all to modern authors, gives no citations, no footnotes and no list of references. The work is entirely his opinion and stands or falls on the strength of his case alone. Apart from common sense, he offers no justification. It consists of a long (300 pages), impassioned onslaught on a widely held view in philosophy, psychology and human affairs which, "with deliberate abusiveness," he labelled "the myth of the Ghost in the Machine" [1, p17]. His goal was to "deconstruct" (as they now say) that myth but not through science, or psychology, or established authorities in philosophy because at that stage, there were none:

> The descriptions given by philosophers of their own objectives and their own procedures have seldom squared with their actual results or their actual manners of working. They have promised, for example, to give an account of the World as a Whole, and to arrive at this account by some process of synoptic contemplation. In fact, they have practised a highly proprietary brand of haggling ... [1, p303].

Having decided that philosophy of mind until then had led us astray, he was essentially starting again on an entirely new project of writing the ghost out of the machine. Although he doesn't mention it, this was consistent with the Vienna Circle's 1929 doctrine, outlined in *The Scientific Conception of the World* [2]. It was a revolutionary move, which seems at least partly responsible for the impact his work had. This was rather ironic as, in some senses, he did not regard himself as a philosopher of mind but chose the topic to demonstrate the power of analytic philosophy—and, quite likely, because the sheer silliness of a lot of "philosophical talk" irritated his well-developed sense of intellectual decorum.

In the final chapter, entitled *Psychology,* he muses that, by insisting we can only study the mind through external behaviour, his volume ran the risk of being "stigmatized as 'behaviourist'" [1, p303], but he was unconcerned as "the entire book could properly be described as an essay, not indeed in scientific but in philosophical psychology" [1, p301]. Psychology should be seen as a broad range of disciplines, particularly as "the researches of psychology's one man of genius, Freud" should really be seen as "(belonging) to the family of medical inquiries...":

> Indeed, so deservedly profound has been the influence of Freud's teaching ... Psychological theories provide, or will provide, causal explanations of human conduct. Granted that there are hosts of

different ways in which the workings of men's minds are studied, psychology differs from all the other studies in trying to find out the causes of these workings [1, p305-306].

His case against the "haggling" of philosophers is based in the notion that, consistent with Descartes' example, philosophers (and psychologists, and priests, and most other people) had fallen into a major error, that of misattributing the causes of behaviour, not correctly to the observable world but incorrectly to a phantom and private inner world. His goal throughout is to explode the myth of what he called "The Official Doctrine" of mind, centred on the Cartesian model, which he introduces on the first page of the first chapter. Held by "Most philosophers, psychologists and religious teachers...," it says that the human consists of two parts, an objectively public, material body and a private, subjective inner life called the mind to which the owner has direct access. He believed this was completely wrong, a myth, but, as he warned in the introduction:

> A myth is ... not a fairy story. It is the presentation of facts belonging to one category in the idioms of another. To explode a myth is not to deny the facts but to reallocate them [1, p10].

This was the basis of his attack: that the official doctrine is an enormous "category error." While there are many possible errors in philosophy, a category error arises when properties or entities belonging to one category are presented as though they belong to another category. This has led, he said, to a complete misunderstanding of the nature and role of mind.

Despite its popularity, there are problems with this book, not least its highly personal approach to the ancient question of whether the human mind exists as a natural, causally-efficacious entity that we can understand. Compounding this is the point that large tracts of the book are of descriptive value only, and often repetitious at that. The next problem is his idiosyncratic style of pursuing a number of themes, often in the same paragraph, if not in the same sentence, freely jumping back and forth between them with little or no warning. Theme No. 1 is to set out what he believes his opponents believe, the Official Doctrine, aka "the Ghost in the Machine." Theme 2 is to show what he believes are the failings of that doctrine. Theme 3 is to advocate for his particular viewpoint and the last is to point out any weaknesses in his own position. All this is delivered in an old-fashioned syntax (with many quaint examples) and a liberal use of subordinate clauses.

It must also be remembered that, while arguing against the notion that the mind is a separate metaphysical entity somewhere in the head, he is not, like some behaviorists, claiming that it can be ignored or even that there is no mind. He repeatedly states that we have causally-efficacious minds, that minds are somehow related to brains, and he routinely uses practically every verb relating to mental function in the English language—thinking, reasoning, perceiving, sensing, deciding, learning, recalling, forgetting, planning, hoping, realising, predicting, enjoying, musing: you name it, he uses it. We humans have minds, we have mental properties, that much is beyond doubt, the only questions being how to approach the question of its nature and mode of interaction with the body:

> People can see, hear and jolt one another's bodies ... (but we are) irremediably blind and deaf to the workings of one another's minds and inoperative upon them [1, p15] ... How can a mental process, such as willing, cause spatial movements like the movements of the tongue? How can a physical change in the optic nerve have among its effects a mind's perception of a flash of light? [1, p21] ... In some ways which *must forever remain a mystery*, mental thrusts, which are not movements of matter in space, can cause muscles to contract [1, p62; emphasis added].

Finally, although he does not offer a theory or account of mind himself, he sets out the only types of evidence that can and must be used in building a rational philosophy and psychology:

> Those human actions and reactions, those spoken and unspoken utterances, those tones of voice, facial expression, and gestures, which have always been the data of all the other students of men, have, after all, been the right and the only manifestations to study ... Psychological research work will not have been wasted, if the postulate of a special mind-stuff goes (the way of phlogiston) [1, p302-303].

All this is offered with no biological arguments and (mercifully) not a mention of evolution. Summarising his case is notoriously difficult as it is built upon a sequential linguistic analysis of how we use mentalist expressions. It is highly detailed, articulate, erudite, abstruse to the point of opacity—and eventually tiresome, just because it is a case of what the mind is not, not what it is. Major presumptions, such as the mystery of mind-body interaction, are presented as facts, with no argument. Also, the strengths of his case have often been absorbed into modern opinion, they have become the new orthodoxy so it is sometimes difficult to know why he is bothering with some objections. However, as I will argue, because of his obsession with showing how Descartes got it wrong, he tangentially makes a vital point about dualism, but doesn't capitalise on it. From this oversight has arisen both the absurdity of functionalism, the doctrine that tries to tell us that torture and rape are nothing to get excited about, and the dead end of physicalist (biological) reductionism. Those are certainly fighting words for most philosophers, most psychologists and practically all psychiatrists, so we will see who is left standing.

13.2. To defenestrate Descartes: the Official Doctrine.

Most people who have ever lived accept the idea, formalised to a large extent in Descartes' work, that we humans consist of a body and a mind. By majority vote, he deems this view "about the nature and place of minds" the Official Doctrine. The body is a physical machine located in space, subject to the laws of mechanics, which can be inspected by others, same as with animals, trees and planets. The mind is private and is not located in space so it is not available to others to inspect. Thus, "transactions" between body and mind ...:

> ... remain mysterious, since by definition they can belong to neither (entity)... It is assumed there are two different kinds of existence or status ... What has physical existence is composed of matter, or else is a function of matter; what has mental existence consists of consciousness, or else is a function of consciousness ... each of us lives the life of a ghostly Robinson Crusoe [1, p14-15].

If the mental contents are conscious, the owner can't be wrong about them because "the consciousness which irradiates ..." the mental states and processes leaves no room for error. Here, he touches on the major point mentioned above, namely, the problem of the infinite regress: if mental events become conscious because they have been illuminated, or conducted past a particular point or any similar analogy, that has to be for the benefit of some observing entity, meaning the mind. But how does the mind observe? By another mind, and so *ad infinitum*. Ryle was aware of this problem:

> All this is meant ... to deny that the execution of intelligent performances entails the additional execution of intellectual operations ... (Supporters of the Official Doctrine) postulate an

internal shadow-performance to be the real carrier of the intelligence ordinarily ascribed to the overt act... [1, p14-15] ... the dogma of the Ghost in the Machine maintains that there exist both bodies and minds; that there occur physical processes and mental processes; there there are mechanical causes of corporeal movements and mental causes of corporeal movements. I shall argue that these and other analogous conjunctions are absurd... I am not ... denying that there occur mental processes. Doing long division is a mental process and so is making a joke ... the phrase 'there occur mental processes' does not mean the same thing as 'there occur physical processes'... [1, p23].

He has set himself a number of questions. Firstly, what is the nature of mind and how does it arise? Second, how does it interact with the physical body and third, if we are to avoid an infinite regress, what is their formal relationship? Essentially, these are the same problems Descartes took on some 300 years before Ryle: *Encore une fois, plus ça change, plus c'est la même chose.*

In Chapter 2, *Knowing how and knowing that,* starts abruptly:

> In this chapter, I try to show that when we describe people as exercising qualities of mind, we are not referring to occult episodes of which their overt acts and utterances are effects; we are referring to those overt acts and utterances themselves [1, p26].

This startling claim rests on the fact that if an act has to be considered before it can be acquitted, then the consideration itself must be considered, and so *ad infinitum.* The only way he sees out of this regress is to deny there is any internal agent to perform the occult episodes, thereby refusing to take the first step on the slippery path to infinity. If we talk about a duality of an outer self and an inner self, we automatically set up in the inner self the very issue we had to explain in the outer self, for which the inner self was the proposed explanation. What evidence do we have that people act intelligently? Their behaviour, of course, so, according to the principles of positivism, in striving for "neatness and clarity" of explanation, all "dark distances and unfathomable depths" (such as inner selves) must be rejected: "In science there are no 'depths' there is surface everywhere... Everything is accessible to man; and man is the measure of all things" [2, p9]. This leaves us with just "their overt acts and utterances" on which to build a science of mind.

Does that explain intelligent behaviour? No, of course not. Describing the behaviour does not explain it. That's why we invoke the concept of an inner entity in the first place, as in: "She's only acting dumb, she's actually much smarter than he is," or "That politician thinks he's being clever but he's actually a dumb man's idea of how a clever politician would act" (as in "I am a very stable genius"). He concludes the chapter with a comment on solipsism:

> I find out most of what I want to know about your capacities, interests, likes, dislikes, methods and convictions by observing how you conduct your overt doings, of which by far the most important are your sayings and writings. It is a subsidiary question how you conduct your imaginings, including your imagined monologues [1, p60].

On the face of it, it would appear that "your imaginings (and) imagined monologues" (whatever they are, he doesn't say) are just the sort of "occult episodes" that the Ghost in the Machine was invoked to explain. Most people are aware that "... 'there occur mental processes' does not mean the same thing as 'there occur physical processes'...", that's why they have different names, but it demands explanation. His dismissive conclusion ("a subsidiary question") is misleading and, in such a scrupulous author, I can't see it as an accident. The crucial point for which positivism must account is the nature of the "mental processes," including imagined monologues, pain, recollections, despair, doing long division, getting a joke, and so on. It must explain how these very peculiar things arise in the physical brain, and how they control behaviour, if they do. But he had already decided that the "transactions" between body and mind "remain mysterious" [1, p14] while a few pages into Chapter 3, he attempted to shut down the debate by declaring that the relationship between mental events and subsequent physical events "must forever remain a mystery" [1, p62]. That is akin to a boxer declaring himself the winner after they have just shaken hands. Ryle does not give any reason for this dogmatic statement, and I don't see any reason to accept it.

For a modern reader, Chapter 3, *The Will*, directed at "refut(ing) the doctrine that there exists a Faculty, immaterial Organ or Ministry" called "The Will" is an historical curiosity but I presume Ryle's analysis had a lot to do with that (even psychiatry has dispensed with the idea). He accepts that "mental thrusts ... can cause muscles to contract" [1, p62] but on the next page, contradicts this by denying that "overt actions ... are results of counterpart hidden operations of willing..." In fact, he is correct on both counts but his lack of a theory of mind prevents him seeing this. It is true that cerebral activity precedes peripheral motor activity; that none of this is random; that the locus of control resides in the head of the actor, not in his liver and not in the environment; and we know that people can exert control over their brain activity. Correct on the first point. But he is also correct on the second point, which is easily demonstrated to people (I have done this hundreds of times with patients):

> Author: "Lift up your right arm. Fine, now how did you do that?"

> Patient: "I don't know, I just did."

> Author: "Correct, and if you try it a thousand times, you will never be able to catch yourself in the act of deciding to do it. That's how the mind works. It's very fast and most of the really important stuff takes place outside our awareness, we can't access that sort of brain activity."

But since Ryle didn't have a theory of mind, he was led to the conclusion: "Transactions between minds and bodies involve links where no links can be ... minds, as the legend describes them, live on a floor of existence defined as being outside the causal system to which bodies belong" [1, p65]. And this exposes the weakness in his entire case: he is arguing that since positivism insists on material evidence as the basis of all knowledge, and there can be no *material* evidence of minds, therefore everything we think we know about minds must be wrong and it is pointless and misleading to talk of them: we must, as Wittgenstein said, pass over them in silence. But that's like arguing that since nobody has ever seen one sort of animal evolve into another sort of animal, therefore the theory of evolution is wrong. Minds do, in fact, "live on a floor of existence defined as being outside the causal system to which bodies belong," that's the problem. It's called the Mind-Body Problem and it's been around for a long time. Descartes was very familiar with it: "These questions presuppose amongst other things an explanation of the union between the soul and the body, which I have not yet dealt with at all" (letter to Clersellier, 12 January 1646). It will not be resolved by deciding that certain classes of evidence are inadmissible: the observations to be explained were known thousands of years *before* the model of science Ryle was using in his attempt to explain it.

Chapter 4, *Emotion*, is certainly the weakest link in his argument, and not just because large parts of it are simply description. He starts by defining emotions in a way that suits his case but, so far as I know, has not been used by any serious writer in the field since Descartes' *Passions of the Soul* (1649):

> I shall argue that the word 'emotion' is used to designate at least three or four different kinds of things, which I shall call 'inclinations' (or 'motives'), 'moods', 'agitations' (or 'commotions') and 'feelings' [1, p81].

Thus armed, it is relatively easy for him to show that emotions aren't what they seem to be. What are they? Something real and private, that is clear: "... we can induce in ourselves genuine and acute feelings by merely imagining ourselves in agitating circumstances" [1, p103]. However, by the end of the chapter, we still don't know just what "genuine and acute feelings" are or how they fit in the mental economy, as he doesn't offer one. He mixes what we would ordinarily call emotions, such as the moods of fear, joy or sadness, with personality factors (inclinations), transient impulses (motives), physiological arousal (agitations and commotions) and sensations such as pain. Finally, he concludes that he learns of your emotions by watching your behaviour and, in particular, listening to what you say, but "My discovery of my own motives and moods is not different in kind..." [1, p111]. This explains nothing: if I want to know what my "genuine and acute feelings" are, I don't have to wait until I speak about them. I know, from being at one with my own feelings: "*Mes sentiments, ils sont moi*." Anything else sets up an infinite regress.

Chapter 5, *Dispositions and Occurrences,* is an experiment in trying to give an account of the phenomena we normally lump under the term 'personality' without having anything like a model or concept of personality, even a regressive one. A large part of it is linguistic analysis, to show that many words we use in daily speech don't mean what we think they mean, or don't make sense: "A baker can be baking now, but a grocer is not described as 'grocing' now" [1, p114]. After a long exercise in grammatical hair-splitting, he concludes:

> My argument has been intended to have the predominantly negative point of exhibiting why it is wrong, and why it is tempt-

ing, to postulate mysterious actions and reactions to correspond with certain familiar biographical episodic words [1, p147].

The problem he hasn't explained is that we developed the words because the "biographical episodes" demanded a label. Putting that aside, where is his account of what we ordinary mortals would term "an enduring disposition to act in a certain way," also known as character traits or personality factors? There is no account. The inescapable conclusion of this chapter is that his decision to rail against the celebrated Ghost came before he had any clear idea of what was wrong with the idea. The answer, of course, is that a naive ghost represents an infinite regress. There are sophisticated ghosts, as Norbert Wiener indicated in 1948 although, when Ryle was writing his phillipic, it is most unlikely he had heard of them.

"I know my own mind." Self-knowledge has always been a problem for anybody wanting a rational theory of mind, as the very words themselves seem to set up a dualism as the first step on a slide to infinity. Ryle was very aware of this and set out his position at the beginning of the eponymous Chapter 6:

> ... I try to show that the official theories of consciousness and introspection are logical muddles. But I am not, of course, trying to establish that we do not or cannot know what there is to know about ourselves ... knowledge of what there is to be known about other people is restored to approximate parity with self-knowledge. The sorts of things I can find out about myself are the same as the sorts of things I can find out about other people, and the methods of finding them out are much the same ... in principle ... John Doe's ways of finding out about John Doe are the same as John Doe's ways of finding out about Richard Roe [1, p149].

The idea that "theories of consciousness and introspection," official and otherwise, are "logical muddles" would not have been news to Descartes; that's probably why he spent so much time on them. The notion that there is no difference between my access to my own mental states and my access to yours would certainly have been news to him, as it is news to anybody but die-hard, resolute positivists who are required to reject "dark distances and unfathomable depths" in favour of observable behaviour in conditions of bright light. This is taken to extreme when he indicates that self-knowledge comes from observing one's own behaviour in the third person:

> No sleuth-like powers are required for me to find out from the words and tones of voice of your unstudied talk, or even from my own unstudied talk, the frame of mind of the talker ... We eavesdrop on our own voiced utterances and our own silent monologues ... I can pay heed to what I overhear your saying as well as to what I overhear myself saying... [1, p176].

Just who is the "I" that overhears "myself" and what is their relationship? The tangles of trying to explain self-reference without slipping into an infinite regress prove too much, and the chapter slithers to a halt on the question of the "systematic elusiveness of 'I'." Yes, the notion is elusive, but pretending that the evidence I have for my sense of being me is of the same order as the evidence I have for my sense of you being you is no solution. As he had already conceded "I am not... denying that there occur mental processes" [1, p23], what we want from him is an account of *how* those processes arise in a physical universe such that I can access mine but not yours. That isn't forthcoming, as he is determined to prove that we don't have an inner life in any sense that we ordinarily recognise.

This is clearer in Chapter 7, *Sensation and Observation,* where he argues against "... the dogma that minds are special status things composed of a special stuff" [1, 195]. Here, he sets the groundwork for functionalism, the contrary and counter-intuitive dogma that, yes, we have something going on in our heads but no, it isn't/can't be what it seems to be and no, we can only find out from objectively listening to and watching our actions because nothing else is admissible as evidence. Now that's a perfectly valid stance to take, just as it is valid to promote the free market over social welfare, or the financial needs of mining companies over the conservation needs of the Tasmanian devil, or prioritising freedom of speech over one's duty to tell the truth, and so on. The catch is that these are ideological decisions, not scientific, and are taken *prior* to the adoption of a scientific program. They determine the form of the program that one adopts, and govern what will be seen as evidence.

Seventy-five years ago, Ryle was acutely aware that there was something seriously wrong with the generally-held concept of mind, that, under the rules in force at the time, it involved inadmissible evidence so he was trying to write an account that could wriggle between the rock of mysterious stuffs and the hard place of infinite regresses. Again, that's entirely a valid program except that, after 75 years, nothing much has changed. It is therefore necessary to look at the basic concepts he is opposing, as in: "... the dogma that minds are special status things composed of a special stuff." Agreed, there are major problems with the idea of a substance that isn't subject to the laws of physics, while the idea of some sort of cryptic inner being is no improvement but, as he concedes in the last sentence of this chapter, linguistic analysis probably isn't going to resolve them:

> I do not know what more is to be said about the logical grammar of such words (i.e. sensations), save that there is much more to be said [1,p 231].

After some forty pages of critique, this amounts to an admission that his chosen approach to the question of mind was not going to deliver. This much is elementary: the mind-body problem will not be resolved without considering the relationship between mind and body (although he had decreed at the outset it couldn't be done: "must forever remain a mystery"). There has to be an attempt to give some account of mental phenomena, of how information gets from body to mind and back again. What was needed was a formal, structured model that allowed the analysis of matter-energy flows in the brain as a precursor to an account of information flows; what he needed, one could say, was a *model analysis* instead of his *linguistic analysis*.

But Ryle didn't know any biology, and what little psychology he did know was in thrall to Freudian pseudoscience. He didn't have a theory of information and so couldn't see the role of information in the emergence of mind as "a special status *thing*," as distinct from the mind as "special *stuff*." This is the trap of positivism: it decrees that there is only "objectively determined evidence" or "all that magical stuff." Even though Ryle said "I am not ... denying that there occur mental processes," he did nothing to explain them: his linguistic positivism still manages to throw the mentalist baby out with the subjective bathwater. Say what you like about Descartes (as Dennett, Ryle's student, did, see Chap. 8), at least he made an honest attempt to reconcile Watson's "two incommensurable orders of being." So, lacking any sort of theory or account of mind, there was no possibility of Ryle being able to explain imagination. And this is what happens in Chapter 8, *Imagination*. Nothing.

Ryle accepts that we can "see things in the mind's eye," or have tunes "running through the head," or even recall the smell of something burning, but there is no attempt at an account of these experiences. This leads him to an error, that of assuming that a "hypochondriac" (i.e. person who complains of certain symptoms of illness without any physical basis to them) is simply pretending to be ill "from morbid egotism" [1, 246]. This is completely wrong. In fact, hypochondriacs are making a category mistake, that of assuming certain bodily symptoms are due to physical illness when, in fact, they are caused by their anxiety—about being ill. It happens that for many in civilian life, anxiety (the response to the perception of a threat) is caused by the thought that the person is suffering a serious illness, for which the evidence is the symptoms of anxiety themselves, in a self-reinforcing or vicious cycle. The symptoms are not made up or pretended: the heart really is racing, the sweat is real, the bowels really are explosive, the knees are visibly tremulous and the voice quavering. But they are not thereby symptoms of a physical illness. The psychological explanation is that the presence of the symptoms (of anxiety) is reinforcing the very anxiety which is causing the symptoms. That, however, is wholly a mentalist explanation which positivists, who dismiss the causative role of mental perceptions, are incapable of seeing. But their blindness is pure ideology, a willed act, you could say, maybe even "morbid egotism," but it is not due to lack of intelligence, the topic of Chapter 9.

This can be brief. In this Age of Information, the Easy Problem of Consciousness (see Chap. 9) seems to be tractable, albeit not yet fully domesticated. The concept of computation as the general basis for goal-directed behaviour is now second nature to us; simply, Ryle's linguistic approach has been overtaken by events. Seventy-five years ago, as a major recently demobilised from military intelligence, it is quite possible that Ryle had heard of Alan Turing's pioneering work on the basic principles of machine-based computation, but he gives no indication of it, nor of Claude Shannon's mathematical approach to communication (a great deal of the work of Shannon and of Turing was still classified Top Secret). Ryle was still arguing, correctly, I believe, against naive concepts such as Organs of Reason, although it is worth noting that the same notion has been resurrected by Chomsky in the guise of a "language organ" (see Chap. 7). In any event, large tracts of this chapter are descriptive with no explanatory content. It is one thing to say *that* humans have intellectual powers; what we want is an account of *how* such powers arise from the physical brain, how they are implemented and how they transact with the world. All this is nowhere to be seen, meaning nothing Ryle says about the intellect bears on the question of mental disorder, or of mental order. And so we turn to the last and, at eleven pages, the shortest chapter in the book, Chapter 10, *Psychology.*

He starts with a blunt assertion of his notion of what constitutes valid enquiry in psychology and philosophy. This is critical to his case so I will quote it at length:

> Abandonment of the two-worlds legend involves the abandonment of the idea there there is a locked door and a still to be discovered key. Those human actions and reactions, those spoken and unspoken utterances, those tones of voice, facial expressions, and gestures, which have always been the data of all the other students of men, have, after all, been the right and the only manifestations to study. They and they alone have merited, but fortunately not received, the grandiose title 'mental phenomena' ... Psychological research work will not have been wasted, if the postulate of a special mind stuff goes the same way (as phlogiston) ... I have argued that the workings of men's minds are studied from the same sorts of data by practising psychologists and by economists, criminologists, anthropologists, political scientists, and sociologists, by teachers, examiners, detectives, biographers, histories and players of games, by strategists, statesmen, employers, confessors, parents, lovers, and novelists [1, p302-4].

This is a clear and indubitable statement of positivism, as set down by the Vienna Circle (see Chap. 1). Applied to human affairs, it amounts to an ideological behaviorism. Humans are to be studied from the same point of view and with the same intellectual tools as rats and blowflies. Apart from a nod in the direction of Sigmund Freud's psychoanalysis, which, he insisted, should be classed as medical, not psychological or philosophical, he argues that psychological research "cannot be defined as the search for causal explanations" [1, p308]. In the last few pages, he discusses the new field of behaviorism as a "progressive science" of "revolutionary importance to the programme of psychology" [1, 310]. Yet having defined psychology's raw data, he gave precious little indication as to what it was intended to achieve. As it happens, behaviorism achieved nothing much, if anything at all, but he expected that biological sciences would fill in the gaps:

> Man need not be degraded to a machine by being denied to be a ghost in a machine. He might, after all, be a sort of animal, namely, a higher mammal. There has yet to be ventured the

hazardous leap to the hypothesis that perhaps he is a man [1, p310].

That is, he offers nothing to explain how a brain could generate not just an entity that experiences pain, but one which can also study and then understand the processes by which that experience is generated by its brain. Chimps, for example, can stand upright, and there is no doubt they know when they're standing upright. But it is something else again to be able to determine the role of the cerebellum in maintaining upright posture, to write a textbook about it, and then apply that knowledge to other animals, to robots, and to humans in space. This is what a theory of mind is about. Language is a function of mind but, by itself, it can't explain mind.

13.3. Conclusion: Ghosts one, philosophers nil.

In his polemic, Ryle did not address any of that, and I think the reason is that he was deeply confused. His adoption of the positivist credo came before he had worked out whether it was appropriate to the subject matter. There was never any doubt that he accepted that mental events occur but he offered no explanations of their provenance and nature (I have argued that their nature is determined by their provenance [3] but that's a separate issue). Throughout, was he saying that:

> 13.3.1: Mental events exist but they are objectively unobservable; science only studies objective data so we'll have to settle for a behavioral analysis as second-best, or was he saying ...

> 13.3.2: Mental events must be dismissed because they are *ipso facto* evidence of the presence or workings of ghostly stuff, or ...

> 13.3.3: Mental events are epiphenomena, superfluous to a scientific account of sensation, intellect, etc, which, in due course, will be explained by biology, or ...

> 13.3.4: Mental events have to be excluded because they are the inevitable first step of an infinite regress, or, for all cases ...

> 13.3.5: Mental events and physical events cannot conceivably interact so they can't be included in a physical science of nature?

Yes, he was. All of them, at different times or even all at once. In the absence of any understanding of neurophysiology, and with no theory of information, there wasn't much else he could do than describe the weaknesses of the existing concepts of mind. But he still hadn't *explained* anything. With the benefit of three quarters of a century of the most explosive development of science in human history, this is clear to us but I'm quite sure it wasn't then. He was doing the best he could with the limited material at his disposal. Even today, the overwhelming majority of humans generally have no idea of the nature and extent of innate informational systems in our lives, of how we *are* perambulated informational systems. Fish don't know they live in water.

It is abundantly clear that Ryle spent a great deal of time and diligent effort on providing a formal framework for a positivist philosophy of mind, so what is his legacy? After this review of half a dozen authorities on philosophy of mind and/or psychology, his work hasn't had the constructive influence that must moved him to take up the task. His "deliberately abusive" expression, the "ghost in the machine," grabbed attention and, I believe, misled many people into thinking that the hard intellectual work of providing a formal basis for a monist account of mind had already been done. In particular, Daniel Dennett's contemptuous attitude to the "green slime" of mentalism has been noted (Chap. 8). In fact, the essential work hadn't been done. Ryle's argument in this book does not rise above opinion—really, ideology. It is an elaborate and elegantly-phrased example of how, when confronted with evidence that doesn't fit its model, science discards the evidence. Summarising Ryle's contribution for *Stanford Encyclopedia of Philosophy*, Julia Tannay said: "It seems then that the two ontological aspects of the Official Doctrine—finding a place for the mental in the physical world and the problem of mental causation—still survive today" (2021).

Perhaps I'm biased. As a psychiatrist, I spent nearly half a century dealing with people in pain, both physical and mental, and people in the grip of bizarre beliefs. I admit I am super-sensitive to any suggestion from anybody, especially people of privileged status, that pain either doesn't exist, or is made up, or is "weakness leaving the body," or is a moral failing, or is trivial or risible or any other attempt to discount or dismiss its significance. Because that is what a theory of mind has to explain, and Ryle's account of non-mind doesn't even grasp that fundamental point.

References:

1. Ryle G (1949). *The Concept of Mind.* London: Hutchinson. Reprinted Penguin University Books, 1973.

2. Hahn H, Neurath O, Carnap R (1929). *The Scientific Conception of the World: The Vienna Circle.* Ernst Mach Society, University of Vienna.

3. McLaren N (2021): *Natural Dualism and Mental Disorder: The biocognitive model for psychiatry.* London, Routledge.

14 Carrier's Natural Metaphysics: dispensing with God ...

It is better to ask some of the questions than know all of the answers.

James Thurber

14.1. ... and with philosophers ...

After a long list of professional philosophers, we turn to a more modern writer whose blog shows he is a "natural philosopher, historian, and author, PhD in Greco-Roman intellectual history and Coast Guard veteran" [1]. As mentioned in Chap. 11, in *Sense and Goodness without a God*, Richard Carrier gives his clear ideas on the role and place of philosophy in these types of questions:

> Philosophy is not a game or hair-splitting contest, nor a grand scheme to rationalise this or that. Philosophy is what we believe, about ourselves, about the universe and our place in it. Philosophy is the Answer to every Big Question ... Our values, our morals, our goals, our identities, who we are, where we are, and above all how we know any of these thing, it all comes from philosophy ... it is odd that people give it so little attention. Philosophers are largely to blame. The have reduced their craft to the very thing it should not be, a jargonised verbal dance around largely useless minutiae ... The have retreated behind ivory walls, talking over the heads of the uninitiated, and doing nothing useful for the everyman ... [2, Introduction; note that the e-copy of this book is not paginated].

He stakes his position with admirable clarity: "I am a first-order physicalist (I believe everything that exists is solely and entirely caused by physical things and events ...), so I must be able to reduce moral facts to physical facts in some way" [1]. Specifically, he endorses the metaphysical position of naturalism and extends its writ in all directions:

> I build and defend a complete worldview by covering every fundamental subject—from knowledge to art, from metaphysics to morality, from theology to politics... (and) discuss free will, the nature of the universe, the meaning of life and much more ... (using) sound reason and scientific evidence ... Nature is all there is ... Metaphysical Naturalism satisfies all our concerns—about existence, meaning, right and wrong—without need of any gods or mystical secrets [2, Introduction].

The particular interest for psychiatry in this fairly audacious program is clear: in order to justify its existence, biological psychiatry requires a clear reductionist pathway, from symptoms all the way down to brain disease. Without this, modern psychiatry lacks any credible scientific basis, meaning it is nothing more than an ideology of mental disorder [3]. Even though biological psychiatrists have never troubled themselves with theories, a clear-talking, confident physicalist philosopher is more or less made to order, so we need to spend a bit more time on this, psychiatry's last hope for salvation via philosophy.

Carrier's book is set out in similar style to those of Ludwig Wittgenstein, except Carrier starts at the beginning and carefully builds a foundation for his project. In Section I, he offers an unusually detailed autobiographical account of how he reached his present intellectual position, before moving to *How We Know* in S.II. After accounts of concepts such as meaning, including words, and reality, he positions himself on the opposite pole from Davidson's coherentism by arguing that "experience is the font of knowledge" (S.II.2.1.3) In S.II.3, *Method*, he expands on the reliability of sources of knowledge. The most reliable of all is the method of logical-mathematical reason, followed by (in descending order of reliability) the methods of science, of experience, of history (his own field), and of expert testimony, with the methods of plausible inference and of pure faith bringing up the rear. The method of logical-mathematical reason tells us what to believe; the faithful are told what to believe: at these extremes, there are no options, no ifs or buts, but between the limits, there is a degree of choice.

14.2. ...but not with philosophy.

S.III brings us to the actual philosophy, *What There Is*. In S.III.2, *A General Outline of Metaphysical Naturalism*, he develops the foundations of his case:

> ...all metaphysical naturalists believe that if anything exists in our universe, it is a part of nature, and has a natural cause or origin, and there is no need of any other explanation ... by "nature" we mean a non-sentient universe, with all its properties and behaviors. Basically, we mean nothing more than space, time, material, and physical law ... there is neither evidence nor need for anything else (a view that is generally called "physicalism").

Now he starts to build his case that, at fundamental levels, our non-sentient universe is populated entirely by "mindless things." His goal is to show we can lead moral and satisfying lives without relying on the supernatural for justification. Topics such as S.III.3, *The Nature and the Origin of the Universe*, S.III.3.3, *Modern Multiverse Theory*, S.III.3.6, *Time and the Multiverse*, lead to S.III.4, *The Fixed Universe and Freedom of the Will*. Here, he adopts the rather surprising view, that a rigid physicalist determinism is not incompatible with free will; rather, the religious or libertarian concept of freedom of choice is at fault:

> Even though the universe and its future is most likely fixed and unchangeable ... Determinism does not justify fatalism—the view that we cannot change our future no matter what we do in the present. Determinism actually entails the opposite: it means we decide our future *precisely* by what we do in the present ... our choices still cause our future, directly and indirectly ..... determinism does not really mean we have no free will. For what we call "free will" is really nothing more than the ability to choose and do what we want, an ability we can have (and have taken away) even in a deterministic world.

At first glance, the notion that free will can exist in a deterministic universe is an antinomy. Formally, his view is known as compatibilism, the idea that determinism and free will are mutually compatible, that it is *not* logically inconsistent to hold both opinions at the same time:

> But all our experiences, all these moments, already exist in the fullness of time, and they are fixed there forever [S.III.3.6]. I

believe determinism is true because it is simple and has great explanatory power ... 'responsibility,' both moral and legal, actually requires determinism [S.III.4.1].

This rather lengthy and, at times, convoluted argument starts to clarify his agenda, partly of establishing his own position but, at the same time, forestalling any possible religious counter-arguments. By S.III.4.5, *What Free Will Really Is*, his case is starting to lose itself in the various contrary positions:

> Even if my choices are entirely determined in advance, I still make decisions, and my decisions are still caused by who I am and what I know—my thoughts and desires and personality... free will is doing what you want—nothing more, nothing less. And being responsible is being the cause—nothing more, nothing less ...

So: Is the future fixed, or is it not? We will come back to this point because S.III.5, *What Everything is Made Of*, takes us in the direction of a concept of mind that may lead to a model of mental disorder. Starting with the blunt assertion that "Everything is a physical arrangement of matter and energy in space-time," he quickly concludes that "... consciousness is among those things that *only* exists as an extension of matter and energy over a span of time" [S.III.5.1]. However, a few lines before, he had said dimensions are:

> ...essentially the existence of extension, and probably constitute the fundamental ground of all being. By definition, wherever there is more than one place something can "be," there is extension, and the entire range of that extension is a "dimension"[S.III.5.1].

Quite clearly, he is using the word 'extension' in two different ways as, also by definition, consciousness cannot be located and it certainly doesn't extend out of the head. Normally, we would say that consciousness is a higher order property of the brain but he doesn't, and there is a reason why he doesn't, which we will come to. Instead, he opts for a general statement:

> Current cutting edge science is already suggesting that everything else about the universe (matter, energy, physical law) derives solely and entirely, in some way or other, from the geometry of space-time ... for now, this is the most plausible conclusion:

matter and energy are geometric properties of space-time, and all physical laws follow therefrom [S.III.5.1].

This is not quite right. The direction of modern science was set in 1929 in the Vienna Circle's Posivist Manifesto (see Chap. 1). Science as we know it was built upon this foundation; the issue of mentality remains as problematic now as then. In Carrier's position, we presume that "everything else" means "besides consciousness," but if it doesn't, then the value of his claim turns on being able to give some substance to the expression "derives … in some way or another." For psychiatry, of course, it doesn't matter whether matter is ultimately just intricate patterns of energy wave forms, or even congealed angels' breath, this is the reality we're in, this is what we have to deal with, so let's deal with it.

Moving ahead in the account of *What Everything is Made Of*, we come to that hoariest of topics, *Abstract Objects* [S. III.5.4]. In his view, abstractions are something the brain grasps because abstract objects, or "universals," as they are sometimes known, "… don't exist apart from … pattern recognition by the brain and our naming that pattern." Surprisingly, the brain soon loses its grip as abstract objects have some sort of reality independent of humans:

> Even if a particular abstraction is never experienced in any way (not even imagined by anyone), it does not follow that the repeatable pattern it corresponds to does not exist. It may exist somewhere, at some time, past, present, or future. And even if a particular universal property, a particular pattern of matter and energy in space-time, is actually never really manifested any-where, ever, the abstraction that would correspond to it could still be manifested… through someone's imagination, as an idea that is never realised … as the brains that do this are a physical part of the universe, so are abstractions.

This is not his clearest section. It's true that, regardless of whether they are recognised by sentient beings or not, patterns exist in nature. And those same beings can imagine patterns that have never been seen in nature or have never existed in physical reality and never will. However, Carrier goes a lot further by arguing that when patterns are either recognised or imagined by a "minded" being (such as ourselves), then that pattern exists as an abstraction in the being's brain and because it exists in a physical brain, it therefore exists as a physical thing itself so all abstractions are physical things. This echoes Dennett's approach of reducing everything to matter but appears to make the same mistake of equating the abstraction (the idea) with the mechanism (the brain) that instantiates it. We will come back to this point.

More important is the question of whether the physical structure of the brain is sufficient to explain all the abstract concepts a brain can hold. He uses a number of examples to show how naturalism can account for abstract concepts, including the number two and redness. These examples are, of course, of central importance to his thesis so they get their own sections. In S. III.5.4.1, *Numbers, Logic and Mathematics*, he explains that:

> ... for this number (two) to exist "in the abstract," all that is required is that there be a potential (real or imagined) for two discrete things of any sort to exist. The word "two" thus means something like "the repeating pattern of two distinguishable things," and to say it "exists," is to say that this pattern is somewhere, at some time, manifest in the world—and nothing more.

It's true that pairs of things existed before humans appeared on the scene, but the implication is that the *concept* of two existed long before humans, e.g. as Platonic forms. Later, he qualifies this, indicating it depends on "a process of coming to know and understand the different patterns that can be formed ... out of the stuff of the universe, and deducing their consequences..." This tends to suggest there is something above and beyond the matter-energy stuff of the universe that does the "knowing and understanding," and apprehends the consequences, but he quickly corrects this possibility:

> In short, logic and mathematics are human creations, just like English or German, and like English or German, logic and mathematics describe both real and potentially real things: repeatable patterns of matter-energy in space-time.

When it comes to colours and processes [S. III.5.4.2], the same is true: "Thus, color is physically real, a difference in rate of vibration in a barrage of real tiny particles, a form of energy." Two "red" objects have in common the property of causing photons of a certain frequency to strike our eyes from which the brain recognises patterns and identifies similarities. He soon concludes:

> Already we can see there is no need for any other explanation for the existence and nature of abstractions. In order for there to be patterns of matter-energy in space-time, we only need there to be matter, energy and space-time... some of those patterns will be repeated, and ... (the brain) will naturally be able to distinguish (those repetitions which) can be assigned a name. That name is what we call an "abstraction," which refers to a real pattern in experience... [S. III.5.4.2].

Now we come to the crucial point:

> I believe this because in every case I have examined, I have been able to reduce an abstraction to some repeating or repeatable pattern of matter-energy in space-time ...more and more it appears that all of sociology can be reduced to psychology, all of psychology can be reduced to biology, all of biology can be reduced to chemistry, and all chemistry to physics, which is the study of matter and energy in space-time. Therefore, everything is matter-energy in space-time [S. III.5.4.2].

In S.III.5.4.3, we learn that modal properties are the causal consequences of a particular pattern of matter-energy in space-time, leading to a discussion of reductionism [S.III.5.5], which is of central importance in biological psychiatry so I will quote it at length:

> ... "reductionism" is the view that everything can be reduced to the same, one thing. Physicalism is thus a variety of reductionism in which everything can be reduced to matter and energy in space and time: quarks and other sub-atomic particles and their behaviors are all that there is, out of which everything without exception is made. And this fits with the fact that society can be reduced to humans, and humans can be reduced to cells, and cells can be reduced to chemical systems, which can be reduced in turn to sub-atomic particles. So therefore societies can be reduced to sub-atomic particles. The natural corollary of this view is that the sciences follow the same pattern: sociology can be reduced to psychology, psychology to biology, biology to chemistry, and chemistry to physics. So, theoretically, all of sociology and psychology can be described entirely by physics [S.III.5.5].

This is a somewhat idiosyncratic definition of reductionism, putting the cart before the horse. Most definitions see it as a method by which the behaviour and properties of a higher order entity are explained wholly in terms of the behaviour and properties of the lower order entities of which it is composed, such that no questions are left unanswered. The physical entities are present in the first place, reductionism is the method adopted to investigate them. His account of reductionism is descriptive, not explanatory. The assertion that societies can be reduced to sub-atomic particles is not, in fact, a "fact," as it begs the question, i.e. the assertion assumes the truth of that which requires proof, that societies are of a nature that they can be wholly reduced to particles, with no loss of function. Or is something lost along the way? He can't say, as his method excludes the possibility. He leaves intact the larger question of whether psychological processes (hopes, sensations, memories etc.) are of a nature which is fully explained by the actions of (say) sub-atomic particles or even neurons, i.e. can a physical structure or process explain a psychological event?

Bearing in mind the controversy that trails in the wake of any reductionist claim, Carrier is adopting an extreme position which most philosophers would find difficult to defend (extreme does not mean "a fair bit," or "more than me," it means "at the limit of human experience, the point beyond which there is no return"). He recognises this later in adding that the patterns of arrangement of the matter-energy also count: a person who falls into a meat grinder will weigh the same after the experience as before, but is no longer capable of thought, let alone higher order abstractions:

> Thus, how matter and energy are patterned, arranged, within space and time is itself a defining aspect of a thing, and this pattern has causal and other distinct properties... *reductionism does not entail that everything is 'just' matter and energy in motion* [S.III.5.5; emphasis added].

If "reductionism does not entail that everything is 'just' matter and energy in motion," we may ask "Fine, so what's the extra thing or component?" As he explains, "patterns of arrangement" assume critical importance as it is just this feature that bestows novel properties or "new causal powers" on the piles of chemicals, which is another way of saying novel properties emerge from the structures. That is, "theoretically, all of sociology and psychology can be described entirely by physics" [S.III.5.5] but that would require an entirely new understanding of "physics." Carrier doesn't use the term emergent or talk of the concept of emergentism, and there is a good reason for this, which we will see later, but is adamant that, given the computing power of a "super-mind," physical causation will be fully explanatory:

> ... a psychological phenomenon is never regarded as completely explained until it is explained biologically—likewise, a biological phenomenon is never considered completely explained until it is explained chemically, and a chemical phenomenon likewise requires a fundamental physical explanation at the most fundamental level. That scientists regard things this way, and the fact that things have been this way and are becoming more so with every passing decade, is proof enough that reductionism is a reality [S.III.5.5].

Nobody is disputing that reductionism works, the only question he needs to answer is whether it will work for *everything*, particularly the ancient problem of how mind arises and how it interacts with the body. Carrier now introduces another qualification to this emphatic credo which, in this computer age, comes as no surprise:

> ... mental and biological phenomena are the outcomes of *patterns of activity* that could be manifested by several different materials ... Psychology would apply equally to a mind produced by a biological or an electronic brain, if the *patterns of activity* were sufficiently the same. If an alien arrived whose brain used entirely different chemicals and structures to perform what are otherwise the same aggregate functions as our brains, our science of psychology would describe both minds, even though their underlying biology was different [S.III.5.5; emphasis added].

Here, he loses his case for a physicalist, determinist universe: there is more to the mind than can be explained by its ultimate particles. Yes, the particles count but what they do counts more. At this point, biological psychiatrists searching for a philosophical justification for their ideological claims would turn away in disappointment because, for them, disturbances of biology are both necessary and sufficient to explain mental disorder. Ephemera such as "patterns of activity" immediately open the door to psychological causes of mental disorder. For them, mental disorder *must* reduce to brain disorder with no other variables involved. But for Carrier, the physical elements of the brain are important, then the physical organisation, and now the final link in the causative chain is in place, patterns of activity, or the controlled manipulation of information which, he states, is *independent* of its implementing (physical) mechanism. That is, he is arguing that human psychology depends on something *more than just* chemistry and physiology, it depends on information and, as we have previously seen, "Information is information, not matter or energy. No materialism which does not admit this can survive at the present day" (Norbert Wiener, *Cybernetics,* 1948). Having revealed he believes there is something more to humans than can be explained reductively, it appears Carrier is endorsing some form of dualism.

14.3. Philosophy persists.

In discussing a reductionist approach to chess, he says "The entire game is reducible to nothing more than binary mathematics." In computer chess, "... nothing is going on except a vast stream of electrons changing places in a web of components according to the physical structure of a tiny computer chip." Now he dismisses substance dualism, but immediately argues that a game of computer chess is "something more" than "just" electrons in a grid. What is that "something more"? A pawn in such a game exists but it is certainly not a magic substance and "just as absurd to say that the pawn exists in some higher abstract reality... it only and entirely exists as a pattern of electrons in motion on a grid of transistors. Yet *that pattern is causally different than any other...*" (emphasis added).

But the pawn does exist in some higher abstract reality, the only proviso being that it's just not in the computer. The computer is simply a dumb machine designed to implement a set of rules in an electronic medium. The "higher abstract reality" that designed those rules hasn't evaporated, it existed in the programmer's mind when s/he devised the particular set of rules, aka program, for the computer to follow, and it's still there. The "abstract reality" of chess is a genuine reality, not spurious, but it's a mental reality, and that is what Carrier has to explain. He has to answer the question "What is the nature of mind that it can dream up abstract things like games, and symphonies, and political manifestos, and religions...?" Carrier believes he has offered a non-mentalist explanation of behaviour but, like Skinner, he hasn't eliminated the mental element at all, all he has done is hide it in the environment. And that just is dualism, albeit not necessarily a substance dualism.

With this rather shaky foundation in place, we move to S.III.6, our major interest, *The Nature of Mind.* In his introduction, he equates the common perception of "soul" with what "scientists and philosophers have long called a 'mind'":

> ...a soul appears to be nothing more than the functional outcome of a particular kind of brain. Since your mind is your soul, to discuss the nature of the soul means discussing instead the nature of mind. Accordingly, the following takes scientific fact and fills in the blanks according to the predictions of Metaphysical Naturalism [S.III.6].

We have to be very careful of that word "functional" as functionalists use it to explain away mind (see Chap. 7) and biological psychiatrists use it to mean "psychological but not dualist." As his definition stands, it is lurching perilously close to meaning "dualist." Moving on, Carrier defines his field:

> The word 'mind' refers to a particular pattern of brain content and activity, which includes not only the input and processing of data (sensation) but also the recognition of patterns in that data (perception), the analysis of relationships among those patterns (reason) and, above all, the ability to recognise a *particular* pattern, that of a *self*. ... distinguish(ing) us from possibly every other animal on earth ... [S.III.6.1]

He insists there is no supernatural element to this as the "self" gives us "magnificent though perfectly natural powers generally not shared by other animals," including self-reflective identity, a rational will, and self-referencing memory, which combines with the first two abilities to produce identity. But this is all a brain function: the brain (specifically the cerebral cortex) is a storage medium for "everything that we are" such as memories and abilities:

> ... its activity generates our continuity of perception and thought, our 'consciousness' ... its self-perception generates entirely new kinds of information that... like all information, affects the behavior of the whole being, changes that are in turn perceived. And so on. *That* is a mind [S.III.6.1] ... I believe the mind is solely the product of a functioning, physical brain, an active pattern of matter and energy in space-time [S.III.6.6] .

After briefly discussing virtual reality, he concludes that "the brains of *all* higher animals are ... virtual reality machines," but the human brain also constructs "an even more astounding virtual construction: that of a self":

> The brain constructs this "self" out of the brain's real values, memories, abilities, calculations and choices. These control the brain's highest functions and they collectively correspond to "us." The virtual self includes the sensation of being at the centre of it all, of observing it all. And this perception of a self is the observation, not something distinct from it. It is a construction of use to the brain of use to *us*. This is what consciousness actually is... the brain (knowingly or not) creates *fictional* models, using remembered data in creative ways ... to work out possible scenarios and choices... This is what permits us to consciously reason, to imagine and plan and to think in our heads using the same language we speak... we can practice and experiment and think through countless scenarios and possibilities, gaining tremendous experience without actually risking anything or exhausting our resources [S.III.6.2]

And it is at this point that we must part company, as that is not a reductionist account of mind, it is unalloyed dualism. By its defining parameters, a "virtual self" *just is* dualist. As Carrier uses the word, virtual *means* an unlocalised, insubstantial, causally-effective entity which emerges from and then exerts control over the physical machine (brain or computer) from which it arose. However, and crucially, it is *not* constrained by the very laws of physics, including the laws of thermodynamics which, as Carrier insists, govern the entire universe in every respect with no exceptions. Why is it not so constrained? Because the laws of physics relate to matter and energy in space-time, and an immaterial "mind/soul/virtual self," generated in an unnamed medium by unknown mechanisms is not made of matter-energy located in space-time. Granted, his "self" is cast in physicalist terms, not as classic Cartesian substance dualism, but dualism is as dualism does: if you invoke an insubstantial, unlocalised, causally-effective entity which is not bound by the rules of the physical universe, you have *ipso facto* created a dual system. Or should I say "recreated," as Descartes got there first.

Similarly, "patterns of activity" are above and beyond the arrangements of physical structure, they need a separate account according to an agreed theory, while "fictional" means "made up, not real." Of course, his case for virtuality may have been strengthened if he had given some indication of how the virtual body arose or emerged from and then acted back on its physical substrate but that would entail an entirely separate and irreducible theory of information. However, because he was committed to the belief that matter-energy reduction is the only valid scientific explanation, he didn't and couldn't have such a theory and was thus unable to incorporate emergence [4].

All of this is description masquerading as explanation (the same complaint as was levelled against Skinner and against Dennett) but dressed in physical terms: *how* does the brain create fictional models? What does it *mean* "to consciously reason, to imagine and plan and to think", how are sensory experiences generated, what are emotions, how are they implemented, on and on? We see this repeatedly throughout this section and in others, for example, S.III.6.4.1, *Thoughts*, consists of a lengthy description of visual perception and how it is processed and fed to "brain centres that are the 'eyes' of the brain itself..." Immediatetly, this establishes an infinite regress (as in "And what perceives the signals from the 'eyes' of the brain?" "More 'eyes'."), so it has no explanatory power. To cap it all, his "virtual self" also sets up an infinite regress, as in: "The virtual self includes the sensation of being at the centre of it all, of observing it all." That is exactly what Skinner railed against, half a century ago [5]. As we see, all the talk about "the brain does this and the brain does that" is a smoke screen, an intuition pump, in Dennett's words (Chap. 7), meaning a first or superficial reading leads to an impression (of physicalism) which is not supported by the literal meaning of the section. He implies "It's all brains, brains, brains," but then smuggles in a "virtual self" at the end to complete the causal chain, as in "It's all brains, brains, brains, except when we need something non-physical to make sense of it." Once again, and precisely as Daniel Stoljar warned, physicalism fails (see Chap. 1).

Returning to the text, in S.III.6.5, *The Nature of Knowledge*, Carrier says:

> Such a network of information possessed in the brain is mutually reinforcing, strengthening the level of emotional and motivational "confidence" or "belief" the brain will generate in connection with any piece of information... It follows that belief is a material property of the brain, a pattern of neurons and neural connections distinct from that of disbelief or uncertainty, a pattern that has causal powers... Knowledge and belief are thus physical realities, physical distinctions... (humans) have such large and intricately developed brain centres for processing

symbolic thought, a "language." By being able to make more (and more precise) distinctions among the patterns in our perception, in our *virtual* models... we are able to acquire far more knowledge... (emphasis added).

Several points: beware of smuggler's quotes. Essential terms are introduced in scare quotes but this is to convince the reader that they are only *façon de parler* when, in fact, they cannot be explained further just because they are being used as description, with no explanatory value. The next time we see "belief," it has been sterilised of its mentalist connotations and is just plain belief, equating to "a material property of the brain," a physical reality that does everything mental beliefs do but without the metaphysical baggage. Except "belief" only works "..in our *virtual* models..." by which means the mentalism is smuggled back into the account. Normal mentalist language has been recast in what are essentially pseudo-biological terms which seem to assign the phenomena to the biological camp as though the question is settled when, in fact, we need full explanations of such terms, e.g. the use of symbols. The essence of a symbol is that it is *not* identical with its physical token; symbols require a separate explanation in non-physical terms but he can't provide one: "I believe the mind is solely the product of a functioning, physical brain, an active pattern of matter and energy in space-time." Granted; that is not in dispute (except by the seven billion people with religious ideas) but that credo is the *starting point* of a philosophy of mind, not the end point.

Take another example from his essay *Moral Ontology*, from 2011 [6]. In discussing fear, he states:

> ... the scariness of an enraged bear is not a property of the bear alone but a property of the entire bear-person system. And it is a physical property (it reduces entirely to the physical facts about bears and people and what the one can physically do to the other) ... This scariness is also not simply subjective. Our emotional experience of fear is subjective, but the ability of the bear to harm us is an objective fact of the world ... So we can understand the ontological status of a bear's scariness and how it derives not solely from the bear but from the whole physical system it is in...

First, we want to know what the word "subjective" means. What is the nature of the brain that it can generate subjective experiences? Who experiences them? How do they work back on the body, and so on?

Second, "the ability of the bear to harm us" may be "an objective fact of the world," but it's non-explanatory. Actually, bear attacks are quite rare so let's use a much more common example of fear: fear of frogs. Frogs would be among the most harmless creatures on earth yet at least 5% of the population are seriously frightened of them. Where is the "the ability of the (frog) to harm us ... an objective fact of the world"? There is no such "objective fact of the world" as it isn't real, it's purely a mental thing [7] and he offers no mental explanation. Pushed, all he can do is invoke unexplained and, in physicalist terms, inexplicable "virtual models" to try to complete the causal chain. That's not good enough, we need some detail, some explanation of how the physical brain generates and manipulates symbols, of how subjective experiences arise in a physical, non-magical organ [8]. Simply rephrasing everything as biology explains nothing. If everything can be explained as biology, then it explains nothing.

Now Carrier may object to this but as soon as he tries to give some account of the "patterns of activity" that his model relies on, he will end up with some form of emergent informational model which is ontologically distinct from the physical structure of the brain that implements it (see above: "in our virtual models"). He tries to escape this by fiat: "... there is nothing a brain does that a mindless machine like a computer can't do even today..." [S.III.6.4.3]. Seeing blue and feeling pain are not brain functions, they are irreducibly mental experiences. He disagrees? Fine, so now we wait for him to prove his point. But he can't: in discussing qualia, the sheer experience of a sensation, he says: "I can't make any sense of such a thing. So I don't see anything here that needs explaining" [S.III.6.4.4]. It is important not to mistake the limits of one's imagination for the limits of reality. What we want from a science of mind is a considered explanation of all the stubborn bits that lurk at the limits of reality, not a blanket dismissal of their importance.

14.4. Conclusion: And philosophy wins .

Carrier does not offer an explanatory model of mind, all he does is give a list of mental functions, redescribe them in biologised language and assign them to the brain. But to no avail: in the end, he has to invoke a "virtual" entity to complete the explanation, just as Descartes did, 400 years ago, just as we have seen with Dennett and with Ryle. Without discussing the concept of emergence, he covertly introduces emergent phenomena such as a "virtual self," yet there is no account of the brain structures or mechanism by which these ghostly entities somehow come into existence, no suggestion of a medium in which they are instantiated and certainly no indication of their nature. Reeling after a blizzard of assertions that mind = brain and that everything is "matter/energy in space/time and nothing more," the reader is led to assume that the "virtual self" is also, in some vital sense, physical, but this is a common error. The fact that "virtual machines" can be programmed into a desktop computer doesn't mean they are physical *in nature*. Because virtual machines run according to the rules of whatever logical system was used to devise them, and they not located in the time-space, matter-energy universe, they therefore do not run according to the laws of the physical time-space, matter-energy universe.That is, regardless of the mechanism by which they are implemented, they are of a different and *incommensurable* order of being. In one word, dualist.

Richard Carrier uses the expression "and nothing more" so often that it makes me think there is something more. And as he shows himself, there is: in the end, he invokes an insubstantial mind or soul to complete the chain of causation.

References

1. Carrier R. *About Dr Carrier.* Available at: https://www.richardcarrier.info/about. Accessed May 29th 2023.

2. Carrier R (2005). *Sense and Goodness Without a God: a defence of metaphysical naturalism.* Bloomington, IN: AuthorHouse.

3. McLaren N (2013). Psychiatry as Ideology. *Ethical Human Psychology and Psychiatry* 15: 7-18.

4. Humphreys P (2016). Emergence: A philosophical account. New York: Oxford University Press.

5. Skinner BF (1978). Why I am not a cognitive psychologist. In: *Reflections on Behaviorism and Society.* New York: Prentice Hall.

6. Carrier R (2011). Moral Ontology. Available at: http://richardcarrier.blogspot.com/2011/03/moral-ontology.html.

7. McLaren N (2018). *Anxiety: The Inside Story.* Ann Arbor, MI: Future Psychiatry Press.

8. McLaren N (2021). *Natural Dualism and Mental Disorder: The biocognitive model for psychiatry.* London, Routledge.

15   Nagel's Third Way

> I don't want there to be a God; I don't want the universe to be like that.
>
> Thomas Nagel. *The Last Word* (1997)

15.1. Against reductionism.

In a critique of Daniel Dennett's *Bacteria to Bach*, (see Chap. 8), New York philosopher Thomas Nagel proposed that "...science will have to expand to accommodate facts of a kind fundamentally different from those that physics is designed to explain" [1]. While undoubtedly one of the most influential philosophers of mind of the past half century, Nagel is unusual (and a relief) in that he doesn't have a personal barrow to push. His position on the nature and provenance of mind is "Mind is a reality that we must explain, but neither theism nor reductive physicalism is up to the task."

His program took off many years ago with the highly-regarded paper, *What is it like to be a bat?* [2]. In this, he gave one of the more enduring definitions of consciousness (on which Chalmers, for one, relies):

> ... fundamentally an organism has conscious mental states if and only if there is something that it is like to be that organism— something it is like for the organism [2, p166].

Note the qualifier: the perception of self will vary from one organism to another. Bats, for example, don't have the perception of hanging upside down and urinating on themselves all day. To them, that's normal. It would only seem that way to us if, as humans, we tried it ourselves. But leaving bats out of it, what does this say? My answer is: Not very much. It's descriptive, not explanatory, and tells us that if we can describe an inner state, then we are conscious. This is not far removed from Descartes' conclusion that thinking (and experiencing, etc.) was the defining feature of a sentient being. But that's all we have and the question is to account for it within a rational intellectual system. The main difference between Nagel's position and that of Dennett and so many others is that Nagel doesn't believe the laws of the physical universe can amount to such a "rational intellectual system":

> Physico-chemical reductionism in biology is the orthodox view, and any resistance to it is regarded as not only scientifically but politically incorrect. But for a long time I have found (reductionism) hard to believe... almost everyone in our secular culture has been browbeaten into regarding the reductive research program as sacrosanct, on the ground that anything else would not be science [3, S.1.1; c.f. quotes by Daniel Stoljar, Chap. 2.6].

He notes that science has made massive progress by the fairly simple step of "excluding the mind from the physical world" but, we can't keep this going indefinitely. As our concepts, methods and tools of physical science have been developed to suit a mindless universe, rearranging science as we understand it to include the unseen mind will force a major change in our perception of the universe and our procedures for studying it. He favours a form of neutral monism, the idea that mind and body are different aspects of a third, unknown state but he doesn't push this idea hard. Rather, his goal is to show the failings of the alternatives, physicalism, idealism and theism.

Theism he dismisses in fairly short order, as a pseudo-explanation: "Theism ... is to be rejected as a mere projection of our internal self-conception onto the universe, without evidence" [3, S2.6]. It should be understood that that is an opinion, not an argument. It extends to all attempts at a supernatural "explanation" of mental life, but that doesn't mean we must submit to a doctrinaire physicalism. If science can't account for the sheer experience of having a mental life, the *being* part in human being, then our concept of science is deficient and we need to do better. That, however, is not his role: "My aim is not so much to argue against reductionism as to investigate the consequences of rejecting it—to present the problem rather than to propose a solution" [2, S.2.1]. He sees an ordered universe, of which mind is a natural part:

> Nature is such as to give rise to conscious beings with minds; and it is such as to be comprehensible to such beings. Ultimately,

therefore, such beings should be comprehensible to themselves. And these are fundamental features of the universe, not byproducts of contingent developments whose true explanation is given in terms that do not make reference to mind (i.e. physics) [2, S.2.2].

In Chapter 3, *Consciousness,* Nagel outlines some of the many attempts that have been made over the past century or so to provide a physicalist alternative to the Cartesian "ghost in the machine." "Here," he says, "begins a series of failures." We've covered most of them in earlier chapters, including various forms of behaviorism, psycho-physical identity theory, functionalism, eliminative materialism, etc, all of which fail for .... :

> ... the same old reason: even with the brain added to the picture, they clearly leave out something essential, without which there would be no mind ... The multiple dead ends in the forward march of materialism suggest that the (mental/physical) dualism introduced at the birth of modern science may be harder to get out of than many people have imagined ... I believe we will have to leave materialism behind. Conscious subjects and their mental lives are inescapable components of reality not describable by the physical sciences [2, S.3.1].

Despite its manifest failure to produce results, he noted wryly that "Many—perhaps most—philosophers are still committed to the reductionist project..." Subsequently, he explores the concept of a monist universe, in which all elements have a dual nature, physical and mental, that can combine to produce a physical entity with a mental component, a doctrine commonly known as panpsychism: "... all the elements of the physical world are also mental ... Any further consequences of their more-than-physical character at the microlevel remain unspecified by this abstract proposal" [2, S.3.4]. However, he allows that the "protopsychic properties" of matter, while needed in an explanatory role, are outside the pale of science: "completely indescrib-able and had no predictable local effects..." He concedes this is really just an idea, "... the form of an explanation without any content..." After considering a number of other possibilities, he concludes:

> I believe that the role of consciousness ... is inseparable from perception, belief, desire and action, and finally from reason. The generation of the entire mental structure would have to be

explained by basic principles, if it is recognised as part of the natural order. Philosophy cannot generate such explanations ... we should not renounce the aim of finding an integrated naturalistic explanation of a new kind [2, S.3.7].

It has to be understood that he has not offered a knock-down argument against psychophysical reduction. He describes *that* it has failed but does not explain, in a general sense, why. In this respect, his case is incomplete: was it just their bad luck that behaviorists or functionalists or identity theorists pulled a bad card from the pack, or was there something systemically wrong with the whole pack? Should we just keep waiting for a resolution of reductionism, as Richard Carrier suggests? Carrier's view is that reductionism is correct, we just haven't yet got the laboratory tools to demonstrate its truth:

> But if physicalism is true, shouldn't science have proved it by now? No. That we haven't done that, is not because physicalism is false. It's because we don't have the means to get there yet. ... What we need to answer these questions is better instruments. ... we can't really understand consciousness without instruments capable of resolving brain activity at the nearly atomic scale [4].

Strictly speaking, Nagel has no answer to Carrier's supremely optimistic promissory materialism. He just doesn't believe it will work so we should also be looking at other options rather than putting all our eggs in the materialist basket. In considering cognition (Chapter 4), the same problem arises:

> The questions is how to understand mind in its full sense as a product of nature—or rather, how to understand nature as a system capable of generating mind [2, S.4.1].

His approach stands in contrast to Carrier, quoted above. Where Carrier has no doubts that in the fullness of time, science will deliver, Nagel looks at the assumptions on which his confidence ressts and finds fault. Not just one fault, but many, including the need for materialists to show how our cognitive and linguistic capacities had intrinsic survival value in the evolutionary sense. For example, using reason to justify our capacity to reason as having inherent survival value is a circular exercise. He can see how conscious elements such as "perception, emotion, desire and aversion" can have survival value, because we can see the same abilities in animals, but our cognitive abilities extend far beyond these primitive performances, such as "...

the avoidance of inconsistency, the subsumption of particular cases under general principles, the confirmation or disconfirmation of general priniciples by particular observations, and so forth ... it does seem to be something that cannot be given a purely physical analysis (or) explanation..." [2, S.3.4].

He is right to raise these objections, but relying on what is no more than an eloquent argument puts his views in the same class as Carrier's, above: opinion. He ends this section with a startling suggestion: "Each of our lives is a part of the lengthy process of the universe gradually waking up and becoming aware of itself." Shortly, he reverts to the idea of a monist, panpsychist universe, on the basis that, compared with standard evolutionary speculations on the emergence of consciousness and rationality, it seems "relatively credible." Surprisingly, he takes the view that a reductive account of reason...

> ... is even more difficult to imagine than a reductive account of consciousness. Rationality ... cannot be conceived, even speculatively, as composed of countless atoms of miniature rationality. The metaphor of the mind as a computer built out of a huge number of transistor-like homunculi ... could account for behavioral output, but not for understanding [2, S.4.5].

This is a direct challenge to Dennett's account of rationality but relies on a shifting definition of "understanding." A wit once said that insisting computers can never understand is like saying aircraft can't fly because they can't land gracefully in trees. Even in the ten years since Nagel's book was published, artificial intelligence has made huge advances. Betting against the future is always risky. Finally, he turns to the question of value, which means what we understand. After a lengthy debate on the virtues and weaknesses of moral realism vs. subjectivism and their relationship to evolutionary pressures, he states:

> Nevertheless, I remain convinced that pain is really bad, and not just something we hate, and that pleasure is really good, and not just something we like. That is how they glaringly seem to me, however hard I try to imagine the contrary, and I suspect the same is true of most people [2, S.5.4].

The debate winds on, eventually grinding to an inconclusive halt which amounts to little more than saying that he finds the arguments in favour of "... the prevailing naturalism, a reductive materialism that purports to capture life and mind through its neo-Darwininan exension

... antecedently unbelievable—a heroic triump of ideological theory over common sense" [2, Ch.6]. Surprisingly, there is no mention of where this ideology arose: in the positivist ambitions of the Vienna Circle (see Chap. 1). In this respect, his survey is not just deficient but really a waste of time. Why are scientists trapped in a failed ideology? Why don't some of them see what, to Nagel, is increasingly obvious? If reductive materialism can't deliver the goodies, what are the steps toward building a new approach to science? Who will start the ball rolling, who will provide the intellectual push to expand our concept of science to include the most complex matter of all, the human mind? Well, certainly not Thomas Nagel.

15.2. Conclusion: There is no conclusion.

While arguments over the nature and place of human values in our lives go back to time immemorial, becoming ever more convoluted and indecisive with each pass, attempts to establish some sort of universality and/or functional independence of values go nowhere. Just as Descartes said, that for every opinion expressed in one of the Great Books, he could go to another and find the opposite opinion expressed with equal conviction, it is true that for every human rule and value, we can easily look around and find contradictory views. Pain is bad. Childbirth? Choosing to have an operation? I don't think so. Pleasure is good. Rape? Corruption? War? Sexual abuse and/or murder of children? There are people who really enjoy those things. Murder is bad? Not when it is ordered by our government for the purpose of furthering their interests. Incest is bad? Not when you're Lot's daughters and all the men in your city have been incinerated by a vengeful God, you need a child to carry the family name and the only man available is your father, so you get him drunk and bed him, naming the resultant sons Moab and Ben-Ammi (Genesis 19:1-38).

Values are what we say they are. Each society is different, each family is different, and each generation. The powerful set the values to suit themselves and savage anybody who challenges them: telling the truth about terrible crimes against humanity is virtuous, except when your name is Julian Assange. Values are just ephemeral social rules, based ultimately in our most primitive drives [5]. We are social animals, therefore we need rules to keep the peace so the first society didn't tear itself to bits. Who makes the rules? The biggest and strongest (nothing has changed). What makes them decide they need rules? The dominance drive, the insatiable human urge to create dominance hierarchies with me and my supporters on top and everybody else grovelling in submission [5]. Add to this the territorial urge, the omnipresent drive to grab property and hang on to it, and we need nothing more to explain values.

A value is whatever will help me survive in the ultra-competitive world of human affairs. Yes, that's a crude and demeaning assessment but do you know how many nuclear weapons there are in the world today and what they're intended to do? How much money is allocated for renovating them over the next thirty years, and how many people will starve as a result, or be driven from their homes by climate change because the money was spent on bombs, not on new technology that would replace fossil fuels? We can easily deconstruct values to show that we are functioning at much the same biological level as a bull elephant seal protecting his harem, that most of our intellectual justification ("the rules-based international order") is no more than face-saving window-dressing [6].

While Nagel is weaving intricate webs of ideas and theories in a cloud of examples and counter-examples, the world is heading to climate catastrophe. His analysis of values does not and cannot address that point and is a clear example of what happens when people try to discuss the concept of mind without having a theory of mind as a starting point: "pain is really bad ... pleasure is really good ... That is how they glaringly seem to me." Seem? Is that the best he can do? Yes, it is, because without a theory of mind, he is stuck at the level of description and opinion.

I agree that physicalist reductionism and theism have failed but, as he himself acknowledges, given the choice of reductionism or theism, panpsychism is not an answer. The knock-down argument against reductionism is clear: The mind deals in symbols. Symbols cannot be reduced to their material substrate; if they could, they would cease being symbols. There is no material way around this impasse; only a theory of information can do that (Wiener: "Information is information, not matter or energy. No materialism which does not admit this can survive at the present day"). However, Nagel made no moves in that direction. In the search for a theory of mind to provide a model of mental disorder, his work stands as an argument against the ideology of reductionism, but is otherwise of no value.

References.

1. Nagel T (2017) Is consciousness an illusion? Critique of Dennett's Bacteria to Bach. *NY Review of Books*, March 9th, 2017.

2. Nagel T (1974). What it is like to be a bat? *The Philosophical Review*, 83 (4): 435-450. Page numbers above refer to his collection *Mortal Questions*, from 1991.

3. Nagel T (2012) *Mind and Cosmos: Why the materialist neo-Darwinian conception of nature is almost certainly false.* New York: OUP (the e-version is not paginated).

4. Carrier R (2018). The Mind Is a Process Not an Object: On Not Understanding Mind-Brain Physicalism (29.06.18) https://www.richardcarrier.info/archives/14282

5. McLaren N (2023): *Narcisso-Fascism: The psychopathology of right wing extremism.* Ann Arbor, MI: Future Psychiatry Press.

6. McLaren N (2021): *Natural Dualism and Mental Disorder: The biocognitive model for psychiatry.* London, Routledge.

16   Reclaiming the mind
from metaphysics

I know that most men, including those at ease with problems of the greatest complexity, can seldom accept the simplest and most obvious truth if it be such as would oblige them to admit the falsity of conclusions which they have proudly taught to others, and which they have woven, thread by thread, into the fabrics of their lives.

Leo Tolstoy.

16.1. Psychiatry's intellectual vacuum.

After that quick stroll through theories of mind and models of mental disorder from the twentieth century, what do we know? Answer: Not much. Next question: How come? With this immense intellectual effort by so many highly intelligent, highly-educated, well-connected and highly paid people on the job, how come we really don't know much more than a hundred years ago? When it comes to the brain itself, we know a great deal but this has not translated into understanding mental disorder. We even have "translational centres" but they have achieved nothing.

The reason is that positivists have spent the past hundred years trying to eliminate all traces of the mentality of the human mind, just because it didn't fit their concept of how science should be conducted. In the process of cleansing science of any traces of metaphysics, they have destroyed anything of interest. All we have is a shell where a major figure can say "I learn about myself the same way as I learn about you, by watching (my) behaviour and listening to (my) utterances" [1, p149]. That is, while we have inner access to our feelings and beliefs, our memories and hopes, they are not proper evidence to use for a theory of mind. But who is the I that does the watching and listening to myself? Immediately, Ryle was locked in an infinite regress, exactly what he said he could avoid by *not* talking about ghostly inner perceptions.

But having spent all that time and effort trying to eradicate the mentality of mind, what happens? Correct. At the first sign of their path running into the sand, they put in an order for a "virtual machine" to swoop down and helicopter them out of the ordure. If it weren't so serious, it would actually be quite funny, but it is important to remember that professors are often in error but they are never wrong, so we need not expect them to recant or apologise for having led us down the garden path.

The time has come to announce to the world: Positivism has failed. It is incapable of providing a plausible account of mind, and thence of mental disorder. The reason it has failed is because it was not built on a theory of information. In order to see this point, we need to look again at the reasons the various theories on offer failed. With biological psychiatry, some might argue it hasn't failed yet because nobody has attempted to write a plausible theory reducing mind to brain (Chap. 1). I disagree: it's over 150 years since Henry Maudsley in the UK announced "Mental disease is brain disease," and nothing has come of it. We can take absence of proof as proof of absence: they haven't written it because they can't. In any event, Daniel Stoljar's conclusion [2] puts the burden of proof well and truly on the biological psychiatrists. If they wish to be taken seriously and, more to the point, if they wish to dominate the institution of psychiatry and control the funding, they need to produce some sort of model of mental disorder as a biological disturbance of the brain. David Kingdon, professor of psychiatry at Southampton, UK, put his finger on it:

> Biological research has produced major advances in our understanding of our bodies and, where systems go wrong, is producing remedies to address these, but it has yet to do the same for the mind. This is because no causative biological evidence has been found for the major mental disorders in contrast to the wealth of psychosocial findings. This disparity in regard and resource needs to be addressed [3].

Before we, as a community, authorise another penny of taxpayers' money be spent on biological research in psychiatry, and certainly before we spend another $20billion, the researchers need to answer this question: "What is the proof that your approach can work?" Generally, when asked that question, biological psychiatrists redden and start spluttering about genes and neurotransmitters and drugs, a bit like devout religionists who, when asked for the proof of their god's existence and benevolence, point to the world and say "You're standing in the evidence." But "proof" is not "evidence." These are distinct epistemological categories. If asked for proof that the square on the hypotenuse is equal to the sum of the squares on the other two sides, you do not find half a dozen right-angled triangles, measure them, calculate all the squares and say "There you are, there's the evidence." Yes, that's evidence but it's inductive evidence and therefore it isn't proof. The overwhelming majority of biological psychiatrists do not understand this point.

But the real question, which Andrew Scull discusses [4], is why were reductionist biological psychiatrists able to snatch the field of psychiatry away from their psychologically-minded colleagues? Part of it was practical: psychodynamic psychiatry, as practised by Freudian analysts, was hugely expensive, it was going nowhere and had become a laughing stock (Chap. 2), but part was ideological. Positivist science, including medicine, was roaring ahead on a hundred fronts so psychiatrists could either jump on the train or be left to slug it out with roving bands of psychologists. It was an easy decision. As psychiatry quickly discovered its "biological roots," the Freudians soon died of irrelevance.

By using a shield bearing the legend "More positivist than Thou," psychiatry was able to keep the psychologists at bay, long enough to grab the bulk of the research money—and the legal authority to enforce treatment. But it was ideology: where is the authority for saying that early life experiences are not, and cannot be, causative of mental disorder? Common sense says they are, but they didn't fit the rigid positivism that psychiatrists had unknowlingly adopted, so out they went. Where is the evidence to say that detention and involuntary treatment causes more good than harm? Every day in every city in the world, without any hint of due process, people are wrestled to the ground, locked up, stripped of their clothes and identity, injected and shoved into solitary confinement ("seclusion") or into yards full of seriously distressed people. There is no evidence for this, it is all on the basis of an ideology of mental disorder that no psychiatrist in the world has ever attempted to develop to the level of a model.

A psychiatry based on behaviorism, the other wing of positivism, never really had a chance (Chap. 3). Sensibly, psychologists didn't attempt to explain the whole of mental disorder on the basis of learning theory. They chose as their field anxiety, well aware that psychiatrists had very little interest in it, then sat on the sidelines carping and complaining that nobody took them seriously. Possibly, "peak psychology" came and went by about 1974, after the popular magazine *Psychology Today* serialised Skinner's *Beyond Freedom and Dignity*. However, had you blinked, you would have missed it.

That leaves only "psychiatry as a gallimaufrey" (that's a polite word for 'mishmash'), a mixture of this and that which, ideally, would be to satisfy the patient's needs but, in practice, meant indulging the psychiatrist's prejudices. First there was eclectic psychiatry, which meant choosing from a range of approaches and treatments but quickly became a matter of "anything goes." That didn't last long. Next was the more durable biopsychosocial (BPS) model, attributed to the late George Engel, which was technically still born but refuses to lie down (Chap. 5). Decades after it was pronounced dead on arrival, this zombie model is kept upright by bands of determined supporters.

One of the most determined is Professor Derek Bolton, whom we met in Chapter 6. His full title is Emeritus Professor of Philosophy and Psychopathology at the Department of Psychology; Institute of Psychiatry, Psychology and Neuroscience; King's College London (he trained in philosophy and psychology). In a lecture delivered to the Royal College of Psychiatrists, Prof. Bolton revealed he is "Looking forward to a decade of the biopsychosocial model" [5]. Using the examples of chronic stress and the perception of pain, he demonstrated how biological, psychological and social factors influence the state of health. Due to the wealth of evidence relating to the effect of psychosocial influences on the precipitation and course of illnesses, both physical and mental, he felt it would be highly appropriate to declare a "decade of the biopsychosocial model" along the lines of the "decade of the brain" from twenty years ago. He ended with a call for the rest of medicine, not just psychiatry, to embrace a BPS model.

To be clear, his paper was an opinion on the direction psychiatry (and medicine) should take. It was not original research and the author gave scant references to the scientific literature. But it illustrates clearly how the illusion of the BPS model is kept alive. In the first place, he referred to "vocal criticisms by experts a decade ago." In fact, the first and most serious critique of George Engel's BPS model was published twenty over five years ago [6], namely, that it doesn't exist. Bolton elected to ignore this paper but acknowledged a number of critiques dating from more than ten years later which focussed on the vagueness and lack of form of the BPS model. He omitted to mention that its vagueness and lack of form is due to its non-existence. He also did not refer to the steady stream of papers which have elaborated on the theme of the first paper, for example, exploring the possibilities for how Engel could have been so seriously mistaken over his own model [e.g. 7].

Now to my mind, if you're going to advocate a particular model, and somebody has published a long series of papers over a quarter of a century arguing that your favourite model doesn't exist, you can be expected to take note of the objections. Bolton didn't do this. Instead, having spent many years telling everybody what a wonderful future the BPS model has, everybody who says Engel never wrote it must be airbrushed out of the narrative. And that is precisely what he has done. He said "Vocal criticisms were voiced by experts." The clear implication is that the BPS model is a reality that simply needs a bit of work to bring it up to scratch when, as a matter of demonstrated fact, it doesn't exist.

The second point is that, just as Engel did 45 years ago, when Bolton talked about the form of a BPS model, he used the future conditional tense ("... a theorised biopsychosocial model would include core concepts ..." [5, p2]), not the present tense. This is a clear statement that it doesn't exist, but he immediately switched to talking about such models (now plural) as real, articulated entities: " ...major new explanatory theories that integrate biopsychosocial factors across very wide ranges of health conditions have been developed in the past few decades ..." [5, p2]. There is no shortage of statistical papers showing an association between psychosocial factors and disease outcomes, but association is not causation. It is simply false to state that there are explanatory, integrative models of mind and body, but this is all part of the expansive narrative of psychiatry surfing high on the crest of a mighty wave.

This suggests Bolton's paper is wilfully misleading and is symptomatic of the debased standard of theorising in, and the general culture of, psychiatry. The standard of what constitutes scientific fraud (the "sniff test") is much looser than criminal fraud ("Beyond reasonable doubt"). One would think the mere whisper of fraud should be enough to put any academic on tenterhooks. I have argued that the standards of intellectual honesty among our "key opinion leaders" are far from what the general public would want, but that's up to the general public to decide. If the editors of the *British Journal of*

Psychiatry and the powers-that-be in the Royal College of Psychiatrists are happy being party to a serious scientific deception then, until it becomes a public concern, it is a matter for their consciences. However, the only evidence available to the public comes from the people who are crafting the narrative and who have most to lose from having its faults exposed.

There is, however, one point in Bolton's short paper that needs emphasis, namely, the profound influence of psychosocial factors on the precipitation, presentation, course and outcome of physical and mental disorders. The evidence, from multiple sources, is such that only positivist ideologues would try to deny it, but the *evidence* that illness is influenced by psychosocial factors is not and never will be *proof* that a model of mind-body integration exists. All it says is "We need one." The only proof that such a model exists is to produce it. There is only one model of mind-body integration available to psychiatry, but George Engel didn't write it [8], it owes nothing to his work, nor did Bolton refer to it in his lecture.

16.2. To fill a vacuum.

Discouraged but undeterred by psychiatry's lack of progress in matters of the mind, we turn to the professionals. As described in Chap. 6, the linguist Noam Chomsky split mental function in two, keeping the cognitive element and throwing the rest to poets and philosophers. In his model, the cognitive functions serving language reduce to two operations, Move and Merge, which are biologically-based and sprang into existence in current form after a single, small mutation some 60-80,000 years ago. Prior to that, there was no language. From the biological point of view, this is vanishingly unlikely; it is far, far more likely that language evolved slowly, albeit with a few jumps or saltations along the way. There is now evidence from palaentology that this is correct, that characteristics we regard as quintessential features of *Homo sapiens*, in particular, funerary rites, were also associated with a recently discovered line of hominins. Excavations from what is known as the Rising Star cave system of South Africa have indicated that *Homo naledi*, a small, gracile hominin with upright posture and a brain about one third the size of *H sapiens,* undertook ritual burial of their dead. This was some 200,000 years ago, long before the previous earliest evidence of burial rites in *H sapiens.*

Can there be funeral rites in animals with no language? Certainly, many mammals and even birds show an awareness of death but digging circular holes deep in barely accessible caves (which implies control of fire and being able to plan ahead to take food, water and fuel for the light), placing bodies in certain postures and then carefully burying the remains is many orders of complexity removed from such simple behaviours. I don't believe it would happen without language: the burden of proving that it could be done without language rests with those who make the claim. Researchers have documented artwork carved on the walls of the caves although it isn't certain that this dates from the same period or was added later by a different species. But the major point is that we did not descend from *Homo naledi*. It seems another and very different species of *Homo* also had some level of language, so how many more were there? This is the sort of evidence that argues that Chomsky's rhetorical question, "Why Only Us?" was misconceived: it wasn't just us, and it wasn't suddenly one day, 70,000 years ago. Time will tell, but I doubt even Chomsky's greatly shrunken ideas will be part of the debate for much longer.

When we turn to the other authors, Donald Davidson definitely has something to offer psychiatry although perhaps it wasn't what he intended. As mentioned in Chap. 12, Davidson's starting point is that the mind is a real thing and, even though it seems contradictory, we have to make sense of it. I'm unconvinced by his resort to a form of identity theory. Identifying mind and brain resolves the question of the mind-body junction by declaring they are one and the same. However, it is not an explanation as it doesn't touch the question of how a physical organ implements non-physical, mental functions. The identity theorist replies that this is a misapprehension of the nature of mental functions since, as a matter of contingent fact, mental functions just are physical in nature. The national anthemn is physical in nature? Specifically, just which part of the physical brain or of its physiology implements mental functions? It has to be a physical part; it can't be neuronal *function*, as that would immediately tell us mental functions are emergent, i.e. that they are not identical with the brain as they have new or novel functions. I submit that mind-brain identity is an example of what Moritz Schlick had in mind with his broadside against metaphysics:

> There are consequently no questions which are in principle unanswerable, no problems which are in principle insoluble. What have been considered such up to now are not genuine questions, but meaningless sequences of words. To be sure, they look like questions from the outside, since they seem to satisfy

the customary rules of grammar, but in truth they consist of empty sounds, because they transgress the profound inner rules of logical syntax discovered by the new analysis [8].

On this basis, the question "How can brain and mind be seen as identical?" is a "meaningless sequences of words," not so much an attempt at explanation as an evasion. However, Davidson's idea that the cause of a belief is another belief does not fall into the same trap. Even though he offers no explanation of the nature of belief as an informational state, it has traction in psychiatry. Beliefs do not exist in isolation, they are nested in prior beliefs, but these are necessarily broader and less developed. Instead of seeing all beliefs as essentially equal, with lines of beliefs joined head to tail like a train, we can envisage them as like small, refined cups, each nested in larger, cruder cups. As we do down the line, our beliefs become broader, more general, less sophisticated but, this is critical, more tightly held because so much more depends on them. At base, I identify totally with my fundamental beliefs: I can't change them without changing who I am. It is by this means that rational people come to believe nonsense.

This is critically important because apparently rational people who believe palpable nonsense have a firm grip on our destiny. There are, for example, powerful people who believe it is possible to fight a nuclear war and win, or that continued burning of fossil fuels will have no environmental consequences. Their doctrine is insane but they are not themselves mad. How can we explain this contradiction? I suggest Davidson's view helps but one way we won't explain it is via John Searle's biological naturalism, in which he states his abiding belief:

> *There is nothing to the causal power of consciousness which cannot be explained by the causal power of the neuronal base.* That is why consciousness ... is an ordinary part of our human and animal biology [2, p170]. ... given the constitution of reality, consciousness has to follow in the same way that any other biological property, such as mitosis, meiosis, photosynthesis, digestion, lactation, or the secretion of bile, follows [9, p177].

The problem is that Searle begs the question, i.e. he assumes the truth of that which requires proof, but in a subtle manner. The central error is his opinion that the underlying processes of mental life are one and the same with the underlying processes of all other biological matters, that the causal power of a neuron as a physical thing also explains the causal power of the mind as a non-physical thing. This is wrong: the "neuronal base" has not one, but two, causal powers. The brain *does not function only* in the same realm as the milk-secreting cuboidal cells in mammary tissue or the epithelial cells lining the renal proximal tubules. That's akin to saying that because I have a mouse trap made of metal and plastic in one hand, and a mobile phone made of metal and plastic in the other, therefore the two things function in the same realm. They do not.

A quick look at any physiology text reveals that while the metabolic (intracellulaar) processes by which neurons operate are essentially the same as all other cells, neurons do not have the same function as other tissues. Governed by its genome, an ordinary somatic cell takes inputs of matter and energy and manipulates them strictly according to the laws of the material realm, to produce a particular output. This may be milk, urine, structural rigidity, motion, a pair of daughter cells, sugars, and so on, all of which have no significance beyond themselves. Given the laws of biochemistry and the particular inputs, the machinery of the cell cannot produce anything other than what its genome determines: there will never be a goose that lays a golden egg.

With a few minor variations, at the level of its biochemical operations, the neuron takes the same matter and energy inputs as all other somatic cells and produces ... nothing. It expends matter and energy in order to return to status quo ante. That is its role and function. In doing so, however, it acts as the mechanism of information transfer, the means by which messages are sent back and forth, which has significance above and beyond the simple action potential and is not reducible to that action potential. If it didn't return to its resting state, if each spike impulse left a trace, the neuron would soon be unable to convey any information.

Crucially, the significance of a message does not lie in the individual action potentials themselves, as they are all identical. The message *emerges* from the interaction of a number of components, as outlined in [9]. In his attempt to escape the central point of mental life, its nature as an insubstantial, unlocalised and causally efficacious entity, Searle errs in conflating the different functions of neural and somatic cells, and then arguing that, because they are the same, so mind and body are of the same nature. In order to prove his case that there is no fundamental difference between neurons and somatic cells, he wrongly assumed that having the same *cellular operations* mandated their having the same *functions* or *roles in the intact human being*. The basic biochemistry of individual muscle cells, for example, is very similar to that of all other somatic cells, but their output (contraction) is different: you will never get milk from a muscle. Most emphatically, consciousness is *not* "... an ordinary part of our human and animal biology" [9, p170]. Searle's claim that "... consciousness has to follow in the same way that any other biological property, such as mitosis, meiosis, photosynthesis, digestion, lactation, or the secretion of bile, follows" [9, p177] ignores the fact that the laws governing information processing are not the laws governing other bodily functions. Searle's attempt at a naturalistic account of mind fails on just this point, so we need to keep looking.

As described, Gilbert Ryle used the mind without offering any suggestion as to its nature, origin, mode of interaction with the world and so on. All he said was "It isn't what you think" while applying his positivist shears to trim it down. From the point of view of explaining mental disorder, his volume is of no value and, having reread it forty years after I was first introduced to it, I wonder what all the fuss was about. The same goes for Wittgenstein, who said of his *Tractatus*: "The whole sense of the book might be summed up in the following words: what can be said at all can be said clearly, and what we cannot talk about we must pass over in silence." Would that that were true. If people don't speak clearly, either they don't know what they're talking about, or they're trying to slip something past you. In any event, our interest lies in his expression "logical space" because that is clearly a mentalist/dualist concept. In the many ways he used it (see Chap. 10), it could mean more or less what the reader wants it to mean, so it's not much use. Had he defined it within the setting of a theory of information, or in informational terms, then the meaning would have been fixed—and useful. As he said in S.3.8 of the *Investigations*:

> It is also possible for someone to get an explanation of the words out of what was intended as a piece of information. [Marginal note: Here lurks a crucial superstition.]

I don't believe the idea of the mind as an informational space is a superstition. Bearing in mind Wittgenstein's ties with the Vienna Circle and their lack of a theory of information, for a lot of very bright people, the idea of the mind as magic was attractive, even compelling. But with the benefit of a hundred years of IT behind us, the value of a formal account of information is that, wholly within a naturalistic ontology, it provides a framework, a mechanism and then a medium, for the emergence of mental functions [10]. It dispels the magic and allows us to see the human mind for what it is, something fairly astounding, but not unique: contrary to our speciesist approach to the world, a theory of information also says that animals have minds. This account of mind also brings with it a model of what happens when informational states go awry: in human terms, mental disorder. But Wittgenstein didn't define his "logical space," so the debates over what he meant rage on and "we must pass over in silence" what he implied but didn't clearly state, an account of information.

So we come to the self-proclaimed "... best scientific theory to date of how our minds came into existence" [11, pxiv], Daniel Dennett's functionalist concept. He invokes the concept of a virtual machine to complete the causal chain in his approach but my view is that the mind as a virtual machine is functionally dindistinguishable from Descartes' substance dualism. We can safely conclude that Daniel Dennett is a prisoner of the antidualism meme that, way back in first year at college, "infested his brain" (I use his term advisedly even though he doesn't). Since then, it has been proliferating and despatching itself hither and thither to infect as many other naive brains as it possibly can, because that's what stripped down, intellectually undemanding ideas do. They spread to naive, uncritical brains, take over and then arrange to capture other victims. That's why stripped down, intellectually undemanding ideas, such as "My country, right or wrong," or "Death to the unbelievers," are so dangerous.

The whole concept of memes is silly: if he claims to be merely the passive host of a parasitic idea, then who wrote his books? But as a child of his positivist times, you could say, he should be pitied, not scorned; he too is a victim, after all. Perhaps we should give him more of the blue tablets to correct his distorted neural-level activity? What rubbish. He chose. Daniel Dennett has had a charmed life, gifted with practically every opportunity known to man. He made his intellectual decisions based on what he thought would allow him to elbow his way up the academic pile. Antidualism licensed contempt for the other side, it authorised and justified using his acid tongue to belittle anybody who disagreed with him. But he backed the wrong horse. He thought his antidualism was biological but it turned out to be a leering, dualist phantom after all. As he said himself:

> Sometimes what seems to be enough smoke to guarantee a robust fire is actually just a cloud of dust from a passing bandwagon [10, p257].

In this case, the bandwagon was the outcome of applying positivism to the mind, antidualism. By his definition, antidualism is a meme; he caught it; and now it's time to let it go. However, unlike the varicella (chickenpox) virus that infected me in 1953 and which lay dormant in my nervous system until a few years ago, or HIV, or Covid, his "virus-like particle" is easily cured. The cure is simply to say "Dire meme, I cast thee out. Take thy sore baggage and be gone from my life." His relatives, friends and supporters can help him through his ordeal by dancing in a circle around him, tapping zills and silver bells while chanting "Let it go, move on. Get over it, be free. Free your dualist Self of the Antidualist meme."

So to return to my original question: Can Daniel Dennett's covert dualism provide a plausible model of mental disorder leading to a viable research program via testable predictions? No, most emphatically not, because he tries to explain away the experience of mental disorder: "No, that's risible. What you call depression is actually just biology, a negatively-signed experience of no moral significance." My view is that mentally-troubled people have enough to deal with without having to listen to that sanctimonious nonsense.

An afterthought:

I will admit that, quite apart from his panting style of writing, Dennett bothers me. For nearly forty years, I have read and reread his stuff, wondering how anybody with such an education and such privilege could possibly believe such an irredeemably self-contradictory and just plain silly notion as his antidualist account of mentality. He set out to write "a theory which is *not* dualism in disguise" but all he did was hide the dualism in plain sight. As far as I can see, his error starts with his antagonism to religion. That's fine, religion certainly gives a lot to object to, but it doesn't stop there. His reasoning appears to be along the lines of:

1. Dualism means magical substances.

2. An ordinary desktop computer is a machine made entirely of physical elements, with no magical dualist substances lurking in its innards.

3. We can implement a virtual machine in an ordinary computer.

4. Therefore virtual machines have no dualist elements.

5. Therefore a virtual machine implemented in the brain has no dualist elements.

6. Therefore a virtual machine in the brain processing information is not dualist.

7. "Conscious human minds are more-or-less serial virtual machines implemented (in the brain)" [11, p218].

8. Despite all the mentalist language I use, my theory of mind is actually a theory of brain events, meaning....

9. There is no possibility of ontologically dual entities in my theory.

10. I therefore proclaim myself the winner of the competition to write a non-mental account of mind. Hooray for me.

11. P.S. Pay no attention to that virtual man behind the curtain.

Or something like that. In any event, his work shows, if further proof were needed, that metaphysical questions are not resolved by empirical evidence. Just to be sure I had not misunderstood him, I emailed Prof. Dennett this question:

> Dear Prof. Dennett,
> At various points in a number of your books, you use the concept of the mind as a virtual machine, e.g. in *Bacteria to Bach*, "Our thinking is enabled by the installation of a virtual machine made of virtual machines made of virtual machines [1, p341].
> You have probably answered this at some stage but it seems to me that a virtual machine is unlocalised, insubstantial and isn't subject to the laws of physics so it meets the criteria for a Cartesian mind/soul. Can you indicate why a virtual machine is somehow different from the "ghost in the machine" your work opposes?
> Thanking you, Sincerely

Within a few hours, he replied:

> Microsoft Word is a VM. So is Zoom. Just tools (or games or ....) made of software. DCD

This, of course, does not answer the question. I submit that, as a closet dualist, he can't answer it without surrendering his position. Historian and natural philosopher Richard Carrier uses the same virtual model albeit not so forcefully. However, it is not the force or flood of detail that decides whether an account of mind is dualist or not, it is the "mere presence" of even a hint of dualism to complete the causal chain. We have to beware of the argument "Aw dad, why can't I keep him? He's such a small puppy," or "But daddy, don't be so upset, I'm only a teensy bit pregnant." As mentioned above, dualism exists wherever an insubstantial, unlocalised entity immune to the laws of the physical universe is used to complete the causal chain. I didn't say "natural universe" because information is also real and natural, just a different sort of real and natural. There are two universes, the physical and the informational [10].

The ability to generate virtual machines is a property of any sufficiently sophisticated data processor, be it carbon-based, silicon-based or anything else. The "mere fact" that a virtual machine arises in a physical machine doesn't somehow convert its ontological status from immaterial to material, because the 'dual' in 'dualism' doesn't relate to substances, it relates to sets of laws. We live in a dualist universe, part of which, the physical part, is governed by the laws of physics, while the rest, the informational part, is governed by what George Boole called "the laws of thought" (he proposed binary logic but it could be some other system we can't yet envisage—and while we have binary logic, we're probably not going to look for another). As we've seen with Dennett and Carrier, anybody trying to give a reductionist account of mind as a physical organ without using a theory of information will inevitably have to invoke some "virtual self" to complete the causal chain. That will destroy the argument just because there is no conceivable definition of "virtual" which means, entails or implies "subject to the standard laws of the physical universe." And that's rather lucky for us because if there were, then we wouldn't have the brain power to write or read books on the nature of mind.

How did Carrier fall into this error? I suggest in exactly the same way as Dennett, Richard Dawkins and others fell into it: from the beginning, they opposed dualism because of a pre-existing antagonism to religion. Everybody knows that all religious systems are dualist; therefore, the best way to avoid slipping into religiosity (or to crush it) is to avoid dualism. Recall Dennett's rancid dismissal from Chapter 7: "...like the little green man in the control room of the man-sized puppet in the morgue in *Men in Black*... an immaterial portion of glowing ectoplasm that oozes around in your brain like a ghost amoeba... an angel whose wings are folded till you are called to fly to heaven." Such open contempt is inimical to a self-critical attitude.

In more formal terms, religiosity is just one member of the set of dualist theories: there is no religion without dualism but there can be—and is—dualism without religion. As mentioned above, dualism doesn't only mean "magical substances": dualism without a supernatural element is called natural dualism. So, with his metaphysical naturalism, Carrier was on the right path, but his program is incomplete. All it needs is an account of how causally-effective "virtual" entities arise in the brain and can act back on it. But for that he needs a theory of information [7] which, of course, opens the door to the dreaded dualism. While there is a dualist entity hidden in the works, his goal to "... reduce moral facts to physical facts in some way" will not succeed unless and until he accepts that dualism is not the enemy of rationality.

16.3: Conclusion: Reality bats last.

On that note, we move to the owner of the natural dualism meme, David Chalmers. It will be clear that I am swayed by his early work on the supervenience (I prefer emergence) of a dualist entity within a naturalistic framework but, when it comes to his latest book, *Reality+* [12], where does one start? Perhaps here:

> La crisi consiste appunto nel fatto che il vecchio muore e il nuovo non può nascere: in questo interregno si verificano i fenomeni morbosi piú svariati Antonio Gramsci (The crisis consists precisely in the fact that the old is dying and the new cannot be born; in this interregnum occur a great variety of morbid phenomena).

Manifestly, I am unmoved by the near-ecstatic accolades showered on *Reality+* . After a quick first reading, my reaction was: Do we clever, educated, healthy, wealthy and assiduously self-involved people in the West have the right to trivialise reality in this way? On Sept.10th, 2022, the Ukrainian composer, Yurii Kerpatenko, was murdered in his home in Kherson by pro-Russian paramilitaries because he refused to support the regime the invading forces had imposed on his city. Was that a simulation? No, that was reality. Are Yemeni children starving because of a virtual Saudi blockade, or is that the real thing? Were the thousands of Gazan children killed by Israeli bombs and missiles in 2023-24 simulacra? Was Fallujah reduced to smoking rubble in a large-scale *SimCity*? Were the piles of skulls raised by the Khmer Rouge simply line items in a computer program, or was Auschwitz *son et lumière*? Some of us regard merely raising these intellectual possibilities as offensive in the extreme. After a slow, laborious second, and then a third reading of Chalmers' latest offering, it is my view that the concepts underpinning his technofantasy *Reality+* are more than just offensive, they are dangerous. They also say a lot about philosophy.

While Chalmers pointedly uses "gender-neutral pronouns" and populates his scenarios with male and female figures of different races in a twee PC (including God as "she" [12, p170]), he asks: "What makes a life good for oneself?" [p316]. That, of course, is the very essence of libertarianism, the doctrine that licensed Margaret Thatcher to screech "There's no such thing as society" while systematically destroying large swathes of British society. In psychiatric terms, such exclusive self-interest is the essence of psychopathy, the personality disorder of heartless domination and amoral self-interest. The whole concept behind *Reality+* is: Indulge, indulge, indulge, there is no tomorrow. If economic libertarianism and militarism have driven the world to destruction, don't worry, just put on your VR helmet, slide into your life support cocoon, flap your virtual wings and fly into a glorious, Technicolor sunset while... While what?

Who will be able to escape like this but, even before that happens, who will protect the "well-protected warehouse"? Who will tend all the machines, squirt the food mixture down the naso-gastric tubes, clean the faeces, diagnose and treat the bed sores and orthostatic pneumonia, grow the food, build and supervise the power plants, and so on? You got it, this is all for the rich to wallow in sybaritic solipsism while the poor, who "lead hardscrabble lives on Earth's wrecked surface, avoiding gangs and dodging mines," all caused by the super-rich members of the Order of Perpetual Indulgence, the poor should find inner peace and fulfillment as a permanent underclass of drudges? I don't think any of this betrays any hint of reality. How ironic, a book about reality is totally unrealistic. It can appeal only to devout believers and/or the impressionable; a reasonably critical reader will dismiss it as an implausible mix of the ludicrous and the dangerous.

Regardless of its technical sophistication, virtual reality is nothing other than a clever technology to feed misinformation into the human brain. It uses the brain's innate sensory-receptive and processing capabilities to mislead the subject into thinking that what is being fed in is not artifice but is "the real thing." The book fails, completely, for the reasons listed above: Virtual is undefined, there is no theory of mind, no theory of information, and it's all rehashed religion anyway, stale altar wine in technobottles, you could say. Thus handicapped, it cannot show how information reaches the brain and acts upon the mind to produce these artificial effects. All Chalmers offers is an enthusiastic, even revivalist, vision of quintessentially religious concepts translated into a science fiction technobabble. To be sure, he is quite explicitly looking at the logical possibilities; at no point does he stop to consider biology, sociology—or morality. But this means there is no boundary between "logical possibilities" and inanity.

For example, in talking of "Solidity, color, and space in virtual reality" [11, p432], he asks: "How can a virtual object be colored?" The answer is quite simple, except we will have to sully ourselves by looking at the ... er... biology of vision. For any real object, light of a specific wavelength is reflected while all the rest is absorbed. Thus, plants appear green because their chloroplasts utilise all the rest of the visible spectrum; for them, the reflected green light of wavelength of about 500-570nm is waste energy. When that reflected light strikes the cone photoreceptors in the human retina, it causes a discharge in just those receptors tuned to respond to this wavelength and no others. These trigger spike discharges in the afferent neurons of the retina which travel via the optic nerve to the brainstem and thence to the occipital regions of the brain. Somehow, by means of codes which we can probably never know, those volleys of spike discharges are manipulated to produce the emergent mental effect we know as "green." Why is this emergent? Because it depends utterly on the structural *and* functional integrity of the brain, but there is no trace of green pigment inside the cranium. This, of course, is wholly a dualist account which gives no traction to functionalism [11].

Virtual or apparent objects are coloured just because the computer program driving them causes a screen to emit light of specific patterns and wavelengths that activate the retina's photoreceptors. But, and this is crucial, without photoreceptors able to send information to a suitably-equipped data processor (in our case, the brain), there is no colour. Colour does not reside "out there," it is wholly an artefact generated in the privacy of one's head. Nature knows nothing about colour, only minded beings do. So one of our most basic and treasured perceptions of the universe, that it's very pretty, is false. No color. It's like those beautiful photos taken by the Hubble telescope: they're artificial. Electromagnetic radiation is invisible. And I can create and eliminate "virtual objects" just by opening and closing my eyes.

So is virtual reality "real"? Only in the sense that a rainbow or a shadow are real, but not in any worthwhile sense of the word. The light rays entering the eyes are perfectly real, as are the soundwaves being generated in the headphones, but the *sense* or *impression* of being in some other place that they generate is, as its designers intended it to be, pure illusion. Is everything in virtual reality phony? Not entirely. As Chalmers pointed out but didn't explain, there is a genuine difference between a virtual cat and a virtual book. The cat is a specific image only, a form on a screen with no other informational significance, of the same nature as a cave painting, whereas the book consists of information with no form. Granted, the book has to be put in a form that can enter the brain (as written or spoken words) before we can use it, but the difference between a virtual cat and a virtual book is of the same order as the difference between the cat that lives in our house and Chalmer's book on my desk (actually, that's my second copy; the first was a virtual or e-book).

The Gramscian crisis in philosophy of mind consists of the fact that positivism is dying but, in the absence of an articulated theory of information, the new cannot be born. This stuff about virtual reality is entirely morbid because it helps nobody. All of this would have been apparent if Chalmers had spelled out the concept of mind, the concept of information [10] and the crucial relationship between mind and information. Without those essential foundations, *Reality+* is little more than dangerous propaganda that will convince excitable 14 year olds they need have no concerns for the world or anybody else because, as rich and privileged Westerners, they can simply plug in, turn on and drop out. Virtuously.

Indeed they can, until somebody, or nature, or AI, does a HAL 9000 [12] on them and switches off the life support.

16. 4 Reality bats last.

As part of that reality, I should point out that, after reading his volume, all the people who think dualism is magical non-thinking fit only to amuse bright but irritating 14 year olds will be greatly encouraged in their convictions. Which is sad because, despite Chalmers' pyrotechnics, it brings us no closer to answering the question: Can there be a positivist psychiatry?

References:

1. Ryle G 1949 *The Concept of Mind*. London: Hutchinson. Reprinted Penguin University Books, 1973.

---

12   The malevolent computer in Kubrick's classic film, *2001: A Space Odyssey*.

2. Stoljar D (2010). *Physicalism*. Oxford: Routledge. See also Stoljar D (2021) . Physicalism, in Stanford Encyclopedia of Philosophy, at https://plato.stanford.edu/entries/physicalism/

3. Kingdon D (2020). Why hasn't neuroscience delivered for psychiatry? *BJPsych Bulletin,* 44:107–109. doi:10.1192/bjb.2019.87

4. Scull A (2022) *Desperate Remedies: Psychiatry and the mysteries of mental illness.* London: Penguin.

5. Bolton D (2022). Looking forward to a decade of the biopsychosocial model. *British Journal of Psychiatry Bulletin,* 46: 228–232, doi:10.1192/bjb.2022.34

6. McLaren N (1998). A critical review of the biopsychosocial model. *Australian and New Zealand Journal of Psychiatry.* 32; 86-92.

7. McLaren N (2020). The Biopsychosocial Model: the end of a reign of error. *Ethical Human Psychology and Psychiatry.* 22:71-82.

8. Schlick M (1930). Die Wende der Philosophie. *Erkenntnis* 1: 4-11. Translated as The Turning Point in Philosophy. Available online.

9. Searle JR (2007). Dualism revisited. *J Physiol Paris* 101: 169–178. doi:10.1016/j.jphysparis.2007.11.003

10. McLaren N (2021): *Natural Dualism and Mental Disorder: The biocognitive model for psychiatry.* London, Routledge.

11. Dennett DC (1991). *Consciousness Explained.* Boston: Little Brown. Page numbers refer to the Penguin edition (1993).

12. Chalmers DJ (2022). *Reality+: Virtual worlds and the problems of philosophy.* London: Allen Lane.

17   Mental disorder and the limits of positivism

> The day science begins to study non-physical phenomena, it will make more progress in one decade than in all the previous centuries of its existence.
>
> Nikola Tesla.

17.1. Who said limits?

In our search for a model of mental disorder, psychiatry is no help and philosophy either evades the question by going in circles or goes backward. This raises the question of ... Why? Why, after a century of the most intense intellectual achievement in human history, do we still have major, unanswered questions about the nature of mind? The answer, in one word, is: positivism. Positivism is the culprit. To explain this, we need to go back to the Positivist Manifesto [1] and Schlick's statement [2] from nearly a century ago.

The goal of the Vienna Circle was to clear what they saw as metaphysical junk from all rational enquiry. They didn't say we have to live sterile, technical lives with no fanciful thoughts—I'm sure they all enjoyed music, novels and drama—but they wanted the clearest of lines drawn between sensible stuff and whimsy. Their starting point had to be what could be seen or measured. That way, there could be no argument. Anything else led to pointless speculation and thence to arguments, schisms, and (they didn't say but I'm sure they understood) to public disdain. So that's it: nothing but the hardest, clearest evidence could be used to build a science. Philosophy was a tool of science but not itself a science. That drove psychology down the behaviorist path until, one day, it ran into the sand.

Meantime, reductionist biomedicine was powering ahead and even psychiatry was on a bit of a winning streak. On one side, there was the ancient tradition of seeing the mind as a biological organ, especially when it started to go wrong. On the other, Sigmund Freud and his followers were loudly trumpeting that, in their objective technique of free association, they had the scientific tool to unlock the secrets of the human mind. They understood the mind as messy but rational; as dispassionate observers, they could see where the problems lay and could intervene to correct them. The way they described it, their psychoanalytic work was almost surgical in its objectivity and precision. Of course, it was nothing of the sort. Psychoanalysis was not new, it was not scientific, it was not universal and it couldn't be separated from fantasy. Eventually it collapsed, leaving the field of mental disorder open to the hard core positivists who wanted nothing to do with metaphysical inventions such as the ego, id and superego. Mental disorder is brain disorder, they announced (and still insist), amenable to a standard, natural explanation using just the tools and techniques of ordinary laboratory science. Despite massive expenditure of money and effort, that too has gone nowhere.

Needless to say, the power elite in psychiatry who control the money are not going to dump their dreams of a perfect science just because a hundred years of positivist ideology has gone nowhere. Inevitably, their answer to failure is "More of the same—more money, more researchers in more laboratories using more powerful equipment." But when it comes to searching for "virtual machines" hidden in an organ of truly cosmic complexity, that approach just isn't going to work, any more than it could help find the end of a rainbow. Or if they believe it will, could they please write a justification (aka model of mental disorder) and give the rest of us some inkling of a time line for their program? No, they won't do that because it would involve admitting they can't do it, and moving to the back of the queue—all of which is anathema to the power elite (that's what "power elite" means).

The problem with positivism is perfectly clear: it cannot deal with information as a natural part of the rational universe. Without an articulated theory of information, an unspecified virtual machine is no better than magical thinking. I need to clarify that point because, without trying to be Delphic, there's information and there's information. Very early in the history of the Vienna Circle, "It became increasingly clearer that a position not only free from metaphysics, but opposed to metaphysics, was the common goal of all" [1, p7]. They continued:

> The scientific world-conception knows no unsolvable riddle.
> Clarification of the traditional philosophical problems leads us

> partly to unmask them as pseudo-problems, and partly to transform them into empirical problems and thereby subject them to the judgment of experimental science... The scientific world-conception rejects metaphysical philosophy ... For us, *something is 'real' through being incorporated into the total structure of experience* ... there is knowledge only from experience, which rests on what is immediately given [1, p10-12; their emphasis].

That closes the door on many issues that some people might see as important but they were trying to find a solid basis for a universal, unified science, uncontaminated by unprovable beliefs and prejudices. Only observable facts can be used in science, anything less must be discarded. Schlick emphasised this in his response to the manifesto, which is worth repeating:

> There are consequently no questions which are in principle unanswerable, no problems which are in principle insoluble. What have been considered such up to now are not genuine questions, but meaningless sequences of words. To be sure, they look like questions from the outside, since they seem to satisfy the customary rules of grammar, but in truth they consist of empty sounds, because they transgress the profound inner rules of logical syntax discovered by the new analysis ... metaphysics collapses not because the solving of its tasks is an enterprise to which the human reason is unequal (as for example Kant thought) but because there is no such task [2, p56-7].

He later specified this more precisely: "... every statement has a meaning only insofar as it can be verified; it only signifies what is verified and absolutely nothing beyond this" [3]. Meaningful questions are those that can be answered by direct observations of the world; those that can't are meaningless. This is important because a lot of apparently wise or important questions are thereby shown to be meaningless: "What is a virtuous life?" "What is the value of truth?" "What is the meaning of the Holy Trinity?" and so on. So they split information in two. On the one hand, they had *closed systems* of information such as syllogisms, theorems, plans, systems of laws, and descriptions of the universe such as Mendeleyev's Periodic Table for chemistry, or the Linnaean system in biology, etc. These are all self-contained and are thereby amenable to their (positivist) system of logical analysis: given the premises, there was only one possible outcome, with no ambiguity, no indecision. That is one sort of information. While they had no formal theory of information, they felt able to use this tamed version (*informationes domesticus*, you could say).

On the other hand, there was all the empty metaphysical talk (religious and philosophical), plus fiction and literature, plus sport, politics and obscenity (not necessarily exclusive), plus humor, gossip and so on, all of which could go on forever and not reach a conclusion. This is a vast and ever-expanding *open system* of information, although they would probably argue it was too disorganised and unruly to qualify as a system (*informationes fera?*). Because it was unobservable, the mind fell in that category and, although they initially had sympathy for Freud's mechanistic and secular psychology, in the final analysis, there was room in their science for only an ascetic behaviorism. What they didn't know, because it was all in the future, was that the mind can be conceived in informational terms, as a fully functional, informational entity [4] (a "virtual machine," as we have read). The seminal papers by Turing and by Shannon were still ten and twenty years away while the Hodgkin-Huxley model of neuronal function wasn't published until 1952. The early positivists of the Vienna Circle simply didn't have the tools to reformulate the mind as something that lay within the ambit of an information-based *science*, so it was dumped with Schlick's "meaningless sequences of words" and "empty sounds."

I'd suggest there was another factor in their relegation of mind to meaningless metaphysics, although I have no evidence. The members of the Vienna Circle and their like-minded colleagues in various parts of the world were all very well educated. They would all have been familiar with the works of Descartes, of Spinoza, Leibniz, Kant and the other great thinkers. There seems little doubt that, as is still widely the case, their understanding of a dualist model of mind would have been heavily influenced by the idea of "substance dualism," that a non-physical mind meant magical properties. They would have understood that a substance has no internal form or structure, no internal mechanism that would allow a reductive explanation of its properties and performance: a substance just is. As an idea, substance dualism offers no traction, it yields no entry point, nothing that specifies "Start here to deconstruct." If the mind is a formless blob, there's no deconstructing a formless blob. All you get is bits of blob with no explanation, so it had to go.

Since then, a hundred years of doctrinaire antidualism has gone nowhere and, as I've argued [5], never will. Therefore, we need to try something else. My suggestion is that the mind emerges from the brain's information-processing capability, that it is *itself* an informational space, meaning there is no conceptual disjunction between the mind and the endless flows of information throughout the body. The body traffics in information and, putting aside its neurosecretory functions, the brain has no other role than to process it. From just that processing arises the informational space we experience as our minds. The value of this approach is that information is not a "blob," it emerges from a precisely-defined physical system with an internal structure imposed by the laws of its calculus. On that basis, we can now understand the emergent mind *as a closed informational system* and deal with it just as we deal with theorems, syllogisms, plans, etc. That is ...

> **An understanding of the origin and internal function of mental life does not involve forays into the enigmatic realms of an unknowable metaphysics/fantasy, any more than does, say, geometry, the traffic code, the periodic table, or knowing why this computer works when switched on.**

There is an obvious caveat here regarding what we can know. Without ever breaching the laws of thermodynamics [4], the closed informational system we call the mind allows us to make stuff up, i.e. to expand the open system of information (the mental contents) without limit. Fiction lies outside the scope of rational enquiry: when we talk of the closed system of the mind, we are talking of its mechanisms, meaning its range of logical operations and their format, not of its content. These are two entirely distinct applications of the word "information." For example, we can have the closed informational system relating to a bus. This would included the plans and designs involved in building it, all the information relating to where the ore for the steel was mined and how it was transported and refined, and so on. Then there is the application of positivist principles to using that bus: how to maximise the profits, when to pay back the loan and all those sensible considerations. What positivism *can't* address is the question of whether, in order to maximise profit, it is *morally* right to reserve the bus for the rich or to make them wait a bit while poor children, who couldn't otherwise get to school, are collected and taken to their classes *gratis*.

There is no place in a positivist analysis for *ought*. All moral talk lies in the open system of information that permeates and distinguishes us as individuals. Morality lies beyond the *limits of positivism,* which is a bit of a shock for hard-core antidualists as they didn't believe their amazing technology had limits. Does that mean we can't talk rationally about morality? Absolutely not: all we do is assemble a closed system of rules of conduct, call it a moral code, and we can deal with it within a formal cognitive system. It's the same as we deal with, say, the football code, i.e. without lapsing into metaphysics. However, asking for a justification *outside* the code, such as a divinity, immediately takes us into the realm of "meaningless sequences of words."

The same applies to the mind: positivism can give a very good account of the emergence from the brain of a dualist (virtual) machine called the mind. As the *science* of mental life, it allows us to conceptualise the operations involved and then to understand how and why the mind malfunctions—but it says nothing about the contents of any mind. To illustrate, positivists can give a complete scientific account of the production of a book; they cannot, however, tell us anything that would allow us to predict the contents of that book. In the case of human mental life, this process is complicated by the fact that the mental contents (what I know and believe, my values and experience) can act back upon the mental machinery to produce mental disorder [4, 5]. A further value of separating the *informational mechanism* of the emergent mind from the *informational content* it generates and manages is that it leads directly to a rational account of the next topic, cognitive distortions.

17.2. Inbuilt irrationality.

This is a huge topic in its own right. The three classes of cognitive distortions are the generic, i.e. those common to all humans [6], those common to a culture, and those unique to each individual. Many generic cognitive distortions or biases are recognised, including the illusory truth effect (people are more likely to believe false material if they have heard it before), confirmation bias (people selectively notice and recall information that confirms their pre-existing opinions, regardless of its validity), *argumentum ad verecundiam* (people are swayed by authority) and, of course, the stereotypes associated with physical attractiveness. We won't dwell on the literature on cultural distortions which would, I imagine, amount to a medium-sized library.

Cognitive distortions unique to an individual are of much more relevance to psychiatry. This work was pioneered by Sigmund Freud, two of whose concepts, transference and ego mechanisms of defence, have more or less entered common language. Transference means transferring repressed emotion from an unresolved conflict in the past to current events, usually relating to interpersonal relations. For example, one person raised by a domineering father may become anxious around all male authority figures, while another from the same background may react aggressively to dominant men. These are examples of transference. Ego mechanisms of defence are readily observable, in clinical practice and in daily life, as recurrent distortions of reality. Freud didn't spend a lot of time on this aspect of psychoanalytic theory but his daughter, Anna, published the definitive monograph on ego defences in 1936 [7]. Examples including intellectualisation, rationalisation, projection, reaction formation, identification with the aggressor, and so on. Shakespeare understood them well.

All these distortions (and many others) occur at the level of the informational or cognitive mechanism which constitutes the mind, *not* at the level of its contents. The mechanism is disordered and thus produces a disturbed output. Generic cognitive distortions or biases are often driven by anxiety, the most common being the anxiety related to the human need for social acceptance, and the separate drive to build dominance hierarchies [4, 5]. Cultural biases are simply learned, explicitly or, more commonly, implicitly, but they can be very powerful, especially when combined with generic biases, e.g. hating strangers. Biases unique to an individual are the product of life experiences, most commonly early life, and may even be acquired preverbally. Again, the learning can be explicit or, usually stronger and more persistent, implicit. The learned material, meaning rules and generalisations, are incorporated in the set of rules known as personality (see [4], Chap. 8). In this respect, what people believe about their early lives becomes very important clinically; it cannot be dismissed as "mere emotion" or, worse, "manipulation." If people are manipulative, there are reasons, and the psychiatrist's job is to find those reasons and bring them to full consciousness, not dismiss them as "pseudo-problems" or "empty sounds" or, worse still, chemical imbalances. They are cognitive imbalances, which have to be understood in cognitive terms.

Crucially, positivism cannot tell us anything about leading a good life. That represents the art of mental life, but leaving it out gives at best half a science, the difference between the shell of a building and a furnished home. Insofar as psychiatry involves disorders of the emergent mind *and* its contents, it must be cognizant of those two complementary aspects of its work, respectively the science and the art of dealing with mental disorder. **The justification for this is the recognition that information is real and causally effective, not "meaningless sequences of words." Information constitutes an explanation in its own right.**

17.3. The end of positivist psychiatry and ...

There is a contradiction at the very heart of the positivist enterprise, namely, that anybody writing on the topic of antidualism is doing so *within* a dualist system. Only a dualist entity can say "I oppose statements of dualism as meaningless sequences of words and empty sounds." The very mind that generates a philosophy of mind is not of the physical realm in which the symbols representing that thought are manipulated and written. It is not possible for us to escape information as it defines us: our very existence is predicated on this inescapable duality. Information is so much part of us that most people don't recognise it: fish don't know they live in water.

The way around this contradiction is to see the difference between closed informational systems, for which positivism is the correct form of analysis, and open, for which it is not. The human mind consists of a closed system that generates the experience of being, as in: "*Je suis une chose qui pense,... et qui sent...*" But that cognitive machinery is continuous with the open informational system it generates, what I think *about*, all of which lies outside the scope of positivism. This includes morality, fiction, talk of the future and all the nonsense with which we convince ourselves that we're acting morally when we're not. Positivism can only apply to the emergent mechanisms of mind, which are closed and finite, not its output, which is open and infinite. Positivism can deal with logical operations but it can't deal with the material those operations are operating on, or the new material they produce. As they didn't have a theory of information, early positivists didn't know that. Thus, they conflated the two functions of information (*how* we know compared with *what* we know) and declared all mental life off limits. Dualism is only a problem for positivists because they lack a theory of information and so it all seems like magic.

Since the Vienna Circle's manifesto in 1929, times have changed very dramatically. We now have an enormous technology built entirely on the principle that "Information is information, not matter or energy," to quote Wiener yet again. The concepts underwriting mind as an informational space, generated by the brain's information-processing capabilities, are no longer "meaningless sequences of words." Yes, it is dualist but no, dualism does not imply magical substances. It means there are two sets of rules at work in the universe, with no points of contact as each set of rules owes nothing to the other. Some people hold that rules or laws exist independently of humans and we simply discover them. Not so: they exist only for minded beings: without minds, there are natural regularities but no rules. Rules are simply our understanding of those regularities.

This duality, of matter-energy and of information, is the essence of our existence as humans. We live and breathe symbols, constantly overlooking that there is an unbridgeable epistemological gap between symbols and the neuronal mechanisms that implement them. Symbols do not reduce to their physical substrate because that's what 'symbol' means. While the tokens in which the information is encoded are physical (carvings on rocks, squiggles on pages, sound waves, radio waves, electronic impulses in microcircuits etc), what they *represent* is a further and insubstantial realm, one which runs by its own rules, completely independent of the laws of physics, *a world of information of which we are part*. We are so used to seeing the world through our information-processing eyes and grasping it with our informational minds that we take this for granted. If symbols did reduce to their physical substrate, they wouldn't be symbols and we would still be squatting on rocks picking each others' fleas. In fact, we wouldn't even be functioning at the level of fleas, since fleas process a lot of information in their dedicated little information-processing systems. Without the capacity to represent states of affairs in a symbolic calculus [4], we would be functioning at the level of cabbages (all of us, not just our politicians).

In order to progress in psychiatry, we need to free ourselves of the prejudice that anything unobservable is necessarily fanciful and/or breaches the laws of thermodynamics. Information is real, natural, insubstantial, unlocalised, and causally effective. Above all, it is *not subject to* the laws of physics but also *not inconsistent with* the principles of thermodynamics as it exists in a different realm. As an informational system, the emergent mind has all those properties and is therefore rational, internally and externally consistent, and can be studied scientifically. Thus it can be understood, not by scanners and molecular biology, because they miss the irreducible point of information, but ... by another informational system with the capacity to represent states of affairs in an internal calculus. Since humans are informational systems, that means "by another human." It is not a solecism to say we can rationally understand each other intuitively.

The central point is this: If physicalist reductionism could give a genuinely explanatory account of everything that we call "mind," then it wouldn't need to invoke immaterial, insubstantial or just plain ghostly "virtual constructions" such as "virtual selves" or "fictional models." The fact that the most determined efforts to to build a non-mental account of mind smuggle in a classic insubstantial Cartesian self to complete the causal chain is, I submit, both the inevitable outcome of trying to explain away the phenomena of mind *and* a frank if unwitting admission of defeat—the *coup de grâce* for physicalism. There will never be a physicalist theory or model of mind and therefore no positivist account of mental disorder. There will never be a biological psychiatry. The era of a pseudopositivist psychiatry is at an end, which leads to ...

17.4. ... the beginning of a spiritual psychiatry.

Before anybody has a breakdown, by 'spiritual psychiatry,' I do *not* mean "Let us pray as we cast out the evil spirits torturing our brethren." I mean this:

1. All attempts to produce a non-mentalist theory of mind have failed, because...

2. The project is self-contradictory and ...

3. There can never be a biological psychiatry so ...

4. We need to build a psychiatry based in the causal mentality of human beings.

My reasons for saying biological psychiatry will always fail are set out above. My account of a rational, natural dualist model of mind and of mental disorder, personality and personality disorder to replace biological psychiatry are set out in [4]. That is, to satisfy Buckminster Fuller's rule, I have shown what is wrong with the existing reality, and built a new model that makes the existing model obsolete. But, and as much as the word is abused, it is a totally new paradigm. It is a shift from the physicalist ontology to dualism, not a magical dualism with celestial choirs or demonic possession but a natural dualism built on the same principles underlying our lives today. Humans are minded beings. Minds are causally significant, meaning we have free will but, as informational states, minds can malfunction wholly at the mental level. We call that mental disorder. A physically-disturbed brain is sufficient to cause a form of mental disorder, but it is not necessary.

"Humans as spiritual beings" simply means we have in our heads a sense of being and self that cannot be explained within the realms of the laws of the physical or material world. There is something above and beyond "mere matter" which we can understand in rational terms. Its reality can no longer be denied. When it malfunctions, we can understand the experience in its own terms. This leads to a novel psychiatry where sufferers are asked to explore their inner experience rather than having it suppressed by drugs or ECT. The difference is stark:

> Mr Jones: I feel so sad and miserable.

> Psychiatrist: What's your appetite like? What time do you wake? What's your level of energy like? And your sexual interest? OK, you're depressed, take these and come back in a month.

Compare that (absolutely normal exchange) with this:

> Mrs Smith: I feel so sad and miserable.

> Psychiatrist: I see. Can you talk about that, can you let yourself experience it now and we will try to find the cause.

That's all. It is the difference between psychiatry as a human experience, and psychiatry as a veterinary practice. Talking of veterinary practice, all this means that animals have minds, too. They're just very polite and don't jabber on about it.

The positivist revolution was intended to separate science from metaphysics but, in the process, it stripped the humanity from the human sciences. It has grossly retarded our understanding of ourselves, to the point where human studies have been left in the dust. After a hundred years, positivism has run its course. Today, we need an articulated model of humans as humans so we can move to a post-positivist future.

References:

1. Hahn H, Neurath O, Carnap R (1929). *The Scientific Conception of the World: The Vienna Circle*. Ernst Mach Society, University of Vienna.

2. Schlick M (1930). Die Wende der Philosophie. *Erkenntnis* 1: 4-11. Translated as The Turning Point in Philosophy. Available online.

3. Schlick M (1932/33) Positivism and Realism. Orig. *Erkenntnis* II-III; Tr. P Heath; Reprinted in Volume II (1979, p259-284) *Philosophical Papers of Moritz Schlick. Eds.* Mulder HL, van de Velde-Schlick BF. Dordrecht: D. Reidel. Available at Sophia Project SophiaOmni, www.sophiaomni.org.

4. McLaren N (2021): *Natural Dualism and Mental Disorder: The biocognitive model for psychiatry.* London, Routledge.

5. McLaren N (2018). *Anxiety: The Inside Story.* Ann Arbor, MI: Future Psychiatry Press.

6. Kahnemann D (2011). *Thinking fast and slow.* New York: Allan Lane

7. Freud A (1936/1977). *The Ego and the Mechanisms of Defence.* London: Routledge.

About the Author

Niall McLaren is an Australian psychiatrist, author and critic. He was born and educated in rural Western Australia, graduating in medicine at the University of WA in Perth in 1970. He completed his postgraduate training in psychiatry in 1977 and subsequently worked in prisons and then in the Veterans' Hospital, with a year's break working in the far southern region of Thailand. From 1983-87, he studied philosophy in order to undertake a PhD jointly in psychiatry and philosophy of science. In 1987, he left Perth city to travel to the remote Kimberley Region of Western Australia as the region's first psychiatrist.

Covering an area larger than California, with no staff, no hospital beds, no clinic and not even an office, nearly 2000km from the nearest psychiatrist, he was the world's most isolated psychiatrist. While there, he continued studying and writing and began publishing work highly critical of mainstream psychiatry. After six years in the bush, he moved to Darwin, the capital of Australia's Northern Territory, first as chief psychiatrist for the Top End, then in private practice, where he was closely involved with the large military population. He has since moved to Brisbane, in Queensland, and is emphatic that there will be no more moves. He retired from clinical work during the pandemic and now has an honorary position with the Dept of Philosophy at University of Queensland.

When he graduated in psychiatry, he was aware that the field was not what it claimed to be. It was clear that psychiatrists routinely made major claims on the nature of the mind-brain relationship and mental disorder that were not justified in the literature and, he realised, could never be justified. This led him to the philosophy of science which established that psychiatry lacked a formal model of mental disorder. In turn, this problem arose just because it had no theory of mind. As a result, modern psychiatry lacks a basis in any known concept of science. It is, in fact, at best a protoscience and, at worst, crude and highly misleading pseudoscience. This author's work is highly original and owes nothing to any psychiatrists, living or dead. Almost invariably, his work provokes bitter antagonism from mainstream psychiatrists.

For nearly half a century, orthodox psychiatry has committed itself totally to the reductionist biological approach to mental disorder, with no possible alternatives. Despite massive increases in expenditure on mental health, there is absolutely no evidence to support the oft-repeated claims that psychiatry is making great advances and people are better off than they have ever been. Every figure indicates that as psychiatry extends its reach, the mental health of the population declines. McLaren argues that this is just because psychiatry is not a science.

Because it lacks a formal model of its field of study, mental disorder, psychiatry is perpetually at the mercy of social and political fads and fashions. He maintains that biological psychiatry is nothing more than a passing fad and must eventually go the way of psychoanalysis, behaviourism and possession theory. In the meantime, it is doing an immeasurable amount of damage.

He recently published the results of a lifetime of work on a model of mind for psychiatry, the biocognitive model, which leads directly to a model of mental disorder. This is the first time in the history of psychiatry that such a model has been available. The present work, a survey of all theories available to psychiatry, provides a solid critical foundation to complete the project. Since theories in psychiatry are so weak and poorly developed, this volume also surveys a group of well-known philosophers, concluding that none of their work can be extended to provide a model of mental disorder. The clear implication is that their work is insufficient to the task of providing a general account of mental life, but this needs further analysis on a much broader scale.

As a test of its scope, the biocognitive model of mind has been applied to the unrelated world of politics, to see if it can make sense of human activity. That study has been published as a separate work, *Narcisso-Fascism: the psychopathology of extremism*. This gives an entirely novel understanding of the politics of extremism which confirms what has often been said, "The fascist is within me." It also offers a means of controlling the phenomenon. Given the present state of world politics, this is definitely needed. This strengthens the case for the biocognitive model of mental disorder to replace the current approaches in psychiatry.

In Anxiety--The Inside Story, the author takes a critical look at modern psychiatry's twin notions that all mental disorders are biological in nature, but anxiety is hardly worth worrying about. By the simple process of taking a careful, detailed history, Niall McLaren shows that anxiety is far more common and far more destructive than mainstream psychiatry realizes. Detailed case histories chart how anxiety arises as a psychological disorder and how it reinforces itself to the point where it destroys lives. McLaren concludes that anxiety is a major factor in most mental disorders, especially depression and bipolar disorder. This book will change your understanding of mental disorders.

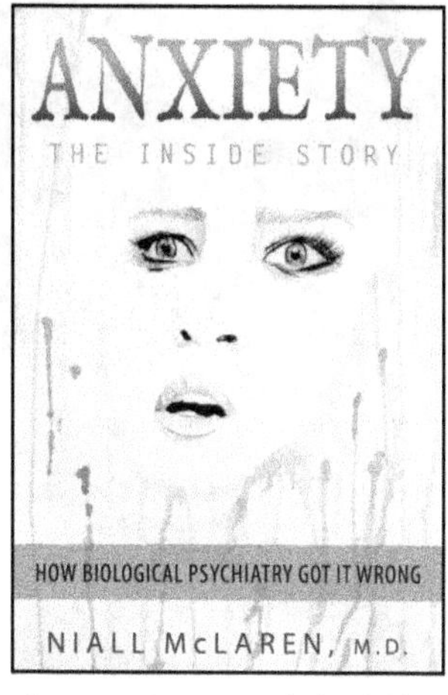

Niall (Jock) McLaren writes as he speaks and he pulls no punches. I love this. People should listen to what he has to say about the academic corruption of his specialty, psychiatry. Read this book. The man is unique. And funny, as well.
-- Prof. Peter Gotzsche, Director, Nordic Cochrane Centre, Copenhagen

Debilitating anxieties are frequently misdiagnosed as "depression" by GPs and specialists alike. In this wonderfully accessible account of anxiety, Dr. McLaren demonstrates with great clarity--and very movingly--how a case history approach can help patients confront and overcome their psychological demons. He provides compelling evidence that instead of drugging people, listening to them attentively and analytically has to be the beginning of the healing process.
-- Dr. Allan Patience, University of Melbourne

This book offers readers a devastating, blistering critique of psychiatry, together with a provocative exploration of how anxiety, so often dismissed as a "minor" difficulty, should be understood as the root cause of so much suffering—which manifests in a diverse range of behaviors that get wrongly categorized as distinct psychiatric "illnesses." Niall McLaren presents a compelling case that psychiatric care in Australia and beyond needs to be completely rethought.
-- Robert Whitaker, author of *Mad in America* and *Psychiatry Under the Influence*

From Future Psychiatry Press

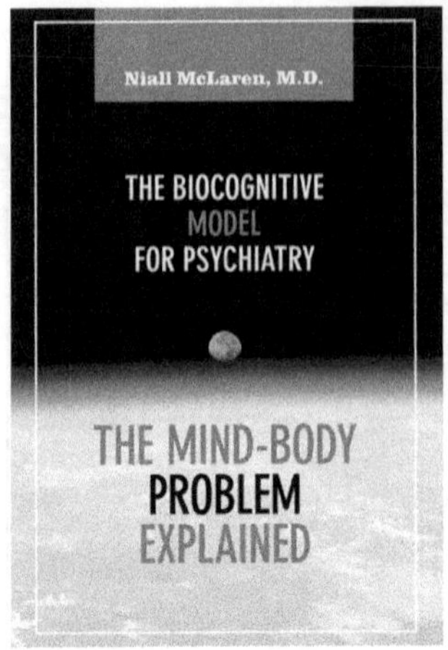

Cracking the Mind-Body Cipher

Dr. Niall (Jock) McLaren is an Australian psychiatrist who uses philosophical analysis to show that modern psychiatry has no scientific basis. This startling conclusion dovetails neatly with the growing evidence that psychiatric drug treatment is crude and damaging. Needless to say, this message is not popular with mainstream psychiatrists. However, in this book, he shows how the principles of information processing give a formal theory of mind that generates a model of mental disorder as a psychological phenomenon.

This book shows...

- How, for ideological reasons, modern philosophy misses the point of the duality of mind and body;

- How to resolve the mind-body problem using well-defined principles;

- Why the entire DSM project is doomed to fail;

- Why the ideas of Thomas Szasz have failed to influence psychiatry;

- Where we go from here.

"*The Mind Body Problem Explained* is a thoughtful, insightful and provocative exploration of the nature of the human mind, and sets forth a powerful argument for rethinking the medical model of mental disorders. The current paradigm of psychiatric care has failed us, and Niall McLaren's book will stir readers to think of new possibilities."

--Robert B. Whitaker, author *Mad in America: Bad Science, Bad Medicine, and the Enduring Mistreatment of the Mentally Ill*

"It is impossible to do justice to this ambitious, erudite, and intrepid attempt to dictate to psychiatry a new, 'scientifically-correct' model theory. The author offers a devastating critique of the shortcomings and pretensions of psychiatry, not least its all-pervasive, jargon-camouflaged nescience."

--Sam Vaknin, PhD, author *Malignant Self Love: Narcissism Revisited*

From Future Psychiatry Press

Narcisso-Fascism: The Psychopathology of Right-Wing Extremism

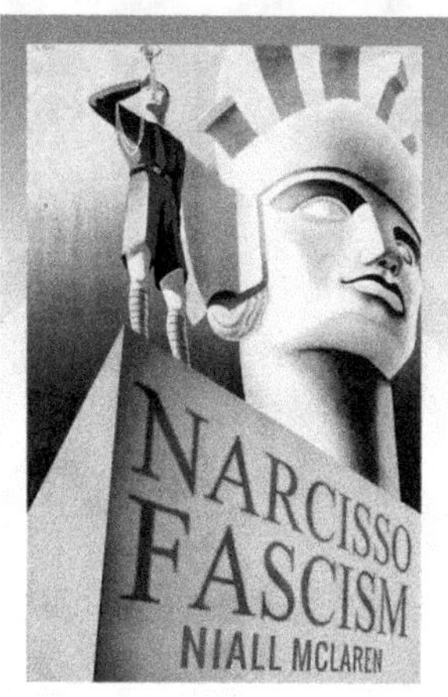

This book examines the biological, social and psychological influences driving one of the most important, and frightening, trends in modern international politics, right-wing extremism. It is radically unlike anything written on the topic before and its conclusions should make all of us stop... and worry about the world we are leaving to our children.

Niall McLaren is a recently-retired Australian psychiatrist with a particular interest in the application of the philosophy of science to psychiatry.

Of this work, Prof. Alan Patience, of the School of Social and Political Sciences, Melbourne University, said:

> "Niall McLaren's new book weaves the disciplines of psychiatry and political science into a highly original approach to the political psychology of fascism... (His) book takes the analysis of fascism to another level, warning how genetically and psychologically ingrained the fascist urge is in human nature generally. In revealing this with rare clarity, this book will help counter the deeply disturbing drift towards neo-fascism across the contemporary world."

From Modern History Press